Medicine, Science, and Making Race
in Civil War America

Medicine, Science, and Making Race in Civil War America

Leslie A. Schwalm

The University of North Carolina Press CHAPEL HILL

Open access edition funded by the National Endowment for the Humanities.

Set in Merope Basic by Westchester Publishing Services
Manufactured in the United States of America

Library of Congress Cataloging-in-Publication Data
Names: Schwalm, Leslie A. (Leslie Ann), 1956– author.
Title: Medicine, science, and making race in Civil War America / Leslie A. Schwalm.
Description: Chapel Hill : The University of North Carolina Press, [2023] |
    Includes bibliographical references and index.
Identifiers: LCCN 2022029934 | ISBN 9781469672687 (cloth ; alk. paper) |
    ISBN 9781469672694 (pbk. ; alk. paper) | ISBN 9781469672700 (ebook)
Subjects: LCSH: United States Sanitary Commission—History. | Racism in medicine—
    United States—History—19th century. | Scientific racism—United States—History—
    19th century. | United States—History—Civil War, 1861–1865—Medical care. |
    United States—History—Civil War, 1861–1865—African Americans.
Classification: LCC E621 .S355 2023 | DDC 599.97097309/034—dc23/eng/20220714
LC record available at https://lccn.loc.gov/2022029934

Portions of chapter one were previously published in a different form as "A Body of
'Truly Scientific Work': The U.S. Sanitary Commission and the Elaboration of Race
in the Civil War Era," *The Journal of the Civil War Era* 8, no. 4 (2018): 647–676.

In loving memory of Olive Fewell Schwalm, Henry Raymond Schwalm, Grace Brooks Stormoen, and Orin Stormoen. We remember you.

Contents

List of Illustrations ix

Preface xi

Introduction 1

CHAPTER ONE
Militarizing Race 12

CHAPTER TWO
Commissioning Race 21

CHAPTER THREE
Narrating and Enumerating Race 48

CHAPTER FOUR
Anatomizing Race 69

CHAPTER FIVE
The Afterlife of Race 93

Conclusion 115

Acknowledgments 121

Notes 125

Bibliography 185

Index 209

Illustrations

2.1 Organization chart of the U.S. Sanitary Commission, 1864 24

2.2 Political cartoon and limerick by William Emlen Cresson, 1864 30

2.3 Sanitary Fair poster, 1864 33

2.4 "For this are we Doctors" sketch, 1864 38

2.5 "Special Diet" sketch, 1864 42

2.6 "The Old Nurse" 45

3.1 Sanitary Commission's individual inspection form (Form EE) 61

Preface

Medicine, Science, and Making Race in Civil War America is about medical and scientific racism during the Civil War. It explores the actions of Northern whites that directly and adversely impacted the lives and deaths of thousands of enslaved and freeborn African Americans. This project had its origins in my research for an earlier book, when I encountered deeply disturbing stories of medical mistreatment of the soldiers of Iowa's Black regiment. From there I found my way into the harrowingly thick archives of Civil War medical and scientific racism. What I found was part of a longer historical trajectory of medical racism and also a critical part of the story of the Civil War. I found as well an important window into the wartime racial politics of Northern white Unionists. In focusing on white ideas and practices around race and people of African descent, this became a project that required me to shift away from my previous interest in the fullness of Black lives and particularly the impact of Black men and women on slavery's destruction and their insistence on a more expansive freedom after the war.

This has been a difficult history to work with, and I want to recognize that it will be painful to read. While the book's focus is on the white men and women whose actions, beliefs, and behaviors advanced the ideology and impact of white racism during the Civil War, I wish to acknowledge that the targets of their actions — the people whose bodies they probed and whose dignity in life and death was rejected or ignored — are the ancestors of people living today. The traumas I describe here remain largely unacknowledged and unaccounted for by historians of the war, and their exposure here is offered in hopes of initiating the process of redress.

Medicine, Science, and Making Race in Civil War America draws heavily from a one-sided archive: tables and statistics, specimens, skull collections, endless reports, questionnaires, surveys — evidence of an unflagging and sometimes seemingly "libidinous investment" in the hunt for "Nature's law" establishing Black people as members of a biologically inferior race. The search, inevitably, was for the proof that Black bodies were different from and inferior to those of whites.[1] It is an archive that attempts to teach fellow whites a fiction, as Christina Sharpe has noted, of "what blackness looks like and how to look at blackness."[2]

This is a painful archive to encounter, both in its virulent intent and its abundance. The archive bears similarities to the "violent and violating" archive created by slave traders and slave owners.[3] The records of the slave trade are both narrow in what questions they easily allow a researcher to pursue and those they hide from and disallow. These records are also similarly overwhelming in volume and affective impact. Because of these similarities, I have looked to and benefited greatly from those scholars, especially Black feminists, who have theorized the archives of racial slavery, scholars who have pushed slavery's historians to think carefully about how to enter this archive without replicating its commodification of Black lives and bodies.[4]

Similarly, knowing what questions this archive was not created to answer—in particular, the experience and resistance of those subjected to these endeavors, and the critique offered by antiracist critics at the time—did not prevent me from asking those questions and seeking paths to answer them. Most often, however, I have taken care to flesh out the white actors portrayed here—not to redeem them as "people of their time" but rather to locate racist action and thought in the lives of fully dimensional actors.

Some readers will find the white actors and actions they encounter here unrecognizably distant from the white abolitionists they are probably more familiar with—the civilians and soldiers who came to see enslaved people as fellow humans, worthy of freedom from the shackles and torture of bondage, and freeborn African Americans as entitled to the same rights of citizenship enjoyed by white Americans. Still, the study of Northern white racism during the war years has for too long fallen short, victim to the "treasury of virtue" that Robert Penn Warren once described as the North's misguided cultural inheritance from their victory in a war that ended slavery.[5] I hope that this book will be read alongside the important and growing body of literature that reclaims the work of Black and white Americans in the long struggle for freedom and equality. For those readers wondering what happened to the allegedly benign or paternalistic racism that some historians have portrayed among mid-nineteenth-century Northern whites, I hope to offer persuasive evidence that racist ideas and actions do not exist without harm.

The racial project of the Civil War was complex and contradictory. This book studies that history by focusing on the endeavors by white medical and scientific practitioners and researchers to master what they thought was knowable about Black bodies: what whites saw as their peculiarities, their distinctiveness, their possibilities, their limitations. In these white Northerners' wartime efforts to create and possess exclusive bio medical and scientific authority over African American bodies and to commodify that knowledge, there is a deep correspondence with the commodification of Black bodies by slave traders and slave owners. I approach these wartime developments as part of the enduring violence of slavery, even during the war that ultimately ended slavery. The medical and scientific endeavors documented here show how racist ideology born out of slavery survived slavery's destruction, securing an afterlife that we contend with today in the killing abstractions that stretch from police brutality to the failure of white physicians to take seriously the pain reported by their African American patients.[6]

Medicine, Science, and Making Race in Civil War America

Introduction

The Civil War's greatest achievement—the emancipation of four million African Americans and all their descendants—was shadowed by another, largely unacknowledged outcome: Northern white Unionists' deepened investment in medically and scientifically reinforced ideas about race and racial hierarchies. This venture was clearly evident in a host of developments, such as the provision of health care that presumed race-based disease vulnerabilities. It included the mistreatment of Black troops, evidenced in their exploitation as laborers, as well as in a wide range of medical abuses. It was also apparent in the Army and Sanitary Commission's investments in research devoted to identifying and documenting indisputable racial characteristics in Black troops and civilians. Finally, it was also evident in the exploitation of the human remains of African Americans, revealing one of the key contradictions of racial thought—that Black bodies, presumed to be so markedly different from those of whites, could nonetheless be used as "stand-ins" for white bodies in studying anatomy and disease pathology.

For white medical practitioners, scientists, professionals, and aspiring laypeople, their common familiarity with medical and scientific racism meant that they believed they could locate race in seemingly corporeal, indisputable, and quantifiable facts—facts that could be observed, measured, dissected, weighed, tabulated, statistically averaged, and reported.[1] Scientific racism gained professional and popular authority in the nineteenth century because of its alleged reliance on empirical data but also because its political, social, and cultural conclusions appealed to white scholars, practitioners, and laypeople.[2] The notion that race had scientific and clinical legitimacy as a means of ranking human society was integral to midcentury developments in the nature and authority of scientific medical knowledge. It was interwoven with an emerging culture of science and professionalized medicine that included medical education, popular periodicals, public lectures, local scientific and medical societies, museums, widely circulated reports of government-funded research, and the common role of scientists and physicians as popular public intellectuals. When the wartime Army Medical Department rejected all but "regular" physicians for appointment, it confirmed the professional ascendancy of science-based medicine over homeopaths (who relied on the idea that "like cures like" and used diluted preparations to create symptoms similar to those created by disease), Thomsonians (who rejected more orthodox physicians and their medicines, relying instead on "nature's apothecary" in the treatment of illness), and other practitioners using alternative medical approaches. That development contributed to the legitimacy and authority of (what was then) scientific knowledge, including assertions about the biology of race that were already deeply interwoven within a number of fields of study, from gynecology to ethnology.[3]

It is important to note that some of the men and women portrayed in this book were opposed to slavery and wrote with sensitivity and even horror about what they learned about slavery during the war. They observed the physical impact of slaveholders' violence and torture on the bodies of male and female refugees from slavery, and they condemned the system of slavery as immoral and inhumane. Nonetheless, they saw no contradiction in being antislavery and embracing the idea that science and natural law separated humanity into superior and inferior races. During the war, when opportunities arose or could be created, they put those beliefs into action. As a result, the war destroyed slavery but emerged with white Northern commitments to racial hierarchies not only intact but also deeply entangled in the postwar turn toward modernizing and professionalizing medicine and medical sciences.

White medical practitioners and enthusiasts for science—Union men, aiding in the effort to destroy the Confederacy and end slavery—were in this way strengthening the power and impact of racial ideologies so that during and after the war anti-Black racism emerged with stronger rationales and more vocal advocates, and it was more closely tied to postwar medicine as well as the policies of the reconstructed nation-state. Neither emancipation nor the military defeat of the Confederacy liberated the Black body from the efforts of Northern white scientists, researchers, and other self-regarded "learned men" to reveal, catalog, analyze, and address the implications of the "physical character of the negro race."[4] As a result, an increasingly intransigent notion of biological race and racial essentialism were among the outcomes of the war.

This book looks to the social and cultural history of medicine and science to help explain why the destruction of slavery failed to more fully undermine American anti-Black racism, especially among the white Northerners who were willing to sacrifice so much in the Civil War. Its central concern is how and why the conditions of war and the Union's war effort increased, rather than reduced, Northern white investments in the utility and advancement of ideas about racial difference. The Union's wartime medical and scientific investments went well beyond the organization and delivery of health care and the development of new surgical techniques and treatments of injuries and disease; they also created specific and concrete opportunities to advance the ties between the making of race and the making of medicine and science.

Although today's scholars make a clear distinction between race medicine and race science, during the Civil War those distinctions were not especially clear and certainly were not always relevant to the conglomerate approaches through which professional and lay practitioners attempted to not only to differentiate humans from each other, but more specifically to identify what separated out Black humanity from white.[5] While we are learning much more about the lived experience of medical racism in Black regiments, contraband camps, and hospitals during the war, we know far less about how the war itself impacted the intellectual and cultural history of American racial ideologies, and the agency of white Unionists in that process.[6]

ONCE IT HAD embraced emancipation as a war goal, the Union military finally permitted the wide-scale enlistment of African American men into the armed services. Many Americans, white and African American, viewed Black military service as a forceful assault on slavery and on racial discrimination as well as an opportunity for Black men to make an irrefutable claim to expanded citizenship rights. As soldiers and as civilian military laborers, Black men and women demonstrated their courage, their capabilities, and their determination to bring an end to slavery. Many whites who commanded them, employed them, and fought and worked along with them recognized Black men and women's enormous contributions to and sacrifices for the war effort. Concurrently, however, the war and Black enlistment was also used as an unprecedented occasion for the Union's professional men in medicine, public health, and science to advance racial science — that is, their belief, as white men of science, that people of African descent were physiologically, anatomically, and sociologically distinct and inferior to whites.

The bodies of Black soldiers — at the point of their enlistment, in hospitals, on battlefields, during fatigue duty, and as cadavers — became fruitful sources of white inquiry into "racial knowledge" during the war. Rather than falling into irrelevance with wartime emancipation, racialized medicine and science gained authority, popularity, and professional appeal among Northern whites. To many, racial science offered a new logic for a new nation where Black subordination was no longer secured by the bonds of slavery.

To others, expertise in racial science offered a clear path toward professional recognition and acclaim. Moreover, the war's production of cadavers that could be disassembled without white reproach was a convenient and welcome development.

Medicine shouldered many new burdens during the war. The scale of carnage created unanticipated challenges to medical knowledge, medical practice, and military organization, and these topics have been and continue to be well studied by Civil War historians and historians of medicine. Two recent surveys of wartime medical care and research have emphasized the many advancements in emergency care, wound treatment, and hospital design and care that resulted.[7] New surgical techniques were developed, new tools were circulated to encourage medical research that might curtail the spread of disease, and medical research and experimentation were encouraged to promote the development of more effective treatments of disease. Recent scholarship has also investigated the horrific failure of military, civilian, and Freedmen's Bureau medical authorities to address the medical needs of Black soldiers and civilians during and immediately after the war.[8]

Less understood is the wartime recruitment of medicine and the allied sciences by Northern whites in the service of creating firmer, irrefutable racial ideologies based on characteristics that could be cataloged and enlisted to distinguish and rank human races. These wartime developments formed an important bridge. They linked the physicians whose antebellum education was steeped in medical racism, the natural scientists who debated polygenism versus monogenism, those who studied craniometry and placed people of African descent outside of historical change and development, the "skull collectors" and craniologists of the postbellum Army Medical Museum and the Smithsonian, men like Frederick Hoffman who argued an impending Black extinction, and the military racial anthropometry of World War I Europe and the United States.[9] In addition, the commodification of African American human remains for personal, professional, and national fame, which accompanied wartime investigations of "racial science," suggests an afterlife to Daina Ramey Berry's revelations of the antebellum trade in cadavers of enslaved people.[10] The "science of race" persisted despite robust challenges, both within and outside the field of medicine and science, at meetings of learned societies, from the pulpit, in the parlors and lecture rooms of Black communities across the nation, and in widespread print culture.

Black Northerners were no strangers to science and medicine before or during the Civil War era, nor should they be viewed only as victims of the wartime rise of medical and scientific advances. Skillful Black medical practitioners and science educators had a loyal Black following in the North. Rebecca Lee Crumpler, the first African American woman to graduate from a medical college in 1864, had learned healing at a young age from her aunt who raised her and worked as a nurse. Prior to her formal medical training, she worked as a nurse among Boston's Black residents, and after the war among Richmond's former slaves as a physician with the Freedmen's Bureau.[11] Sarah Mapps Douglass, the abolitionist and advocate for Black women's leadership, taught anatomy, physiology, and natural sciences to Philadelphia Black schoolgirls for four decades, prepared her own extensive collection of natural science specimens, took several courses at medical schools, and participated in the city's several lyceums and Banneker Institute's lectures and presentations on science.[12]

African Americans were not only popular medical practitioners and science educators in their Northern communities but also used their expertise to challenge whites' efforts to deploy science as a tool of racism. Douglass armed her students with the ability to challenge racist science and medicine and the particular objectification of Black women's bodies. Dr. James Mc-Cune Smith (a Black physician who trained in Glasgow) challenged the racial environmentalism that appeared in a widely circulated report on the Colored Orphans Asylum in 1839 as well as in a wide range of writings; Frederick Douglass challenged the racist proponents of ethnology in his 1854 commencement address at Western Reserve College; William Craft, born enslaved in the United States and living in Liverpool for many years, challenged the authors of two papers presented at the inaugural meetings of London's Anthropological Society for their assertions about the biological basis of racial hierarchies.[13]

Historians including Gretchen Long, Mia Bay, Britt Rusert, Vanessa Northington Gamble, and Melissa Stein have pointed to an important Black response to the uses of science to support racial inequalities as well as the efforts of Black medical practitioners to gain formal training and professional status in a white-dominated profession.[14] While this book provides additional insight into the experiences of African Americans as wartime recipients of medical care and objects of scientific consumption as well as health care workers, its primary concern is with how and why white Northern scientists and physicians created and used the opportunities presented by the war to more deeply invest in race medicine and race science. To the extent that this study considers "race" as a lived experience, readers will find the work presented here largely focuses on the emergence of whites' aspirations to professional recognition and authority as imagined experts on Blackness.

It is important to clarify that the white investigators studied here were not engaged in an open-ended search for something they understood as "race." They did not seek to discover and catalog biological race in white bodies.[15] To them, white bodies—those of white men—were naturally and unremarkably superior to Black bodies. Although there was some limited interest in ranking the aptness of different national "stock" among whites for soldiering, those efforts largely understood "nation" as a subclass of whiteness, and more importantly, those efforts lacked the scale, consistency, intention, and impact of their interest in Black bodies. In describing their approach to measuring white soldiers, commission agents focused on a "race-neutral" accumulation of knowledge: "to ascertain the effect of climate, locality, & mode of life upon men, the difference in size of men from the States of America & countries of Europe, also what form & weight of men are best adapted to the different branches of the Service & which branch of the service is the most unhealthy. Also to collect statistics relating to the habits & mode of life of soldiers previous to enlisting, etc. etc."[16]

While far more white soldiers were biometrically measured during the war than Black, investigators were not concerned with proving white superiority by studying white racial characteristics so much as they were intent on identifying, measuring, and confirming the inferiority of Black embodiment. Both while in progress and in the published version, Benjamin Apthorp Gould's discussion of the compiled and tabulated measurements of Black soldiers conducted under his direction for the U.S. Sanitary Commission was consistently framed with rhetoric pointing to the deviation of those measures from those of whites—never are the "white" measures similarly rhetorically presented as a departure from "Black" measurements. The same is true of the discussion of measurements of the bodies of American Indian men. When Gould asserted the value of his volume as its catalog of information for others to assess and interpret, he was disingenuous; his entire presentation of data on Black men's bodies was discussed in terms of their departure from the measure of presumably normative white bodies.[17] Similarly, there were no parallel social surveys asking military medical staff or commanding officers whether white men of varying nationalities or birth could succeed as soldiers, no queries into the race-based responses to army rations, disease resistances, or vulnerabilities, and no advice solicited on their special needs as dictated by their white "race."

The silent center of a nearly monolithic whiteness illuminated in the chapters to follow was accompanied by a parallel centering of male bodies as stand-ins for humanity. Chapter 2 pays careful attention to the actions of both men and women in establishing the bureaucratic domains of white authority and power during the Civil War, but in the chapters that follow both the agents of investigation and their subjects were primarily men, involved as soldiers, volunteers, and employees in the Union war effort. Women (as refugees from slavery during and shortly after the war) did find their way to hospitals, and they became objects of interest as patients and as cadavers; surgeons, hospital employees, and other medical workers were not especially discriminating when it came to the sex of the Black bodies they gained access to. Still, it would be fair to approach this book as a study of men's pursuit of race in other men; female physicians and hospital stewards were exceptionally rare on the ground during the war. It is important to acknowledge the wartime world of medical and scientific race-making as largely a world of white masculine authority.[18] Even so, white women were important actors in the war's racial politics, as I discuss in chapter 2.

The wartime advance of science- and medicine-based anti-Black racism served many masters. As this book will demonstrate, it sustained a racial hierarchy that lost its key purpose and legal mooring with emancipation. It enhanced the professional status of the white physicians, scientists, public health advocates, laypeople, and organizations who claimed expertise in "racial science." It would also rationalize wartime and Reconstruction era polices that sought to discipline freed people as laborers while ignoring the material conditions that threatened their health. Science-based arguments about Black inferiority also offered a rhetorical basis for criticizing the Reconstruction era extension of civil rights and citizenship. The war provided Northern white medical practitioners in particular with abundant opportunities to assert their own professional identity and authority as racial scientists, but also made the American state a more active participant in generating and circulating a racial science that was rooted in slavery—regardless of slavery's wartime destruction. A racial logic that, before the war, had modernized justifications for slavery by using the language and authority of science would endure well past slavery's destruction—not only through the work of proslavery southern physicians but substantially through the investments and actions of Northern whites.

The wartime devotion to and legitimation of racial science can be traced through the scientific racism that blossomed in the Gilded Age and Progressive Era.[19] Civil War anthropometry became a core feature of scientific theories about racial difference and was widely employed by later nineteenth-century scientists and scholars to develop a vocabulary with which to describe racial difference. It gave legitimacy to racial science and the validity of its conclusions about race and racial inequality.[20] Darwin read and was influenced by Civil War anthropometry in writing *The Descent of Man* (1871).[21] Frances Galton would link anthropometry and eugenics in his *Hereditary Genius* (1869). Social scientist Joseph Alexander Tillinghast, author of "The Negro in Africa and America" (1902), drew on the Sanitary Commission's work. Edward Drinker Cope, zoologist, paleontologist, and for a period editor of the *American Naturalist*, not only relied on the Sanitary Commission's anthropometric measurements to support his own arguments about racial physiognomy but extended his argument to advocate for Black disfranchisement and forced migration.[22] Rudolph Matas, a Tulane University professor of surgery, repeatedly referred to Gould's statistics in his 1896 book *The Surgical Peculiarities of the American Negro*.[23] Frederick Hoffman drew very heavily from Civil War race science and medicine in his 1896 statistical narrative (*Race Traits and Tendencies of the American Negro*), arguing that African Americans were racially predisposed to ill health and high mortality rates.[24] The economist and anthropologist William Zebina Ripley gained widespread recognition for his 1899 book *The Races of Europe: A Sociological Study*, which relied on both Gould and Baxter's work to caricature Black anatomy and physiology.[25]

Anthropometry continued in research conducted by American physical educators, and the U.S. Army's anthropometric study of World War I soldiers was initiated with Gould's Civil War research in mind.[26] Aleš Hrdlička, the prominent anthropologist and advocate of racial science, heralded Gould's work in his 1927 essay, "Anthropology of the American Negro: Historical Notes."[27] Harvard physiologist Henry Pickering Bowditch and the anthropologist Franz Boaz (in the United States) and Rudolf Virchow (in Germany) were among those who followed the Sanitary Commission's innovation in conducting large-scale anthropometric surveys, aided by French anatomist and anthropologist Paul Broca's many refinements to the instrumentation used in racial-science craniometrics and anthropometric studies.[28] The pursuit of bodily proof of race led prominent American eugenicists Charles Davenport and Morris Steggerda to subject the bodies of Tuskegee Institute's students to similar anthropometric measurement from 1932 to 1944.[29]

The wartime monuments to racial science and medicine produced by the Sanitary Commission and the Union army also drew substantial and pointed refutations. The well-known Black mathematician, sociologist, Howard University faculty member, and editor of *The Crisis*, Kelly Miller, critiqued

Frederick Hoffman's use of Gould's flawed data and Hunt's assertions (which drew on Benjamin Woodward's questionnaire) in *Race Traits and Tendencies of the American Negro*.[30] The exhaustive anthropometric and anthropological study directed by W. E. B. Du Bois, *The Health and Physique of the Negro American* (1906), pointed to the many flaws in Gould's work.[31] However, as Du Bois scholar Maria Farland has pointed out, Du Bois lacked the "scientific capital" to gain wide acceptance for his refutation of racial ideologies.

Historicizing race—and making legible the policies, the atrocities, the hierarchies and power relationships that ideas about race served in particular times and places—has curiously evaded the focused attention of many historians of the American Civil War. Wartime racial discrimination, particularly in soldiering and in employment, has long been accounted for, of course. And for good and important reasons, studies of wartime emancipation have focused on the process, conditions, and experience of slavery's final destruction and on postwar struggles—political, legal, social, cultural, and economic—by Black Americans to define the meaning and extent of Black freedom in the postwar, postslavery United States. Mindful of the importance of this scholarship, and indeed as a contributor to it, I hope that by turning our focus more specifically to how Northern whites' ideas about race mattered during and immediately after the Civil War, we might gain greater insight into how and why ideas about racial difference and inferiority survived slavery's destruction.

Taking white Unionists' ideas about race seriously as a subject of historical inquiry requires a careful distinction between ideas about slavery and emancipation, and ideas about race. There has been much scholarly interest in the evolution of Northern whites' ideas about slavery—soldiers, officers, and civilians alike—over the course of the war. This work is important to our ability to understand how Northern whites thought about slavery and the relationship of those ideas to their understanding of the Civil War's causes and consequences. But Northern opposition to slavery was full of curious contradictions and illogic. Some whites opposed slavery because they opposed the political and economic power wielded by the South's planter elite; some feared economic competition with enslaved labor; some believed slavery was immoral and a sin. All these beliefs could be, and were with some frequency, paired with anti-Black racism. As Elizabeth Blair Lee insisted in 1862, she regarded herself as an abolitionist "for the sake of my own race—Contact with the African degenerates our white race."[32] In this book, white Unionists' opposition to slavery is not at issue; instead, we explore their explicit investment in ideas about race and their willingness to act on those ideas—whether in organizing soldiers' aid societies or deciding what to do with a cadaver.[33]

The army and the Sanitary Commission's shared commitments to the project of race-making capitalized on several intersecting cultural forces that had gained considerable momentum and legitimacy by the time of the war. First, medicine and its allied sciences had already identified clinical expertise and empiricism as the definitive characteristic of medical science and as the path forward for professional uplift and authority. As John Harley Warner has noted, by the mid-nineteenth century, the "clinic and the autopsy table," with their opportunities for firsthand observation and experience, had replaced the philosophical theories of humoral imbalance and other rationalistic systems of medical thought. The Civil War's amassing of huge armies introduced an unprecedented medical and scientific opportunity (including personal professional advancement) for those in a position to take advantage of it.[34]

Second, the history of American medicine and its allied sciences were already deeply entangled with slavery. By the time of the Civil War, a familiar roster of scientists, naturalists, and medical practitioners from Jefferson to Agassiz had tied the pursuit of medical and scientific discovery to the exploitation of Black labor and Black bodies. On the eve of the war, they had created and circulated a widely accepted, ranked, comparative, and corporeal language of race. Civil War research drew heavily on the technology and cultural capital of this foundational work.

Third, the gathering and circulation of information about the American population—even undigested data—had become a function of the nineteenth-century modernizing state. The nineteenth century saw an increase in the creation, publication, and circulation of state-sponsored social and scientific investigations as official, often government-published reports. On the eve of the Civil War, one-fourth to one-third of the national budget supported scientific enterprises that produced mountains of reports, and state-sponsored medical print culture ballooned during and after the war.[35] In the arena of medical print culture, the U.S. Army's Medical Department and the U.S. Sanitary Commission dominated, together publishing more than fifty major volumes in the twenty-five years that followed the start of the war. They competed for proprietary rights over the soldier's body as a source of knowledge and for public recognition as the singular, premier, authoritative source of the war's medical history. Nevertheless, they shared a compelling common interest and engagement in advancing what we might call "racial knowledge," pursued in the form of social surveys, physical examinations, anatomized medical specimens, and postmortem examinations.

Finally, the commodification of the bodies of people of African descent already had a long history in the United States at the time of war's outbreak. It was not only the living enslaved body that was commodified; as historian Daina Ramey Berry has demonstrated, an elaborate trade in the human remains of the enslaved met the demands of anatomy classes at medical schools across the country. Private collectors and museums added to the demand for crania, skeletons, and fresh cadavers as well as photographic representations of living people of African descent, as institutions competed to gain prominence in the growing field of ethnography and comparative anatomy.[36] Museums, circuses, and other purveyors of commercial spectacle also commodified people of African descent, including the P. T. Barnum's displays of Joyce Heath and the unnamed man exhibited as "What Is It?" in his 1860 display.[37] Scholarship addressing this spectacle of race has helped us understand why and how whites commodified the corpses of deceased African Americans. Whether for the spectacle of public dissections, the supply of cadavers for medical schools (an extensive postdeath slave trade), or the increase of cranial and anatomical collections, whites had established elaborate systems for procuring, valuing, transporting, and supplying the cadavers of African Americans for their own uses.[38]

Medicine, Science, and Making Race in Civil War America excavates and analyzes the wartime investments in race among Sanitary Commission and army medical personnel through five topical chapters, followed by a conclusion. Chapters 1 and 2 provide an overview of both agencies and the racist practices that established a foundation for their race work. Chapter 3 explores the narrative and numerical construction of race through questionnaires, social surveys, and biometric measurement. Chapter 4 explains the ways in which both agencies participated in the anatomization of race through the study and objectification of living African Americans and their human remains. Chapter 5 follows the commodification of Black bodies into death and the persistence of racialization in the disposition of human remains. The book concludes by pointing to the afterlife of these wartime efforts to advance "racial knowledge" and white authority in the fields of racial medicine and racial science.

CHAPTER ONE

Militarizing Race

The War Department and the U.S. Sanitary Commission (USSC) had a powerful and lasting impact on American ideas about race.[1] The army and the USSC included abolitionists and advocates for racial equality in their ranks and others whose ideas about slavery or race changed significantly over the course of the war. But members of both organizations also acted to protect white supremacy with a profound impact on how they organized and whom they identified as worthy of inclusion. A careful consideration of race in the formation and operations of both organizations helps us understand how and why they became engaged in wartime efforts to affirm and advance the notion of race as a biological and hierarchical construct. Even with their important differences, these two organizations shared more than a dedication to Union military victory: they shared a commitment to their own position in American racial hierarchies and a corresponding view of African Americans as an immutably inferior people. The Civil War provided both organizations with the opportunity to enact and advance those commitments, and each organization endeavored to contribute to the premise that race was embodied in the human form, character, and intellect.

Why and how did the two largest bureaucracies of the Union, the U.S. War Department and the U.S. Sanitary Commission, become powerful advocates for a definition of race that could be read in the human body? Their civilian and military investments in the science of race were nurtured and sustained by circulating ideas about the body, the anatomical and physiological locations of race, and its currency in explaining and predicting social structures and relationships. Race was not simply what they studied; it was also endorsed by what they did. As the next two chapters demonstrate, both the army and the USSC perpetuated the everyday racism of the midcentury nation, which sustained the structures of white empowerment and Black exclusion.

In their membership, their leadership, their understanding of the meaning of the war, and their approach to the work of war, the Union's military bureaucracy as well as its largest civilian war relief organization held similarly entrenched ideas and practices that ensured racial disparities in the antebellum North. This proved foundational and complementary to their medical and scientific work in pursuit of new racial knowledge during and after the war. They replicated and extended the racial hierarchy that governed public life in the North first by excluding African Americans and then by circumscribing their participation, as soldiers and civilians, in the Union war effort—on the battlefield and beyond. In this and the following chapters, we consider the centrality of race-based practices to how white Unionists and Northerners conceived and led the Union war effort in military and civilian settings.

Race and the U.S. Military: Black Soldiering

Early in the war, congress, the Lincoln administration, and the War Department's leadership first rejected then moved very cautiously toward Black enlistment. By 1863, it was military necessity and the progress of the war, rather than a commitment to Black equality, that ultimately opened the door to Black enlistment.[2] As historian John David Smith succinctly concluded, "The freeing and the mobilizing of Black troops were consequences, not objectives, of the war."[3] With reason, Northern Blacks and radical abolitionists within and outside the army understood that Black enlistment strengthened the war's attack on slavery and their critique of racial discrimination while reinforcing the long struggle among Northern Blacks for full citizenship rights.[4] At the same time, the War Department limited the radical potential of Black enlistment through policies and practices that perpetuated a lasting structure of inequality for Black soldiers.[5] Confining that radical potential in a web of racializing policies and actions amounted to an overwhelming devaluation of Black humanity, one that came at a very high human cost.

Even with Black enlistment, the wartime army was segregated and organized around the premise of Black inferiority and white intolerance for Black authority. For the most part, neither the Lincoln administration nor the nation's leading military commanders believed white soldiers could or would serve with African Americans; until late in the war, many also doubted the ability of Black men to meet the rigors of soldiering, and certainly most whites refused the notion that white soldiers could be officered by Black men.

White prejudices immediately and lastingly shaped Black military service. For the first year of Black enlistment, the army paid Black soldiers at the same rate as Black military laborers rather than the same rate as white soldiers, evoking extensive protest and causing great hardship among the soldiers who refused to accept Jim Crow pay. Yet the pay controversy was only the opening salvo in military racial discrimination. Throughout their service, Black soldiers would be treated unequally. They were conscripted into service through violence or its threat by Union enlistment agents in the border states and occupied South. They were denied commissioned office and were forced to serve under white commanders. They were disproportionally assigned heavy fatigue duty, posted in the South's most unhealthy regions, denied furloughs, deprived of adequate rations, issued second-class weapons, subjected to humiliating and abusive punishments—the list of disparaging and prejudicial treatment was long and costly to soldier morale, their families back home, and the survival rate in Black regiments.

"The color line circumscribed virtually every aspect of Black military life," one historian concluded.[6] The white surgeon Benjamin Woodward, who served with the 22nd Illinois and after the war as an investigator who interviewed white commanders of Black troops about Black soldiering, offered insight into the appalling conditions endured by the Union's Black soldiers. "The whole history of the negro in the South since the war began even his treatment by northern men has been one of cruelty and neglect. He has been trampled on and outraged in every way, and though legally free, it is but in name."[7]

Race and Military Medicine

Among the first white officers and military medical practitioners that Black soldiers encountered were the examining surgeons who performed the requisite physical examinations that determined the fitness of potential recruits and draftees for service. When surveyed at the close of the war about their observations on the qualifications of Black men for military service, 62 percent of responding examining surgeons commented extensively on what they perceived as racial characteristics that marked the anatomy, physiology, and mentality of African American men.[8] Those surveys will be discussed more fully in chapter 3, but it is important to note that even as they offered their lives to the Union war effort, Black enlistees were viewed by white medical men as living proof of the bodily meaning and appearance of racialized anatomies.[9]

There was considerable pressure on examining surgeons to overlook disability, ill health, or suffering in order to increase the number of successfully enlisted men. As observers of the recruitment of three Black regiments in Missouri noted:

The examining surgeons were instructed to examine the men as if they were conscripts, taking it for granted that they [the Black men] would exaggerate all their physical defects. But the negroes were generally anxious to enlist, and as a rule tried to pass themselves off as healthier than they really were. The rejection of a single recruit provoked censure from the General Commanding and the strongest pressure was employed to override their decisions. Rejected recruits were ordered before a Medical board, and passed into the service in defiance of the judgement of the Regimental Surgeon. A vast amount of worthless material was thus incorporated into the Regiments. Some of the men thus sent have never done a days duty since enlistment. Of one squad of 11 thus passed contrary to the surgeon's judgement, not a man survives.[10]

Examining surgeons also underestimated the punishing physical consequences of the wartime flight from slavery. The majority of Black troops enlisted were from slave states: "fatigue and exposure" were a constant threat to their ability to survive the flight from enslavement as well as their enlistment experiences.[11] Formerly enslaved soldiers suffered from the physical consequences of slavery, but many white commanders concurred with the anonymous major general who wrote in one of Washington's newspapers that he was sure he could extract more physical exertion from Black soldiers than white.[12]

In a war where disease felled the majority of soldiers and a far higher proportion of Black than white soldiers, access to medical care at the hands of skilled and knowledgeable physicians could be pivotal to a soldier's ability to survive the war. When Black regiments were finally authorized in the summer of 1863, the majority of white medical men eager to serve had already found their places in white regiments. As historian Margaret Humphreys noted, the new regiments meant 138 new positions opened for regimental surgeons, but the pool of qualified candidates was very small (although now Black physicians had a chance to serve). Humphreys also has pointed out that white applicants for appointment as surgeons to Black regiments were allowed to meet lower standards; some applied simply for the opportunity of promotion—no empathy toward African Americans or opposition to racial discrimination were required from officers in Black regiments. As a result, many Black soldiers served in units with inept, hostile, or absent surgeons.[13] One sympathetic agent of the U.S. Sanitary Commission volunteering at City Point, Virginia, reported in a family letter, "We have had to almost fight the doctors to get them to treat the colored men decently and to give them proper attention."[14]

Black soldiers demanded better care; they protested that their regimental surgeons were inept. As one soldier complained, "They do more harm than good for they Poison the Soldiers. They are called doctors but they are not. They are only students who knows nothing about issueing medicines."[15] Even in the most celebrated Black regiments, white medical officers could be cruel and sadistic toward their charges. Surgeon Charles E. Briggs, who served with the 54th Massachusetts (Colored Infantry), unhappy with a court-martial that found a soldier innocent of charges of bestiality, took it upon himself to punish the man in question. Briggs had the soldier brought to his tent under guard, chained, partially stripped, and gagged so that Briggs could forcibly perform a circumcision on the soldier.[16]

John Allen, a member of the 60th U.S.C.I., explained of himself and his comrades that "we formed a kind of prejudice against the hospital." He had gone once for treatment of his chronic diarrhea, but, as he explained, "the treatment was so bad that I had to get away." Several fellow soldiers also noted their aversion to medical treatment at regimental hospitals.[17] In another regiment, a Black sergeant with sores on his penis was treated by the white surgeon who poured "a bottle of nitric acid over the prone penis, in the presence and to the infinite delight of some of the officers."[18] Not only was this treatment intentionally, publically humiliating, it was harmful: diluted nitric acid was a common nineteenth-century treatment for syphilitic chancres, but full-strength acid was not.[19] Tortured and mistreated for the entertainment of white officers, Black soldiers may have avoided white medical staff not only because of the specific therapies being used but also because of similar examples of dehumanizing and racist encounters.

Certainly, some regimental surgeons identified as abolitionists. Seth Rogers, for example, was recommended to his post as surgeon of the 33rd U.S.C.I. by Thomas W. Higginson, the notable commanding officer of South Carolina's first Black regiment. Yet Rogers—whose subordinate hospital steward wrapped up prescribed medicines in pieces of the abolitionist newspaper, the *Liberator*—described the men in his regiment as "children of the tropics," whose physiology was demonstrably different from and inferior to that of whites, leading to racially differentiated disease vulnerability, which he hoped to prove through his attendance to the regiment's medical needs. In addition, he commented on the "valuable information" he gathered from a proslavery surgeon about what he described as Black physiology.[20]

White hospital nurses were among the abolitionists who advocated for fair treatment for Black soldiers while also regarding the Black women and children they encountered as something less than human. At Benton Barracks Hospital, Emily Elizabeth Parsons wrote home to her family asking if they wanted her to send them a "pretty" pickaninny: "I can have as many as I want," she wrote, in a shocking disregard for family ties among the formerly enslaved.[21]

BLACK PHYSICIANS who were able to gain appointment were few in number. Fourteen African American surgeons are known to have applied and served during the war, but only two gained appointment to Black regiments; most of the others were hired as inferior civilian contract surgeons at hospitals.[22] They encountered harassment and violence both within the service and from a white public that took offense at Black men in uniforms with officer insignia. Alexander Augusta (as an examining surgeon he performed physicals on over 5,000 men and also had charge of a hospital) was the subject of protest by six white medical officers on discovering that Augusta's appointment made them subordinate to a Black officer.[23] He was also attacked by a white mob in Baltimore and his officer's insignia torn off his uniform; in Washington, D.C., he was thrown off a whites-only streetcar.[24] Cortlandt V. R. Creed, an 1857 graduate of Yale, was repeatedly rebuffed and ignored in his application for appointment as army surgeon until early 1864.[25] Dr. Theodore J. Baker served in 54th Massachusetts, but as a contract steward, even though the regiment needed an assistant surgeon at the time.[26]

The other Black surgeons included Anderson R. Abbott, Benjamin A. Boseman,[27] John Van Surly DeGrasse, William Baldwin Ellis, J. D. Harris,[28] William P. Powell Jr., Charles Burliegh Purvis, John H. Rapier Jr., Willis R. Revels, Charles H. Taylor, and Alpheus W. Tucker. Only Augusta and DeGrasse secured commissions as regimental surgeons, and the remaining were hired as contract surgeons—employees, rather than officers, paid less than regimental surgeons and more easily dismissed.[29] As historian Margaret Humphreys noted, "It took exceptional bravery and resolution to brook the army's racism and the barriers to practice it created."[30]

Male physicians were not the only Black medical workers who encountered institutional discrimination and other manifestations of racism as they served the Union cause. African American women, who were about 10 percent of the more than 21,000 female Union hospital workers, were employed in the lowest prestige and lowest paid jobs as cooks and laundresses; the highest status jobs (as nurses and matrons) were 93 to 94 percent white.[31]

According to historian Jane E. Schultz, Black women were most likely to be employed if the work was especially difficult, demeaning, or if the patients were Black soldiers. African American hospital workers endured insult and abuse from white soldiers, white female hospital workers, and white military commanders who presumed that Black women were at best a burden to the army, at worst prostitutes threatening the moral and physical fitness of white soldiers.[32]

In other words, the majority of Union hospitals were highly segregated and racialized spaces that reinforced white notions of Black incapacity and inferiority, regardless of the essential contributions of Black hospital workers to the comfort and survival of Union troops. In their recollections of the work they performed in hospitals, it is easy to see how important their labor was to the comfort, cleanliness, and efficiency of wartime hospitals.[33]

THE MILITARY'S ENTRENCHED RACISM had a high human cost. The shortages, inadequacies, and other challenges that plagued the entire army medical system were intensely manifested in the mistreatment of ill and wounded Black soldiers.[34] When the newly organized 60th U.S.C.I. arrived at Benton Barracks in St. Louis, with sixty men already ill, the white medical director refused to allow the sick men access to the empty hospital beds that were only 100 yards from the barracks.[35] All along the Mississippi valley, hospitals serving Black soldiers were more likely to be headed by hospital stewards (the equivalent of a pharmacist) rather than surgeons.[36] Major General Nathaniel Banks, commanding the Department of the Gulf, was flooded with complaints about the treatment of Black soldiers by unskilled white medical personnel.[37] Medical inspectors reported, sometimes with alarm, the exponentially higher mortality rate in hospitals that treated Black soldiers.[38] Historian Joseph Glatthaar has documented many instances of brutal mistreatment of Black soldiers in hospitals at the hands of white medical officers.[39] Soldiers themselves, along with officers of Black regiments, army medical inspectors, civilian volunteers, and observers, offered extensive testimony and protest about the filthy conditions and the mistreatment of hospitalized African American men by incompetent and racist doctors, as well as the constant pressure that sick men be returned to duty.[40]

In addition to the issues of hospital conditions and the impact of racism on how white surgeons approached their patients, the hospital edifice itself was part of the army's commitment to institutionalized segregation. Hospital directors had to conform to changing army policies about how segregation should be operationalized. After Black enlistment, Benton Barracks

Hospital, for example, was required to shift from a post hospital with segregated wards to a desegregated post hospital and then into a racially exclusive hospital. Operationalizing segregation took time, resources, and effort away from patient care.[41]

Most mid-nineteenth-century Americans were averse to hospitals because of their association with the severely ill, but the formerly enslaved brought a distinct perspective to their encounter with military hospitals. Enslaved people had known hospitals as places of forced confinement, torture, and discipline.[42] As soldiers, their distrust of white surgeons, the crude and filthy arrangements that passed for hospitals, the types of therapies offered, and the derision with which white physicians treated their Black charges left many soldiers averse to hospital care, just as they had been averse to white medical treatment under slavery.[43]

Yet Black soldiers, far more than whites, found themselves in need of medical treatment. A number of diseases took a severe toll on Black troops, including pneumonia, malaria, diarrhea, measles, and the mumps. Black troops were more likely than whites to contract smallpox, more likely to die from it, and in the Mississippi valley more likely to be injected with impure or ineffective vaccine matter as the army tried to curtail the disease as it swept through the troops.[44] The Black regiments that gathered in St. Louis were vaccinated with both. One regiment vaccinated with impure matter was quickly infected with a serious *Streptococcus* infection, and smallpox subsequently spread throughout the unit; another regiment faced frightening consequences when the soldiers were vaccinated with matter taken from a syphilitic donor. As one Black soldier reported, "We all was vaccinated, [and] that killed a good many of them"; his own arm was so swollen he could not wear a coat, and the ulcerations at the site of his vaccination persisted for so many months that the surgeon cauterized them several times; the soldier ended up with an atrophied, lame arm.[45] George Kebo, vaccinated with matter infected by syphilis, would suffer from syphilitic ophthalmia and ulcerations of his palate and throat.[46] Hundreds of troops suffered similarly, along with the invisible victims of infection—wives and children.

Although some soldiers reported good and decent hospital treatment, many soldiers and their families wrote to the president, the secretary of war, and other Union officials to expose the hospital conditions they and their comrades endured and to beg for and demand better treatment. White surgeons and hospital staff discredited the ability of Black soldiers to report their symptoms, made light of their pain and discomfort, and did little to rectify the conditions soldiers encountered in hospitals.[47]

It is nearly impossible to overestimate the radical challenge that Black military service posed to white presumptions about Black inferiority. Skeptical and contemptuous white officers as well as military and civilian observers weakened in their commitments to anti-Black racial ideologies by witnessing Black soldiers' courage, sacrifice, and valor—as well as their humanity. Yet we cannot ignore the weight and gravity of military racism in inflicting considerable and unnecessary harm on the Black men who offered their lives in defense of their nation.

CHAPTER TWO

Commissioning Race

The U.S. Sanitary Commission (USSC hereafter) is perhaps best known as the federally authorized civilian organization that supported the health and comfort of Union soldiers. It solicited donations of cash and supplies worth at least $25 million from local soldiers' aid societies organized primarily by and among women. The USSC also helped reform and modernize the army's medical practices.[1] Together, the USSC and the army became among the largest bureaucracies the nation had ever formed, and both reflected the intersection of modernizing impulses with deep commitments to racial ideologies and practices.

Civil War and women's historians have closely studied the leadership, operations, and legacy of the USSC, and most agree that elite class interests and gender conflict characterized the commission's work. However, additional, important, and unrecognized issues profoundly shaped the work of the USSC. The USSC's medical investigations and pursuit and application of "sanitary science," along with its "relief work," engaged thousands of white men and women affiliated with the commission in implicit and explicit local and national processes of making and remaking ideas about race and their relationship to social practice and citizenship. Through the USSC, scores of Northern white civilians participated in shaping the relationship between race and social citizenship during the Civil War.

The USSC produced and contributed to "racial knowledge" through a web of interconnected and mutually reinforcing behaviors. The commission sustained the racial beliefs of Northern white civilians in several ways. They did so by acts of inclusion and exclusion as they imagined and negotiated their commission-related individual and corporate relationships with African Americans—including Northern civilians, soldiers, and refugees from slavery. They did so in their decisions about whom to empower as providers of relief and which populations were legitimate targets of relief. They also did this in their social conduct, including relationships with other whites and with African Americans. Finally, they sustained anti-Black racism in creating and circulating new kinds of race-based cultural and social authority.

The commission's founders had not envisioned these developments when they first came together. But when slavery, the most powerful marker of difference and hierarchy among Americans, was unraveled by war and when military service—one of the presumptive avenues to citizenship rights was opened to African American men, the nation was forced to reconsider the political and social place of people of African descent in the United States. The example of the USSC helps us see how and why Northern whites embraced the authority and logic of medicine and its allied sciences to reinforce what they understood as the natural laws that supported and endorsed the nation's racial hierarchies. Through their large-scale and quantifiable investigations of the human form, the USSC intended to "discover the types of humanity, as well as the types of the several classes and races of man."[2] Their findings, discovered through medical and scientific study and reified as natural law, helped justify the racial stratification that would be woven into the new cloth of national citizenship.

Organizing the Commission

As Northern men and women gathered and organized local soldiers' relief societies—the precursor to the USSC—they claimed the conflict as a "people's war." Barely a month after the firing on Fort Sumter, loyal Northerners threw their "hearts and minds," "bodies and souls" into the war effort; according to the USSC's own historian, the "rush of volunteers to arms" was equaled by the enthusiasm of women to support them, but "in their ardor to contribute in some manner to the success of our noble and sacred cause," civilian enthusiasm soon overwhelmed any effective or efficient effort to organize them.[3]

The USSC saw themselves stepping in to bring "nationality of sentiment and influence," method and direction, to the otherwise undirected, and (some argued) counterproductive benevolence that threatened to overwhelm the War Department.[4] An unprecedented scale of human organization was needed on both the home front and the battlefront. It is not surprising, given the gendered politics of public life and citizenship, that men and women clashed over who should direct and who would follow those directions. Neither is it surprising, as historians have pointed out, that through their work with the USSC, elite and aspiring-elite white men and women attempted to consolidate their public authority over philanthropy, benevolence, and public health. What is rarely acknowledged, however, is the centrality of race to the USSC's key activities and conflicts.

THE U.S. SANITARY COMMISSION originated in the April 1861 efforts of Dr. Elizabeth Blackwell, the first woman to receive a medical degree in the

United States, to launch and then bring organization and method to the flood of soldiers' aid societies. Blackwell drew on her medical and social welfare expertise administering the New York Infirmary to propose a women's relief organization—the Women's Central Association for Relief (WCAR)—that would centralize and advocate for women's wartime relief work and the training and placement of female nurses. Blackwell invited the Reverend Henry Whitney Bellows to preside over the second organizational meeting and to lead a group of three male physicians to visit Washington, D.C., in mid-May as the WCAR sought recognition and a direct relationship with the U.S. Army's Medical Department.[5]

The recognition that did come, that June, was not for the WCAR or for a relief-centered effort, but instead for a different kind of organization: the male-led Sanitary Commission.[6] Bellows, during his visits to poorly organized encampments in the nation's capital, apparently became convinced that a more ambitious organization was needed. Unsurprisingly, given mid-century gender ideologies, the new USSC imagined by Bellows would be led not by the women of the WCAR but rather by elite male philanthropists and professionals who would lend their medical, sanitarian, investigational, and organizational expertise to the army's Medical Department. It is this organization that received the approval of the Secretary of War on June 9, 1861 (see figure 2.1).[7]

The Work

According to the USSC's own, premature history (published in 1864 before the end of the war), the "intelligent, scientific" members would "methodize" and "reduce to practical service" the "undirected benevolence of the people." With powers of investigation and advice, they would bring "the "fullest and ripest teachings of Sanitary Science in its application to military life" to bear on the army.[8] Despite what quickly became a conflicted relationship with the army's Medical Department, the USSC became well known for its systematic support for soldiers and armies in the field. This included what historian William Maxwell noted as sending agents and stores to 500 battles; developing a relief corps for camps, battlefields, and hospitals; organizing 7000–10,000 local societies; establishing lodges for convalescing soldiers; organizing and staffing feeding stations for soldiers en route to hospitals; and many more contributions to the Union war effort.[9] The USSC would be credited with organizing affiliated societies in soliciting, manufacturing, and distributing supplies and funds for the relief of soldiers and their families.

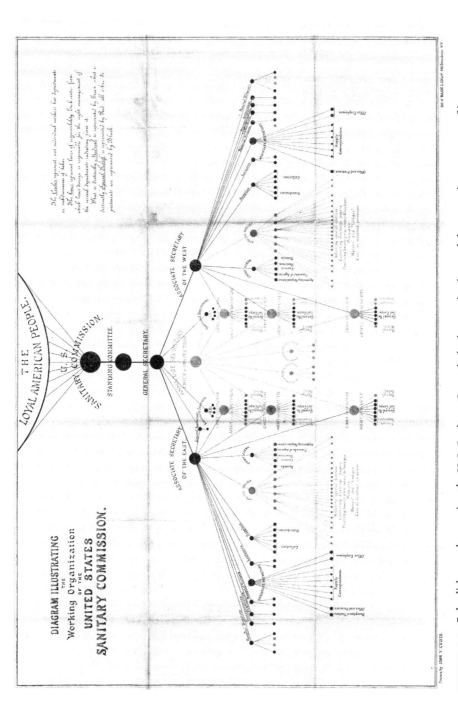

FIGURE 2.1 Color lithograph mapping the U.S. Sanitary Commission's organization and the reporting structure of its many branches. Courtesy of the Manuscripts and Archives Division, New York Public Library.

By July 1861, the all-male executive board broadly outlined the commission's work to include, in addition to the extensive vision of coordinated relief proposed by the WCAR, a host of activities. These included sanitary inspections of the gathering armies in the eastern and western theaters; a Bureau of Sanitary and Vital Statistics; the future publication of "an extended and most valuable series of monographs in medicine, surgery, and hygiene, for the use of Military Surgeons"; investigations into the hygienic and medical condition of military hospitals; and proposals, directed at the Medical Department, for improvements in recruiting, organizing camps, and providing for the comfort of soldiers. The USSC moved quickly to mobilize capital from merchants and corporations (mostly life insurance companies) as well as the cultural authority of "science" to enable their work. A month later, they would also embrace providing relief for discharged invalid soldiers. The USSC's founding association, the WCRA, was brought under the USSC's male administration.[10] Although Northern women would organize in unprecedented numbers, raise astonishing amounts of money, collect and forward to the armies an overwhelming amount of food, clothing, and other goods, they would never regain the primary leadership position that Blackwell and others had proposed as their duty and their right.

The USSC's work expanded as their membership grew and the war proceeded. With characteristic immodesty, the commission regarded itself as "one of the most shining monuments" of the nation's "civilization."[11] The commission opened offices to help soldiers with back pay, bounties, and pensions. They developed a directory of names and locations of hospital patients. They also solicited, funded, published, and circulated dozens of medical tracts, investigations, and reports, and published periodicals for popular audiences.[12] Women would establish a number of subordinate central "branches" along with the WCAR, the Women's Pennsylvania Branch, and the New England Women's Auxiliary Association (NEWAA).

Despite the important work of historians in capturing the extensive work of the commission, a central part of its work has remained unexplored. All the USSC's key goals—its endeavor to modernize American benevolence, to reorganize the army's Medical Department, and to advance the state of medical knowledge—mobilized the dynamic, multilayered social practices of racial segregation and exclusion. By ignoring the critical role and significant impact the USSC had on the popularity and circulation of wartime and postbellum racial practices and ideas, historians have disregarded the important and consequential ways in which bureaucracy and knowledge were leveraged by white Northern wartime actors to sustain white supremacy in a complex and changing landscape of racial inequality.

Race and the Privilege of Commission Work

Much of the work of the USSC, reductively coined "relief work," was carried out by its volunteers in local societies and organized under the leadership of women in the semiautonomous regional "branches" in New York, Boston, Philadelphia, Buffalo, Milwaukee, Cleveland, and Detroit (sometimes alongside separate male-led branches). There were additional male-led regional branches in the nation's capital, in California, and in England, as well as in the eastern and western theaters of war. Other branches organized around specific objectives such as compiling hospital directories, conducting sanitary inspections and medical investigations, aiding veterans and their families with bounties, back pay, and pension benefits, and compiling the history of the USSC. The commission's national leadership consisted exclusively of white philanthropic and professional men, including a general secretary, associate secretaries in the East and the West, and an executive board (later known as the Standing Committee).

"Relief" encompassed a very large category of activities, connecting the work of local societies to the regional and national supply chain of USSC offices, distribution networks, and field agents. Food items, clothing, and other supplies (especially those needed for medical care, from bandages to brandies) were donated, purchased, handmade, or contracted out as charity work among soldiers' wives and forwarded from local societies to branch headquarters. From there the goods were repackaged and forwarded for distribution to soldiers in hospitals, soldiers' homes and lodges, and to soldiers and agents serving in the field. Cash donations were solicited (through various activities, most notably the spectacular and popular sanitary fairs, but also lectures, entertainments, and other public events) and forwarded to branch offices for the purchase of necessary items and to support the work of USSC employees and volunteer agents. Nearly all of the USSC's employed agents and workers—some 450 by 1864, according to historian Robert Bremner—were male whereas the tens of thousands of volunteers affiliated with USSC work were overwhelmingly female.[13]

Race and the Commission

Race—as an idea, as a social relationship, and as a rationale to justify hierarchy, inclusion, and exclusion in social practice and policy—shaped the

USSC's work both explicitly and implicitly. Commission members asserted racial privileges, shaping policy and practice. They were not the only white Northerners anxious about the war's potential to undermine existing racial hierarchies. Whites opposed Black soldiering during the war because they believed that idealized manhood could only be embodied by whites and that men of African descent could not adequately perform the duties of soldiers — and certainly were not entitled to the privileges and recognition that accompanied the performance of military duty to the nation. White women's claims over relief work were similarly racially charged — and were more successful in excluding African Americans. Just as Civil War enlistment and service confirmed a specifically gendered exercise of citizenship and conferred an idealized masculinity on the veteran, so too the participation in the work of the USSC became an opportunity to claim a different but also highly politicized social citizenship for U.S. women. As L. P. Brockett noted in his popular 1867 book exalting women's work during the war, these volunteers "won for themselves eternal honor" as key participants in "the nation's defense."[14] Whites laid claim to those honors as theirs alone.

White women were substantially empowered by their work with the USSC. As historian Judith Giesberg has noted, USSC women "protected the autonomy of women's benevolence work," "kept local-community reform from being absorbed into a men's organization," and "asserted their right" to determine the best uses of vast sums of money raised by women's organizations. They assumed leadership roles, "expected to be treated like professionals," and in so doing challenged the gender conventions of white middle-class and elite men's political culture.[15] The empowerment of white women through their sanitary work (as they challenged efforts by men to contain, lead, and "discipline" them) reinforced the equation of women's exuberant, gendered nationalism with whiteness. Through the women's branches of the USSC, white women also gained access to some of the political and cultural power wielded by elite white men. As Giesberg noted, "The young women who ran the commission branches learned to work with men and the male political process in ways that would further their own interests and that prepared many of them for careers as professional reformers and agitators in the politically charged environment of the postwar years" — but they gained this experience at the cost of cross-racial alliances.[16]

White women excluded Black women from nearly every level of USSC-affiliated work: from joining white societies, from affiliating their own Black-led relief societies with the USSC, and from leadership positions in the women's branches. The November 1862 and January 1864 "Women's Council" meetings in Washington, D.C., of delegates invited from the most prominent women's auxiliaries, excluded representatives from African American relief work. Among those excluded were Elizabeth Keckley, who started the Contraband Relief Association in Washington, D.C., in 1862 and quickly expanded it into a prominent, well-recognized national organization.[17] Black women were also denied the protective shelter of USSC lodging while traveling as volunteers or paid agents.[18] Even when simply visiting USSC lodges as inquisitive fellow aid workers and in the company of white workers, Black women encountered "sneers and side-looks" for trespassing across the color line of wartime relief.[19] And, when contacted by Black women who sought assistance in forwarding donated items to the battle front, white commission women made little effort to recruit or sustain Black women's relationship with the USSC. White USSC work, then, was integral to the wartime and post-emancipation process of white racial formation and the racialization of "modernity."

The racially exclusive work of the USSC extended to its exacting record keeping and its carefully crafted and widely circulated printed reports, which provided public recognition for women involved in war work. The commission maintained lists of donating societies, noting when local societies wished to be considered "auxiliary" to the USSC, naming "associate managers" presiding over local or regional societies, and generally keeping elaborate records of collaborating organizations and donors. Neither individuals or local societies were ever denoted with the traditional "col.," which would have identified them as African American. With the exceptions in Philadelphia and Cleveland noted here, none of the Black women leading or belonging to notable societies are listed in USSC records. And despite the affiliation of African American women's sanitary associations in Philadelphia, none of the officers of those associations are listed among the members or officers of the Women's Pennsylvania Branch.[20]

The spectacular sanitary fairs produced by women's committees and attended by hundreds of thousands from California to Long Island also produced a race-based vision of national service and citizenship. Although some African Americans organized benefits for the fairs, donated goods and cash, offered professional performances, and joined the regimental parades that opened some of the fairs, there were several instances where white organizers excluded or limited Black participation and attendance.[21] This was the case in Baltimore and Philadelphia's 1864 fairs; it was also true for Cincinnati's Great Western Sanitary Fair of December 1863. St. Louis fair organizers reported that although "many" African Americans attended, there were "one or two manifestations of the old prejudice" (but "the prevailing sentiment," they insisted, "was liberal, humane and tolerant").[22] Organizers of Philadelphia's 1864 fair rejected an appeal that Black women be allowed to join the organizing committees or staff and supply their own table. The color line was so rigidly enforced in Philadelphia that even handiwork prepared by African American women was excluded from display.[23] White feminist and freedmen's aid worker Frances Gage criticized New York's 1864 Metropolitan Fair for entirely excluding "a few of the four million poor souls who have been compelled to be the cause of all this need for aid for the soldiers."[24] Occasionally, white commission fairs invited Black regiments to perform drill, but refused to serve Black clergymen and others who wished to attend or be served at the temporary cafés set up at the fairs.[25]

Sanitary fairs also capitalized on the commodification of racist caricature in Northern popular culture—the same fair targeted for criticism by Frances Gage sold, as a fundraiser, a collection of illustrated limericks, *The Book of Bubbles*, which used African Americans and ideas about race as a rich source of satire and caricature.[26] In one sketch, Anglo-Saxon radicals dined with caricatured Black men (a soldier and a civilian) and an Irish man on a meal that featured a "sauce made from Sambo," suggesting that eastern abolitionists were so taken with Black Americans they wished to consume them (see figure 2.2). The meal also included dishes of "Blarney Stone," "Plymouth Rock," and "Nigger Head" (a popular brand of canned oysters), with a dose of "Black Draught" (a laxative) to drink. The room includes artwork such as a classical bust of a Black man's head and a painting alluding to interracial courtship. The image seems to satirize Northern whites whose commitments to abolitionism led to a complete abandonment of appropriate social boundaries between Black and white Americans. "Arcades Ambo" is used here in a pejorative sense: "both fools alike," two people of like tastes, two rascals.

The white Cincinnati board of managers of the Great Western Sanitary Fair (December 1863) resolved the potentially explosive question of whether Black Ohioans would be permitted to staff a table at the fair, or even attend it, by suggesting that they hold their own fair somewhere else and donate the proceeds to the Great Western.[27] Later, in writing the history of their fair, white USSC members failed to acknowledge what Black Cincinnatians clearly understood as a flagrant act of racial exclusion. In Albany, New York, one observer chided that it was an "unexpected honor" for the white Army Relief Association to invite Black women to participate.[28] Black women knew the difference between organizing a fair and being allowed to help. As the

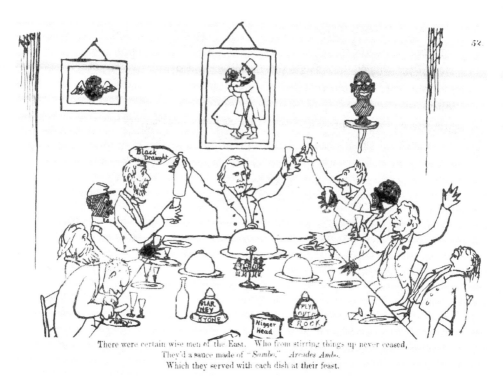

There were certain wise men of the East. Who from stirring things up never ceased,
They'd a sauce made of "Sambo." Arcades Ambo.
Which they served with each dish at their feast.

FIGURE 2.2 One of several cartoons focused on the racial politics of the war included in a collection sold for the benefit of a U.S. Sanitary Commission fair. With Charles Sumner at the head of the table, it appears to poke fun at the allegedly radical racial politics of eastern Republicans—from whom the commission drew several members. "There were certain wise men of the East. Who from stirring things up never ceased, They'd a sauce made of Sambo, Arcades Ambo. Which they served with each dish at their feast." Illustration by William Emlen Cresson, from *The Book of Bubbles, A Contribution to the New York Fair, in Aid of the Sanitary Commission, New York, March, 1864* (New York: Endicott & Co., 1864), 52. Courtesy of the University of Florida Digital Collections.

Detroit Ladies' Freedmen's Relief and Educational Society noted, the Chicago freedmen's fair had "originated with the white ladies assisted by the colored"; they, by contrast, proposed a fair that would "originate with ourselves, and *we will be assisted* by some of the first white ladies of this city" (my emphasis).[29] In these and nearly every form of participation in USSC work, white women's exclusion of Black women was very rarely acknowledged or openly discussed, obscuring their exclusion of Black women in the historical record.

It is not surprising that white women's soldiers' aid societies and the fairs they organized were very rarely integrated. The only secular venues where white and African American women socialized before the war would have been at meetings of radical abolitionists and women's rights advocates, whose political work and commitments brought them together. Indeed, the "amalgamationist" reputation of abolitionists inspired caution among some white women as they contemplated the growth and expansion of USSC work as well as the reputation of those associated with it.[30] The color line was particularly sharp in domestic spaces; local aid societies frequently met in private homes, and most white women would not have wanted or dared to invite Black women into their homes — except as servants.

The most important departure from a color line in wartime relief work occurred in the freedmen's aid movement. The movement originated with the Union occupation of the South Carolina Sea Islands late in 1861 and the army's call on missionaries, abolitionists, and philanthropists for assistance and donations to aid former slaves there. From there, the aid movement quickly took off, particularly among Northern white abolitionists, sympathetic denominations, and among African Americans across the Union. The Western Sanitary Commission (WSC), organized in the summer of 1861 in St. Louis, evolved into a major source of support for troops in the western theater of war. The WSC rejected the USSC's efforts to subsume them under the national organization, and they were far quicker to embrace the imperative of aid to Black soldiers and refugees from slavery. By late 1862, "contraband relief" became a central focus of their work.[31] The relationship between the USSC and freedmen's aid was complicated; even as USSC women excluded African Americans from membership, USSC workers at home and in the field were quick to call on freedmen's aid societies — white, African American, and integrated — for donations in instances where commission aid could not be expected.[32]

At the conclusion of the war and the USSC's work in the South, it was commission women who most strongly advocated for transferring remaining USSC goods and funds to the freedmen's aid movement. Still, there were points of conflict in relationships between these two arenas of wartime relief work, as noted by historian Carol Faulkner. Mrs. Sarah Tilmon was one of several African Americans working during the war to help secure Northern employment for recent refugees from slavery. Tilmon, a minister's widow who lived with her formerly enslaved father, had supported herself at least since 1860 through the fees she earned by helping African Americans find jobs in New York. Ellen Collins, a white founding member of WCAR (and later active in freedmen's relief work), was critical of the federal policy endorsing Black migration northward, and she was especially critical of what Faulkner recognizes as "African American entrepreneurship." Relief work, Collins felt, was properly voluntary—the domain of elite women who could afford to be charitable toward others. She was particularly critical of Tilmon's work (and likely her advocacy of African American self-help and independence) and made a complaint to the Freedmen's Bureau in Washington, D.C. Tilmon, on learning that a complaint had been made, offered to open her office and her records for inspection and challenged Collin's presumed authority, asking who and where Collins was. Collins— whose name was imprinted on the WCAR letterhead—might have been surprised to learn that there were significant arenas of wartime relief work in which neither her authority nor her reputation held sway.[33]

There were both immediate and long-term consequences to white women's insistence on a color line in USSC work. They refused to include African American women in the Union's "imagined community" that connected white women across class and across urban/rural communities, which had profound implications for the civil rights, women's rights, and suffrage movements during and after Reconstruction.[34] Popular and historical memoirs of the war, written by or about white women, would exclude the record of local, state, and nationally networked relief work conducted by and among African American women. The personal connections nurtured among USSC members served to empower only white women, who ignored the struggles that African American women encountered and engaged with during and after the war.[35] As Carol Faulkner noted in her study of the freedmen's aid movement, many white women active in wartime relief work of all sorts viewed the value and competence of their own work as tied to their presumption of dependence and incapacity among African American women.[36]

Black Women's Sanitary Work

Yet Black women were undeniably both independent and capable. They organized in large and small groups and participated in a wide range of wartime relief activities. Still, the USSC held on to its color line. More than thirty-five African American women's Union or soldiers' relief associations were organized during the war in ten Northern and border states and the District of Columbia; only three of these were ever officially associated with the USSC.[37] Two of the latter were in Philadelphia: the Ladies' Sanitary Commission of African Episcopal Church of St. Thomas (an elite institution, reflected in the membership of this auxiliary) as well as that city's Colored

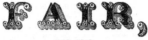

FAIR,

FOR THE

SICK & WOUNDED SOLDIERS!

The Ladies of the Sanitary Committee of St. Thomas' Episcopal Church, auxiliary to the United States Sanitary Commission, intend holding

A FAIR,

for the benefit of Sick and Wounded Soldiers, at Concert Hall, Chestnut Street above 12th, commencing on Monday, December 19th, 1864.

The tables will be supplied with a fine assortment of Useful and Fancy Articles, Refreshments, Confectionery, &c.

Believing it a duty we all owe, to assist in quelling this unholy rebellion of the slave power, and sustaining the U. S. Government in establishing Universal Freedom! We flatter ourselves our efforts will be fully appreciated by the Public, and will cheerfully extend their patronage.

Any donations in goods or money will be thankfully received by the undersigned Committee:

Mrs. Thomas J. Bowers, Prest.,   917 South Street.
Mrs. John Chew, Vice-Prest.,   749 So. Ninth Street.
Miss Ada Hinton, Cor. Sec'y., 612 Locust Street.
Mrs. Thomas J. Dorsey, Treas., 1231 Locust Street.

Mrs. F. Sebastian, C. Miller,   E. Drummond,
E. Boddy,   L. Goines,   C. Christianson,
Mrs. Gibbons,   Mrs. Minton, L. Galloway.

Tickets 25 Cts. to be had of any of the Committee.

G. T. Stockdale, Printer, 117 South Second St.

FIGURE 2.3 Poster, Sanitary Fair organized by the Ladies of St. Thomas Episcopal Church, December 19, 1864. The St. Thomas organization was one of the very few Black female sanitary organizations officially recognized by the U.S. Sanitary Commission. Courtesy of the Library Company of Philadelphia.

Women's Loyal League (see figure 2.3).[38] Besides forwarding goods and donations directly to Black regiments, they donated money and goods to the USSC based on their understanding that the USSC dealt with "colored and white soldiers as men and citizens, entitled to equal consideration and respect."[39] The third officially recognized Black auxiliary was organized in Cleveland as part of a statewide union of local, otherwise white soldiers' relief societies.[40] Some African Americans took the "Sanitary Commission" name as their own; Baltimore and Boston both had such groups, the latter even identifying its work as part of a national, organized effort (yet not affiliated with the USSC).[41]

Of these Black (and female-led) Sanitary Commissions, both of the Philadelphia organizations repeatedly and publically asserted their status as officially recognized USSC auxiliaries. Members of the St. Thomas auxiliary noted that they were "solicited by the ladies of the U.S. Sanitary Commission to become an auxiliary," and along with donations they made directly to Black soldiers and their families they forwarded donations to the Women's Pennsylvania Branch of the USSC, which the branch enthusiastically and publically acknowledged.[42] But the meaning of their auxiliary status remains unclear. Certainly none of the African American women who served as officers of Black auxiliaries ever appeared on membership lists published by the Women's Pennsylvania Branch.[43] Most Northern Blacks organized locally (rather than as part of the USSC's much-vaunted national directive), but they, too, created and participated in a national network of relief—visiting associations, fairs, and institutions located in other cities, publishing their minutes in nationally circulated Black newspapers, and forwarding donations to other Black societies.[44]

Among African Americans, freedmen's aid events and societies significantly outnumbered the more generic soldiers' aid and Union societies. Some cross-racial activism occurred among aid societies organized on behalf of Black refugees and freed people, and in antislavery societies that continued meeting during the war. Until the end of the war, the freedmen's aid movement and the USSC remained separate and distinct, and African American women were far more active in the former than the latter, a development discussed more fully later. Moreover, African American women were not always interested in working alongside whites, given the risk of insult and interference with the work at hand. As historian Janette Greenwood noted, in Worcester, Massachusetts, white women organizing aid societies welcomed African Americans as members—but "Black women ultimately chose to establish their own."[45] In other locations, like St. Louis, white women involved in commission work could prove themselves staunch defenders of their privileges as white women. When the city's Black women organized their own soldiers' aid organization and traveled to the city's military hospitals, their members—among the city's elite—were forced by streetcar operators to ride on the outside of the streetcars. When they protested and secured the right to travel *inside* the cars on Saturdays, white aid workers still met them with resistance, hostility, and "deliberate insult."[46]

In some ways, the work of Black relief societies was very similar to that of USSC societies: members met regularly, solicited donations of cash and needed articles from friends and the greater public, made goods for sale and donation, and forwarded donations to those in need at home and on the battlefield.[47] Prior to Black enlistment, they made donations to support white regiments.[48] Some societies purchased newspaper subscriptions (to the *Anglo-African*, for example) for Black regiments.[49] They staffed diet kitchens for hospitalized Black soldiers and solicited clothing for children and women among the Black refugees from slavery.[50] They forwarded donations to other Black women's fairs and to relief associations located near the front or to where Black soldiers and freed people were hospitalized (the Norfolk, Virginia, Ladies Aid Association requested and received numerous donations in this manner).[51] The majority of their wartime relief work was aimed at two objectives: providing for refugees from slavery (both those who migrated northward during the war and those who remained in the Union-occupied South and border states) and providing for Black regiments and the families of Black soldiers. But that work also sometimes required that they critique segregation and discrimination in war relief activities. The (Black) Philadelphia's Ladies Union Association, unaffiliated with the USSC, used the proceeds of their own soldiers' fair as leverage to persuade the city's white Sanitary Commission women to admit Black soldiers to the soldiers' home.[52] Black commission workers in Philadelphia were joined by Black women in St. Louis and Washington, D.C., in protesting streetcar segregation and its deleterious impact on their relief work, and in commenting on the refusal of the Sanitary Commission's Relief Branch to assist the families of Black soldiers as they did for whites.[53]

With the Emancipation Proclamation and the enlistment of Black men beginning in 1863, the public war work of Northern Blacks expanded. African American communities organized and attended what the Black press described as "war meetings," where Black communities gathered for political speeches and discussion, and encouraged Black men to enlist and Black women to provide support for Black regiments.[54] In addition, African American women increasingly organized around singular events, including fairs, performances, and lectures, where they solicited donations for the aid of freed people and soldiers.[55] Black women organized at least sixteen fairs during the war. More than sixty African American women from Brooklyn, Williamsburg, and New York, for example, organized a fair to benefit freed people and Black soldiers, and this was followed by additional fairs organized by other Black women's organizations in the city; one African American auxiliary in Philadelphia organized a large and successful fair, as did the Boston Ladies' Sanitary Commission (unaffiliated) (and in an interesting reversal, white women were permitted to staff tables there). Women in New Bedford organized to offer two "Literary and Musical Entertainments" to support the Black soldiers of Massachusetts.[56] All these wartime activities were in addition to the rather significant level of ongoing women's community relief and charity work that kept churches, schools, newspapers, and benevolent work afloat in peacetime.[57]

From early in its organization, the white executives of the USSC asserted that in order for relief work to be modern, efficient, and truly nation-building, local societies had to work for the good of the corporate army rather than for local companies or state regiments. Clearly implicit in their view of modern nation-building was a belief that whites would be the architects and beneficiaries of the new nation. African Americans, women and men, challenged these definitions of modernity and nationhood. They insisted on their ability and obligation to meet new demands of Black citizenship but also understood that their citizenship was best expressed by enlisting civilian and soldier alike for the Black community's specific contributions to the war. When the revolutionary present (of emancipation and Black war efforts) became the memorialized past, African American women wanted to be able to "look back upon what we have accomplished" and "feel proud of the part we have enacted."[58] Neither white exclusion nor segregation kept them from "the front ranks of usefulness and benevolence."[59]

The Commission and Black Soldiers

Black enlistment, beginning in 1863, forced a revision to USSC policies. Having committed itself to comprehensive support for an idealized and implicitly white soldier, the commission announced it would now "furnish our troops without respect to color."[60] Agents and workers in the South volunteered to nurse wounded and ill Black soldiers and helped staff the army's segregated hospitals. They donated food and supplies to Black regiments. That work, in turn, led some USSC workers to make fuller commitments to serving the relief needs of Black civilians. Black enlistment meant that Black civilians could make a stronger claim as the relatives of soldiers, not simply as government employees.[61] But the overall success of the USSC's pledge to provide equally for African American troops was limited by both internal and external factors. Commission work occurred in tandem with a military structure that was both segregated and unequal. The USSC could not and did not circumvent the army's practices of segregation in field, regimental, or general hospitals; nor were they responsible for the army's failure to appoint skilled medical men as regimental surgeons for Black regiments. But as close collaborators with the medical officers and regimental surgeons who treated Black soldiers, USSC agents were sometimes vocal reporters (and critics) of discriminatory medical treatment by the army.

It must be noted that some USSC workers were fierce advocates for the Black soldiers they cared for. Helen Gilson, who helped establish a hospital for the Black ill and wounded at City Point, Virginia, and directed a squad of USSC relief workers who tended African American patients, was well known during and after the war for the generosity and rigor of her care and her willingness and ability to circumvent the discriminatory practices of the army. She also quietly worked contrary to USSC policy when she appealed directly to freedmen's aid societies in the North for donations to aid the freed women who gathered at City Point.[62] Gilson was not alone: at New Berne, North Carolina, Dr. J. W. Page and other USSC agents distributed relief to Black refugees in direct contradiction to policy.[63] Yet for every Gilson and Page there were many more USSC agents like Samuel Jayne, who worked on behalf of Black soldiers and civilian refugees along with Gilson. He privately worried about the mistreatment Black patients received at the hands of white surgeons but also commented extensively and pejoratively on what he perceived to be the racial characteristics and inferiority of people of African descent compared with whites (see figure 2.4).[64]

The USSC very quickly expanded its work from providing advice and practical knowledge to the military and relief to the soldier and the army, to providing for soldiers in transit to and from enlistment camps, mustering-in stations, and the battlefront, as well the needs of soldiers' family members traveling to assist the ill and wounded. Dubbed "Special Relief," this branch of USSC work employed male as well as female agents in the South and on the Northern home front.[65] The commission expanded relief work to include creating and updating hospital directories, appointing hospital visitors, staffing the office that assisted veterans and their families in obtaining their bounties and pensions, operating lodges for visiting family, providing relief for the impoverished families of soldiers, and assisting veterans in their pursuit of peacetime employment. The travel of troops (healthy, wounded, and sick) through the major cities of the East Coast demanded particular attention. As the Pennsylvania Branch women noted in 1866, over one and a half million soldiers had traveled through the city on their way to and back from the war. Supporting hospitals, training grounds for regiments, discharge

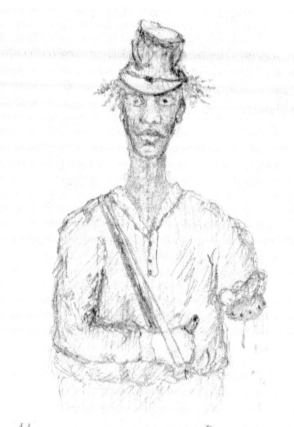

For this are we Doctors,

FIGURE 2.4 Pencil sketch captioned "For this are we Doctors," drawn by "Roberts," a friend of Samuel F. Jayne, in camp at City Point, Virginia, August 1864. The artist appears to propose that the nobility of white physicians was denigrated by the expectation that they treat Black soldiers. Courtesy of the William L. Clements Library, University of Michigan.

camps, barracks, and lodges for family members as well as soldiers in transit all placed heavy demands on the commission.

In the South, the USSC's expanding work of building and renting, staffing, and supplying soldiers' homes, lodges, and parlors (for in-transit soldiers and USSC workers) adopted practices of exclusion and segregation. This meant, for example, that Black soldiers passing through Brashear, Louisiana, were accommodated at the city's Soldiers' Rest but in the rear of the building where they shared their rooms with "colored help."[66]

Here, too, we see the formative impact of ideas about race on relationships of charity and benevolence. White commission women were now, more than ever, empowered to determine who the USSC would regard as a legitimate recipient of relief—especially as the Northern public became somewhat suspicious of the potential of waste, fraud, and malfeasance in the operations (and substantial cash reserves) of the USSC.[67]

Black regiments were organized in each of the three major cities where the USSC's presence was particularly notable and where white women led semiautonomous branches: New York, Boston, and Philadelphia. In New York, home of the largest and most powerful (white) women's branch (the WCAR), African American women, under the leadership of Mrs. Julia W. Garnet, took charge of organizing to meet the needs of sick soldiers from the 26th Regiment, U.S.C.T., at Rikers Island. In January 1864, with the permission of the white commanding general, a donation from the white Sanitary Commission, and the "sanction" of the city's all-white Union League, Garnet's group established a special diet kitchen and cared for some sixty soldiers.[68] Although apparently happy to be relieved of the work of providing intimate care for Black soldiers, the WCAR and the New York City Branch both distributed aid to the families of Black soldiers and to disabled Black veterans during and after the war. In Indianapolis, where local USSC workers were apparently slow to recognize or respond to the needs of the families of Black soldiers, the Reverend William Revels—an active recruiter for Indiana's 28th U.S. Colored Infantry—effectively challenged the white organizers to share sanitary funds among the wives of Black soldiers.[69]

Although the extant record makes it impossible to determine what kind of negotiations over Black agency and the politics of segregation may have been at play in New York City and Boston, a unique record emerges in Philadelphia. There, Black women formed at least four different soldiers' aid societies, two of them officially recognized Sanitary Commission auxiliaries. Not only did they support USSC work with donations, but they also challenged the white women of the Pennsylvania Branch for failing to provide for the families of Black soldiers in the same way it provided for whites. In response, by March 1864 the women's board of managers of the Pennsylvania Branch put into place a unique plan: "It has been ascertained," they noted in meeting minutes, "that one fourteenth of the men entering the army from Philadelphia are colored"; consequently, "one-fourteenth of the time and money of the 'Relief'" would be appropriated to the needs of those soldiers' families.[70] When local Black activists (and husbands of African American commission members) also challenged the USSC's exclusive control over governmental contract work—through which the commission offered charitable employment for needy soldiers' families—they won a concession that government contracts would, in the future, also be awarded to African Americans.[71] The branch also agreed at this time to arrange with charitable associations to find work for those in need, although applicants would have to undergo a home visit and investigation by the white agents to assess the applicant's circumstances.[72] Indeed, within the year nearly 10 percent of the women employed by the branch (either making goods for shipment to the South or working as subcontract laborers on government jobs) were widows and wives of Black soldiers, who were assigned the particular labor of making garments and bedding for freed people in Nashville, Tennessee. There was an important advantage to gaining employment through the Pennsylvania Branch: they paid women twice the rate provided by government contractors.[73] No other USSC branch developed a policy explicitly committing to include African Americans among its constituents.

WHITE RACIAL ASSUMPTIONS AND DEBATES about the USSC's obligations toward Black soldiers, their families, and refugees from slavery were also prominent in the western theater of war. In St. Louis, white Unionists, men and women, began organizing to care for soldiers in the aftermath of a battle near Springfield, Missouri, in the summer of 1861. By September, they had organized the WSC.[74] Although the WSC would reject proposals to merge with the USSC because of their concern that the USSC's eastern focus left the West's demands misunderstood and unmet, the WSC would also confront the question of its obligations to Black civilians and soldiers.

The equivalent of its (white) female branch, the Ladies Union Aid Association, worked closely with the WSC and by January 1863 had already received a number of requests to assist the thousands of Black refugees from slavery in and around St. Louis. When they decided they would not use funds donated for soldier relief for this purpose, several members, joined by additional new members, organized the Contraband Relief Society to provide for the refugees from slavery temporarily housed in camps between Cairo, Illinois, and Memphis, Tennessee.[75]

By November 1863, however, local free Black women ("well-educated and wealthy; lady-like in manners and conversation," according to a white observer) organized their own Union society, to assist the refugees but also to visit and care for the Black troops in camp and hospitalized in and around the city. Unsurprisingly, their work sometimes brought them into contact with white aid workers, women among them, who offered "deliberate" insult. Like their counterparts in Philadelphia, Black women found the enforcement of streetcar segregation a detriment to their work and an affront to their patriotism. They obtained the right to travel unrestricted after filing complaints, but only on Saturdays.[76]

Despite the challenges of relief work in such segregated environs and the publically announced decision by the local white WSC women that the needs of Black civilians were not a proper target of their work, by the spring of 1864 the WSC claimed to be engaged promptly and "with characteristic humanity" in freedmen's relief work.[77] This was a significant departure from the practice in eastern auxiliaries of strictly separating freedmen's aid from Sanitary Commission work.[78]

The Commission and Refugees from Slavery

The race-based prerogatives and status accrued by white women of the USSC came not only from the power to exclude African Americans as suitable colleagues and peers in war relief work. White women (like white men) enlarged their dominion when they assumed the authority to determine whether, and in what circumstances, they would regard African Americans—North and South—as legitimate recipients of USSC-funded wartime relief. With generations of experience in the business of benevolence, many USSC members were not new to positions of authority in client relationships; however, their USSC work allowed them to create a very specific relationship to African Americans, one framed in a racialized hierarchy of provider authority and client need.[79] Even in their annual reports, USSC women emphasized the social distance they claimed from those to whom they provided assistance. They referred to white female commissioners as "ladies" and to their female clients as "women."[80]

In the early months of the war, USSC policymakers insisted on the ineligibility of enslaved or freedom-seeking people for commission support. However, as they discovered, the war could not be fought without disrupting slavery, without enslaved African Americans seizing their opportunities for freedom, and without the invaluable contributions of Black civilian laborers (see figure 2.5). Despite hesitant and contradictory military policy, the Union war effort hungrily incorporated Black labor in the South. "Colored female servants in the capacity of cooks, washerwomen, and laundresses," noted one USSC hospital worker from Nashville, "are doing a great service to our wounded soldiers, and through them to our country, but . . . for some cause are greatly neglected."[81] White USSC workers—onboard

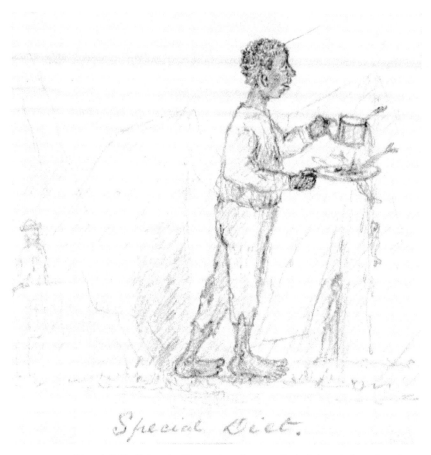

Special Diet.

FIGURE 2.5 "Special Diet" sketch, illustrating the use of Black hospital workers by the U.S. Sanitary Commission. Drawn by "Roberts," a friend of Samuel F. Jayne, in camp at City Point, Virginia, August 1864. Courtesy of the William L. Clements Library, University of Michigan.

hospital transport boats, as part of the supply train of donations to the army in the South, and in regimental and battlefield hospitals and camps— were among those who proved glad to employ former slaves.[82] As historian Jane Schultz has noted, not only were female refugees from slavery hired to do work that the elite white women of the USSC deigned beneath them, they also performed work (such as vegetable gardening and laundry) that USSC workers understood to be valuable and cost-saving while freeing white agents to lend more personal attention to white patients.[83] Freed people employed by the USSC not only gained remuneration (and more reliable wages than those provided by army employment) but also joined the small number of Black civilians that the USSC felt obligated to support with rations and other forms of relief.

THE USSC'S FIRST EXECUTIVE SECRETARY, Frederick Law Olmsted, appointed in the early summer of 1861, saw the need for government oversight on the status of refugees from slavery. From the summer of 1861 into early 1862, Olmsted could imagine no man better situated than himself to direct federal policy pertaining to the slave's transition to freedom. Olmsted claimed his authority on two grounds: his administrative experience supervising 15,000 laborers and a multi-million-dollar budget as architect-in-chief and superintendent of Central Park in New York; and his belief that he had given more thought to the "special question of the proper management of negroes . . . than anyone else in the country," a reference to his time spent traveling in the South and his three widely read travelogues describing slavery and Southern society.[84]

Even after accepting his appointment as executive secretary of the USSC in June 1861, Olmsted continued to pursue a position as a superintendent over Southern freed people. He proposed a plan for this position to Union General George B. McClellan in August 1861 and he pressed Secretary of the Treasury Salmon Chase for an appointment over the South Carolina Sea Islands after their November 1861 occupation by Union forces. He also ordered Dr. Robert Ware, a USSC medical inspector, to prepare a report on the condition of refugees from slavery at Fortress Monroe for his use; and he even drew up a bill outlining a system for federal oversight, which he had introduced to the U.S. Senate (and worked hard to gain public support for). Olmsted also attempted to persuade Secretary of War Edwin Stanton of the unique efficiency and economy of his proposal to coordinate the government's economic interest in a superintendency over former slaves with the religious and educational interests of the freedmen's aid movement in the North. Although Secretary Chase would tentatively offer the position to Olmsted, they were unable to come to agreement on the scope of the position; instead, Chase appointed Brigadier General Rufus Saxton in the summer of 1862.[85]

Olmsted's interest in the transition from slavery to freedom never centered on humanitarian relief (although he certainly made note of the illness and starvation that affected Black refugees behind Union lines). Instead, he sought to prove three things to the nation. First, that free labor was superior to the slave labor economy of the South. Second, that conditions in South Carolina (and other places occupied by Union forces) were an unavoidable consequence of war. Third, that a "true republican plan" of action must be based on an understanding of the "peculiarities . . . of the class in question." To Olmsted, those "peculiarities" meant that "the negro is not a gentleman and a Christian. . . . He is little better than a cunning idiot and a cowed savage." Olmsted believed that former slaves themselves recognized that their dependence on white supervision was so substantial that they "would rather have an owner than no guardianship."[86] He firmly believed that it was not benevolence, charity, or philanthropy so much as efficient and forceful white governance that the formerly enslaved, so marked by "mental and moral peculiarities" as well as "congenital idiosyncrasy," most needed.[87]

When he failed to secure the federal superintendency he sought, Olmsted turned his attention and energy elsewhere, and left the USSC in 1863. However, it is worth noting that despite his intense if brief interest in assuming a position of authority over the disposition of former slaves, it appears he never proposed that the USSC intervene in or absorb Black civilian relief as an additional target of its work. Instead, he saw the "field" of humanitarian aid in the South as the responsibility of the government and of the freedman's aid movement. Certainly, his view held influence over the USSC and especially the men in executive, policymaking positions. This might be why the first history of the USSC, written and published by nurse Katharine Prescott Wormeley, makes no mention of slavery or African Americans among the Union forces served by USSC workers.[88] Prior to 1863 and Lincoln's shift to embracing slavery's destruction as a war aim, the USSC rejected most requests for aid to Black civilians in the South, even as its publications, the widely circulated *Bulletin* and *Reporter*, openly and frequently criticized the failures of the military to provide for Black civilians, noting the high mortality and morbidity confronting that population.[89]

Although scattered evidence shows some USSC agents distributing relief to fugitives from slavery as they saw fit, the closest that USSC executives came to a general policy arose from a May 1863 appeal made by commission workers in New Berne, North Carolina, for "supplemental relief" for Black refugees hospitalized there.[90] After consulting with USSC executives, Bellows approved medical assistance for the Black laborers employed by the government because the commission should address "every source of disease," whether among the soldiers "or the communities in which they may be quartered."[91] Even then, Bellows also asserted that there should be clear limits to the USSC's duty: "We do not wish to commit ourselves to the principle of including the Contrabands in *our* care, but when common humanity is suffering, we do not under any circumstances wish to hoard our stores. . . . The needy Black can only have

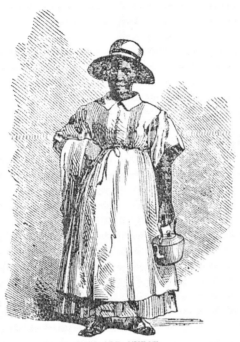

THE OLD NURSE.

HOSPITAL FOR FREEDMEN FOUNDED.

FIGURE 2.6 Illustration captioned "The Old Nurse," portraying an aged Black woman at New Bern who nursed a Black smallpox patient when no white physician or attendant was willing. The drawing was included in Vincent Colyer [Superintendent of the Poor under General Burnside], *Report of the Services Rendered by the Freed People to the United States Army, in North Carolina, in the Spring of 1862, after the Battle of Newbern* (New York: Vincent Colyer, 1864), 41.

a very fortuitous claim, on us, though they have a very certain one on the Government. Would to God that it were met."[92] The commission also applied this policy in Norfolk, where it had "given satisfaction."[93]

A year later, the New Berne correspondence would be recirculated when questions arose again about whether medical care should be provided to African Americans. In this instance, a request had been made for food and clothing for a smallpox hospital for New Berne freed people (see figure 2.6); once again, USSC executives tried to distinguish between aid to Black civilians generally and efforts to prevent the spread of disease to white soldiers. "The commission does not feel justified in assuming general care of civil Hospitals for the Contraband," asserted the general secretary of the USSC.[94]

Bellows—who spoke frequently to freedmen's relief meetings—was sympathetic to the humanitarian needs of refugees from slavery, but as USSC head he was unwilling to affirm any specific duty or obligation on the part of the USSC to Black refugees from war.[95] The WSC women in St. Louis followed a similar path.[96]

The commission may have imagined it could maintain a clear line between aid to soldiers (which it defined as central to the organization's existence) and aid to civilians, but substantial amounts of aid were already provided to the families of white soldiers without generating policy debates, so this was not clearly a debate about the exclusive centrality of soldier relief to USSC work. Furthermore, it was a rare occurrence for the USSC to back away from an opportunity to expand its arena of authority and action. It is possible, and even probable, that Bellows and the larger executive committee were concerned about alienating a white public that was not wholly sympathetic toward either emancipation or African Americans in general. The executive members of the USSC were notoriously concerned with avoiding anything that might interrupt the flow of donations from a supportive Northern populace, particularly when, in the fall of 1862, the USSC came under fire with charges of corruption and malfeasance.[97] At the least, their failure to address the medical crisis experienced by African Americans in the South suggests a failure to acknowledge the medical reality of a civil war, a failure to comprehend the consequences of slavery's wartime demise, and a failure to understand the centrality of Black civilian labor to the Union army and the war effort.

BY THE END OF THE WAR, the USSC's convoluted wartime negotiations over race and relief eased, as white Union troops mustered out and the need for USSC donations ended. Several Black regiments were kept on as occupying forces in some of the most dangerous locations in the postwar South, and they continued to suffer enormously from disease and malnutrition. Nevertheless, the USSC wound down its work supporting soldiers in the field. Several of the leading white women of the USSC—Ellen Collins, Abby May, and Louisa Schuyler among them—imagined a new unity between freedmen's aid and commission work, and they proposed that what was left of USSC stores and property be donated to the Freedmen's Bureau.[98]

Indeed, the new Freedmen's Bureau as well as freedmen's aid societies became recipients of the USSC's remaining donated cash and goods as well as the buildings and rooms in USSC control. The Washington, Boston, New York, and North Carolina branches made repeated donations and transfers of property to the bureau, and the Pennsylvania Branch transferred supplies housed in its lodge to the American Freedmen's Aid Society.[99] These donations made sense—transporting goods north to soldiers' homes, for example, would have likely cost more than their worth—but the ease of this decision stands in notable contrast to the USSC's careful racial policing of its wartime relief work. It suggests that one of the principal motivations behind the USSC's color line in wartime relief work was their belief that support and donations would dry up if the white public understood they were aiding refugees from slavery. This conclusion is strengthened when we recognize that the USSC's core *postwar* work—assisting veterans and their families in securing bounties, back pay, and pensions—brought important benefits to thousands of African American military families. Their work with Black veterans was consonant with the USSC's explicit focus on soldiers, but it also occurred largely after the war when the USSC had stopped fundraising.

However, the USSC's interactions with Black soldiers included far more than supplying fresh vegetables or hospital care. As the next chapter reveals, USSC officials, along with military health care workers, viewed Black soldiers as racial specimens worthy of study. How and why they engaged in race studies makes sense when we understand that race thinking saturated every aspect of their organizations—who was included, who was excluded, who could lead, who could only "help"—and their understanding of the Civil War as a military conflict rather than a revolutionary assault on the system of slavery.

CHAPTER THREE

Narrating and Enumerating Race

During the war, white practitioners recruited medicine and its allied sciences (which, according to one nineteenth-century participant, included "Anatomy, Physiology, Psychology, Ethnography, Ethnology, Philology, History, Archaeology, and Palaentology [sic]") in the service of advancing more certain, irrefutable racial ideologies.[1] Those ideologies—based on the presumption of measurable, stable, observable characteristics that could be cataloged and enlisted to distinguish and rank human races—not only survived the end of slavery but also fueled opposition to the extension of civil and citizenship rights to African Americans.

Of course, the elaboration of racial ideology using medical science was not new to the Civil War era. Historians have closely documented how racialized medicine and science predated the war. Men like J. Marion Sims, Josiah Nott, George Gliddon, Samuel Morton, Louis Agassiz, and Samuel Cartwright—scientists, naturalists, public intellectuals, and medical practitioners—had participated in the growth of racialized science (such as the "American School" of ethnology). Their ideas, research, writing, and public pronouncements had been crucial to proslavery ideology and beliefs about race as an immutable feature of human life with natural hierarchies.[2] Antebellum physicians and scientists looked to natural history, craniology, Linnaean taxonomy, comparative anatomy, and observations and experimentation using enslaved and free Black subjects as well as their cadavers to elaborate, rationalize, and justify racial hierarchies in America.[3]

The war saw Northern whites making even deeper investments in the "scientific and historical researches . . . on this vital question."[4] The U.S. Sanitary Commission (USSC), as well as the Smithsonian Institution, the U.S. Surgeon General, the army's Medical Department, the Army Medical Museum, and the Provost Marshal, contributed to the interdisciplinary study of the racialized human body, often described as the "science of man." In so doing, they committed substantial effort and resources to the scientific and medical knowledge that was capable of sustaining the racial hierarchies threatened by emancipation and Black enlistment. The results of their work—whether in the skull collections of the Smithsonian Institution, the vast displays of anatomical specimens at the Army Medical

Museum, or in the prolific and widely circulated war-related medical and scientific print culture—received popular and professional acclaim.[5]

The medical print culture of the war was notably diverse in form and extraordinarily prodigious, as more than a thousand physicians prepared papers and letters that they submitted to the USSC with hopes of joining the ranks of published authorities on the war's medical events.[6] The army and the USSC saw the soldier's body as a source of knowledge, and the two competed for public recognition as the premier source of the war's medical history. They competed in the realm of medical print culture for authors, audiences, reviews, and readers. Both organizations saw authorship as a means of asserting a new public professional authority in the postwar period, reinforced by the view of many medical practitioners that authorship carried considerable professional and cultural capital. Executive Secretary Henry Bellows called the commission's publications "our only chance for being valued by men of mark in time to come."[7] The museum and print archive of race-related research produced during the war was substantial, well received, and eagerly circulated among popular and learned readers—and it was also long-lived.[8] The cumulative impact was great enough that decades later the young social scientist W. E. B. Du Bois directed his early career toward a refutation of those data and the conclusions based on them.[9]

A careful exploration of the enterprise of creating and circulating medically based "racial knowledge" helps us historicize the wartime process of race-making. It allows us to trace how white Unionists employed medicine and its allied sciences as potent tools for crafting their opinions about racial hierarchy into bodies of knowledge. When white wartime medical practitioners, observers, and investigators pursued the "facts" of race in the bodies, illnesses, wounds, and deaths of African American people, they did so because they already believed that documenting the somatization of race was relevant to therapeutic practice and scientific knowledge.[10] They were also participating in the establishment and exercise of new forms of medical authority and expertise. In pursuing "racial knowledge" with the tools of medicine and science, surgeons, physicians, and aspiring practitioners were able to profit from new avenues of professional advancement and sources of professional authority.[11]

Prior to Black enlistment, the USSC had already recognized the scale of information and potential for new knowledge presented by the war and embraced the fact-finding investigation as one of its primary means of contributing to and influencing wartime medicine.[12] The commission also devised and used statistical data in assessing the medical condition of the armies, beginning with an 1862 report on mortality and sickness, and in the ongoing work of the commission's Bureau of Sanitary and Vital Statistics. By 1862 the commission had also endeavored to send inspectors to visit every recruiting station, camp, hospital, fort, and location through which soldiers passed to assess what improvements might promote a healthier army.

Commission men in the medical profession (female physicians were excluded from this entire arena of work) brought their "rich and abundant" professional experience and authority to bear on studies of camp disease and sanitation as well as medical and surgical treatments. They published and circulated thousands of copies of nearly 100 brief tracts to instruct and aid army surgeons in their work ("The Value of Vaccination in Armies," "Report of the Associate Medical Members of the Sanitary Commission on the Subject of Venereal Diseases," "Report . . . on the Subject of Amputations," "Hints for the Control and Prevention of Infectious Diseases," etc.).[13] The commission also introduced the technology and representational power of social investigation into the war effort, using narrative questionnaires and reports collected by physicians and cooperating examiners of life insurance companies ("accustomed to an exact and searching method of inquiry") to investigate the conditions leading to Union defeat at the Battle of Bull Run in September 1861.[14]

The commission formally merged politics and medicine in the winter and spring of 1862 as it lobbied members of Congress to secure the passage of a bill that reorganized the army's Medical Department, increased the number of medical employees as well as the rank conferred on them, and secured a new appointee as surgeon general who was an active collaborator with USSC work.[15] Another major arena of medical work was in developing better transportation of the wounded (via ambulance and boat) and more efficient hospital design. The commission sponsored the first substantial proposal for a system of veteran's pension benefits and care for disabled veterans. Finally, the USSC also created a Bureau of Vital Statistics.[16]

As a result of two developments that were central to emancipation—the enlistment of 200,000 African American men into the military and the arrival of hundreds of thousands of enslaved people to Union lines—thousands of sick and injured African Americans were examined and treated by the Union's military and civilian medical professionals and volunteers. White military medical practitioners and white civilian volunteers involved in health care and relief work brought to their encounters with African Americans an intense interest in Black bodies as sources of study and a concern with Black bodies as perceived risks to public health. As case studies and as quantifiable populations, African Americans in good and ill health were subjected to investigation, measurement, and speculation. Their severed limbs, tumors, bones, blood, and tissue were photographed, sketched, and taken as specimens. Their cadavers were autopsied, their skulls cleaned and collected, and their brains and lungs weighed, all to substantiate whites' belief that people of African descent constituted an indisputably inferior race with physiological and moral peculiarities that could be revealed using the modern and modernizing techniques of medical science.[17] White medical practitioners and scientists seized on the war's medical crisis as an opportunity to demonstrate their professional status in the form of their astute observations of the manifestation of race in the bodies of people of African descent. Often, it was the male militarized body subjected to scrutiny while civilian refugee bodies were more often (but not always) managed, discarded, and buried as "unknown contraband."[18]

White Authority and the Social Survey

Of all the wartime modalities of producing and circulating medical and scientific knowledge, two—the gathering and use of anecdotal, narrative, qualitative data in the form of surveys and the creation and reporting of statistical data—would become most pertinent to the Sanitary Commission's investment in and impact on the production of racial knowledge. When Black enlistment began, the army as well as the commission incorporated these innovative modalities of gathering, analyzing, and circulating data. Like nineteenth-century social reform organizations, the army and the commission also chose to embrace and deploy the cultural power of "numerical discourse," the association of modernity and facticity with statistical thinking.[19]

The investigative survey stood out as a familiar, well-respected form of state-sponsored reportage, one that elevated the value and authority of personal observation in the economy of wartime knowledge about African Americans. A wide range of observations by military and civilian whites offered curious Northern readers wartime eyewitness accounts of Black soldiers and Southern Blacks in newspapers, periodicals, pamphlets, lectures, and books.[20] The USSC and the army, however, surveyed regimental surgeons, army engineers, and examining surgeons appointed to enrollment boards for their assessment of African American bodies and capabilities.

These surveys accomplished a number of things. They called into being the very part of society they studied: the mere fact of soliciting authoritative commentary about Black soldiers created them as a scientific and medical class in need of study. They also created and reinforced an identity among white respondents as scientific and medical authorities on Black bodies. Because these surveys were conducted on behalf of state or state-authorized bureaucracies, they were identified with the work of governing, and their findings gained the imprimatur of state authority. Finally, they create a body of data that lived on well past the war in terms of utility to racial science.[21]

An army engineer, Major T. B. Brooks, who supervised the work of Black soldiers on entrenchments at Morris Island, South Carolina, was one of the first to use surveys to solicit and document racial characteristics. Here and throughout the South engineer departments relied heavily on Black fugitives from slavery as well as Black soldiers for the hard labor of digging and constructing defense works and entrenchments, often while under fire. In September 1863, Brooks circulated a questionnaire among other officers in the engineering department, soliciting their observations of the relative fitness of African Americans for military service, especially fatigue duty. "As the important experiment which will test the fitness of the American negro for the duties of a soldier is now being tried, it is desirable that facts bearing on the question be carefully observed and recorded," Brooks noted. Six engineers who supervised Black troops responded with reports on what they viewed as the physical, mental, and psychological characteristics that distinguished African American men.[22] They characterized the men as softer, more emotional, and more docile and obedient than whites, and as more enduring and less intelligent, less heroic, and less skilled than white soldiers. One posited that while white men could be likened to horses ("often intractably and balky"), Black men were more like the ox; another characterized the white man as having "bull-dog courage" while the Black man was merely "a pitiful cur." Respondents offers two related conclusions: that racial characteristics rendered African American soldiers inferior in many ways to whites, but at the same time rendered African Americans uniquely—perhaps even more—qualified for difficult fatigue duty. None of the respondents expressed any hesitation or equivocation in their responses; they offered their assessments with rhetorical certainty, understanding from Brooks's inquiry that their opinions and feelings would be received as facts.

The invitation to respond to Brooks's circular and the conviction with which they answered appeared to reflect among these white engineers not only a sense of their authority as astute observers and experts on racial characteristics but also their confidence in the legitimacy of their observations.[23] Neither Brooks nor any of the officers who responded to his queries noted the human cost of the labor performed by African American soldiers who worked on entrenchments and forts. A medical inspector reported that same month that the soldiers who performed this labor did so while being shelled; the wounds produced were so terrible that half of the injured would perish. The inspector also regretted that "the bones are so shattered" that he could not prepare specimens to forward to the Army Medical Museum (more on this in chapter 4).[24]

Two related surveys were conducted at the end of the war and in the months directly following the Confederate surrender. Benjamin R. Woodward, a surgeon in the 22nd Illinois Infantry and a medical inspector in the Mississippi valley, devised and circulated a survey on behalf of the USSC in the last half of 1865. He targeted surgeons in Black regiments and other expert observers — including Southern physicians — for participation in his "scientific" inquiry into "the Physiological Status of the negro as compared with white soldiers."[25] Woodward's questionnaire was far more comprehensive than that of Brooks, asking respondents to comment on hunger, fatigue, nervous diseases, disease resistance, and disease susceptibility. "You are respectfully requested to give the results of your observation and experience on as many or all of the points indicated as may seem best to yourself." Woodward inquired, "Can the negro bear hunger & fatigue as well as the white man? What was the influence of nostalgia on the negro? Did he require a greater quantity of stimulating tonics than did white men? Did he display any instinctive or intelligent care in adding to his rations from what was available in the countryside? Under what diseases does he most hopelessly sink?"

Woodward's survey was also much more widely circulated. Two hundred sixty copies of his questionnaire were printed and circulated, and the respondents were encouraged with a promise of future publication.[26] The responses reveal that white surgeons believed themselves to be authoritative, exacting, and unimpeachable observers of racial characteristics in Black soldiers. Their confidence was unsurprising, given the rise of clinical empiricism among regular practitioners in antebellum medicine, which emphasized the value of direct experience and observation.[27] The war permanently elevated the primacy of experience and close observation over rationalistic therapeutic systems (such as homeopathy and Thomsonianism, which relied on a unified theory of disease origins and treatment, regardless of variation between diseases), in part by providing 12,000 army-appointed medical professionals with unprecedented access to and authority over the clinical material of damaged and ill human bodies. As John Harley Warner has noted, by the second quarter of the nineteenth century, the "clinic and the autopsy table," with their opportunities for firsthand observation and material experience, replaced the philosophical theories of humoral imbalance and other rationalistic systems of medical thought.[28]

At the same time, white medical practitioners also drew heavily on ethnological and other anthropological studies of race when they categorized African Americans as a corporeal species, defined by bodies that were marked by primitivism and inferiority.[29] The responses to Woodward's survey offered detailed, descriptive, and contradictory accounts of racial difference manifest in musculature, flexibility, physiological processes, strength, and vigor. One rare respondent insisted, "I find so few distinctive sanitary traits between the negro and the white man, that I have less to say upon the subject than I anticipated," but dozens of others offered detailed, descriptive, and wildly contradictory accounts of how racial difference manifested, and what the unique characteristics of Blackness included.[30] They variously reported that the Black soldier's muscles were not as solid or substantial as those of whites; his leg muscles were less developed, he had no elasticity in his tread, and tended to slouch; he had a larger abdomen than the white soldier and his colon nearly twice as large. He was a great feeder, and his digestion was rapid; he was more and also less susceptible to disease; by mixing with whites, he had gained mental strength and vigor at the expense of physical power and endurance.[31]

Notably, several surgeons used the circulars as an opportunity to protest the overwork of Black troops and their abusive treatment by white officers. But even those who protested the exploitation and mistreatment of Black troops were firm in recording a host of racial characteristics. As one such respondent noted, the Black soldier's "want of vital energy and constitutional vigor has been made a scape goat for incompetency and neglect to a very great degree."[32]

A third survey was conducted at the close of the war by J. H. Baxter, the chief medical officer of the Provost Marshal-General's Bureau; the results appeared in 1875 as part of a major postwar U.S. government publication, *Statistics, Medical and Anthropological, of the Provost Marshal General's Bureau*. In May 1865, Baxter sent a circular to all the surgeons who had served on boards of enlistment—that is, the medical men (the vast majority of them white) who had examined recruits, draftees, and substitutes for their physical fitness for military service. Baxter's stated goal was to compile an authoritative account of "the physical characteristics and the social and hygienic conditions of the inhabitants of the non-rebellious states."[33]

The circular inquired about the number of men examined, the range of disqualifying illnesses and disabilities they encountered, the character of their district's geography and population, and the successes and failures of the examining process. One of the ten questions asked surgeons to report on "your experience as to the Qualifications of the colored race for military service." This was not a question about how Black soldiers had performed under fire or in carrying out garrison or fatigue duty. This was a query that presumed the existence and significance of observable racial characteristics and took as a given the familiarity of examining surgeons with contemporary medical, ethnographic, and anthropometric literature that espoused the existence and nature of those characteristics. Seventy-two of the 116 respondents offered substantial answers to this question. Twenty used nearly identical language explaining that, although they had examined very few African American men, they nonetheless had extensive observations to offer. Their confidence in expostulating on racial characteristics came from a wide range of sources. Some referred to "well-known facts." Several asserted their observations were based on historical or biblical fact. Some referred to what they described as "universal opinion." Many used the rhetoric of "belief." One referred to his experience as a physician treating enslaved people in Guyana, and another drew extensively on the technical rhetoric of ethnography and anthropometry, demonstrating a deep familiarity with contemporary ethnological literature.[34]

Of course, their findings varied widely. They offered a large catalogue of what they believed to be racial characteristics, from disease resistance and vulnerability to body morphology and gait. Many observed that, as enslaved laborers, Black men trained by servitude, drudgery, and privation functioned well under the conditions of war. One of the respondents offered a detailed cataloguing of anatomical racism, citing racially unique facial angles, buttocks and position of the anus, size and function of the genitals, and jaw, thighs, shoulders, bellies, and feet. One concluded, "There is just enough animal about them to make good soldiers." Several noted that the capability of African Americans for military service depended on command by knowledgeable and skilled white officers; "while there is little doubt that there is some capacity for military service, similarly there is no doubt about the usefulness of the horse when subject to intelligent training." Here we see the same logic offered by Southern slave owners in the decades leading to the war—that specialized racial knowledge of "negro peculiarities" was required to commodify the limited capabilities of people of African descent.[35]

The majority of Baxter's respondents found African American men suitable for soldiering, not because of their equal manhood with whites but rather because their bodies were so evidently created for exploitation. Black men, they reported, were notable for their muscularity. Like draft animals, they could perform labor, endure, and be obedient. The parallels between these descriptions and antebellum notions of "soundness" in the bodies of the enslaved are inescapable.[36] In sum, Baxter's respondents produced the consummate white vision of male-gendered Black "superbodies." Historian Deirdre Cooper Owens, of course, has alerted us to the construction of the female equivalent in her study of the history of American gynecology and its stereotype of enslaved women.[37]

During an era when anti-Catholic Protestants and Anglo-Saxon nativists targeted Irish immigrants with denigrating caricatures, when illustrators could rely on the legibility of these caricatures in their visual representations of Irish Americans, and when anti-Irish discrimination in the workplace was increasingly evident, we might expect Baxter's survey to reflect a racialization of the Irish in American culture and politics. However, Baxter's survey firmly distinguished between the biological racialization of Black Americans and the ranking of white nationalities. Apart from querying his respondents about the racial characteristics that marked Black men, Baxter asked in a separate question, "Which nationality presents the greatest physical aptitude for military service?" Far fewer respondents mention Irish men (51 of 116, or 44 percent compared with 62 percent offering opinions on African Americans). One respondent suggested excluding Irish men from the army, but most simply noted the Irish, among nationalities, as ranking typically below what they described as "Americans."[38] Following the language of Baxter's query, descriptions of Irish difference by respondents were more likely to label those as "national" rather than "racial" differences.

For Brooks, Woodward, and Baxter, and those who answered their surveys, cataloging what they believed to be the racial characteristics of Black men engaged them in a state-sponsored process of race-making while affirming their own learned abilities to observe, identify, and report on what they believed race to mean in the era of emancipation. Even as Black soldiers demonstrated their equal commitments to destroying slavery and defending the Union, and even as the War Department acknowledged their obligation to pay Black soldiers equal wages, many white observers saw Black enlistment as an opportunity to advance rather than challenge their ideas about race and racial inequality.

Measuring the Black Body

Although relief work gained the Sanitary Commission its large and devoted national constituency and secured a major portion of the USSC's financial support, the commission's self-aggrandizing, all-male executive board was never happy being characterized as a "mere relief association." When relief and supply seemed to overtake both the work and public characterization of the USSC, its officers never failed to try to call it back on course. President Henry Bellows warned against the "decline of the scientific part of our labors" because "the truly scientific work we had assigned ourselves" was "our only chance for being valued as men of mark in time to come."[39]

The USSC commitment to a major project of human measurement capitalized on several intersecting cultural forces that had gained considerable momentum by the time of the war. During the nineteenth century, the popularity of racial biometrics or anthropometry—the measurement of human anatomy—reflected the growing investments of medical science in the classification of humanity into a hierarchy of distinct races. Under the influence of Lambert Adolphe Jacque Quetelet (a notable Belgian statistician, astronomer, and sociologist), scientists compiled quantifiable data from which they believed the ideal and average human form could be obtained. Before the war, anatomical measurements and devices for obtaining them were the backbone of racial typology, what scientists argued were observable and measurable physical traits. Facial angles, the cephalic index, craniometry, lung capacity (or "vital capacity"), and bodily proportions and dimensions were measured with the goniometer, calipers, the craniograph, the spirometer, and the andrometer, inventing an inherently comparative and corporeal language of race.[40]

In addition, as nineteenth-century social and anatomical investigators created what Ian Hacking described as "an avalanche of printed numbers," that helped elevate the popularity of "political arithmetic," or statistics.[41] James Cassedy describes statistics as "an essential part of the day-to-day conduct of government and business," the rendering of "torrents of data" about the American population into information that could be mapped, classified, compared, and analyzed to guide public policy and effective governance.[42] Of course, statistics were never simply neutral reports of fact; they created facts, particular in their utility as a mode of comparison and classification. ("The imperative to compare invaded every facet of commission work," Oz Frankel observed about state-produced knowledge.[43])

Finally, the nineteenth century saw an increase in large-scale, state-sponsored social investigations circulated in nineteenth-century print as official, often government-published reports. An eager public read the representation of the nation's social body in the collected and unadorned facts of widely circulated published reports, blue books, large-scale social surveys, and expedition reports, which were understood as both authentic and authoritative. Furthermore, as Oz Frankel noted in his history of print statism, the Civil War marked a turning point in U.S. investments in state-sponsored investigation. The infrastructure was already in place to produce, circulate, and create a popular demand for such reports. On the eve of the Civil War, a substantial one-fourth to one-third of the national budget supported the scientific enterprises that produced mountains of reports; the war, Frankel noted, further "triggered an unprecedented burst of investigative projects for Congress and the administration," including congressional inquiries into the state of affairs in the South.[44] Together, these antebellum intellectual and material infrastructures provided a strong foundation for the race projects of the army and the USSC.

When Benjamin A. Gould, the nation's foremost astronomer, accepted an appointment to direct the work of the commission's Statistical Bureau in June 1864, he was surprised that no study of Black troops had yet been undertaken. More than 8,000 white soldiers had already been measured, a project to ascertain the "physical and social condition of our soldiers" that had begun under the auspices of the Smithsonian Institution.[45] In May 1861, the president of the Smithsonian, Joseph Henry, indicated that he "thought that the measurement of all the troops . . . gathered in and about Washington, would be of value and I have accordingly made arrangements for this to be done," a project that included "a large number of measurements of different parts of the body."[46] Sometime during 1862, Henry turned that project over to Frederick Law Olmsted and the superior resources and staff of the USSC. The Smithsonian continued on in an advisory role.[47]

Once he gained his executive appointment to the Sanitary Commission, Olmsted pursued the measurement project with great enthusiasm, drawing up a lengthy questionnaire ("Form E") and devising two portable versions of the andrometer—an anthropometric measuring device—with the goal of determining what the commission called ethnic taxonomies. Smithsonian president Henry had chosen an experienced, committed successor: in 1859, Olmsted had conducted anthropometric measurements of some 1,000 white, largely immigrant workers employed in the construction of New York City's Central Park. For this reason, Henry had good reason to place his confidence in Olmsted as the USSC's executive secretary to follow through with their shared interest in the "peculiarities of the different nationalities," "stock," or ethnic taxonomies, which Henry expected to find embodied in Union troops.[48] Also, in 1862 Olmsted lobbied hard for the superintendency of refugees from slavery at Port Royal, South Carolina, in the process revealing his deep intellectual commitments to white supremacy and Black inferiority (see chapter 2).

Although USSC inspectors and physicians had relatively easy access to white troops for study, it was the bodies of what one commissioner referred to as the "three races of negroes," as well as those of Iroquois and other indigenous people, that were pursued most vigorously and energetically under Gould's leadership, especially during the closing months of the war.[49] Gould explicitly recognized that some of the data collected "seemed capable of influence by ethnological agencies," a clear indication that he understood the project's ethnological significance had risen greatly with his attention to Black and Native people.[50] His overriding goal was to follow in Quetelet's footsteps in constructing the "typical" or "average" measurements of men of different classes and races — classes, in Gould's usage, referring to subcategories within a single racial group.[51]

Although Gould felt that this endeavor was so obviously important it needed no elaboration, other commissioners were less hesitant to declare its value. The head of the commission's Medical Bureau, Elisha Harris, described it as studying "the future welfare of the colored people & the usefulness of the colored soldier."[52] "The practical value of the branch of inquiries you are directing is readily appreciated by every philosophical student of hygiene and the branches of knowledge on which science depends," Harris asserted.[53] Ever in competition with the army's Medical Department as the most authoritative source for scientific investigations into the soldiers' bodies, the commissioners also believed (mistakenly, as it turned out) that their investigations into Black bodies would set them apart — and ahead of — the army's research and publishing agenda. "*This* field is exclusively ours," declared Harris.[54] The measurement and observation of Black bodies was "worth more than all the rest that the Sanitary Commission was doing."[55]

An astronomer might seem like an unlikely candidate to oversee this project, but Gould, as a precocious undergraduate at Harvard, had focused on mathematics as well as physical science, and the USSC project was deeply influenced by a belief that it was possible to identify the expression of race in human anatomy using statistical averages. In the 1850s, after spending time in Europe where he established a reputation as a first-rate astronomer and built a network of professional relationships with leading men of science and medicine, Gould returned to the United States where he worked to advance American astronomy. He established and published until 1861 one of the first scientific journals devoted to the field, one he insisted was not a journal for citizen-scientists or philanthropists but rather for elevating the rigor of scientific endeavors. He also worked energetically if peripatetically for the U.S. Coast Guard Survey, and for a few months he directed the Dudley Observatory in Albany, New York, only to be fired in a public, rancorous conflict over staffing, management, and the proper culture of science.

The death of his father in 1859 forced Gould into the role of trying to salvage his father's mercantile business. At the time of his appointment to the USSC project, Gould brought with him a national and international reputation as a rigorous scientist, a large network of lifelong friends in the most elite scientific circles, deep commitments to the work of scientific publication and professionalization, and experience working with scientific bureaucracies and personnel management.[56] Although his biographers tell us little about his beliefs concerning race, Gould's closest circle of friends and colleagues included scientists and public intellectuals who embraced and advocated science as a tool for affirming racial difference and racial hierarchy, such as Louis Agassiz and Joseph Henry.

With his appointment to the USSC, Gould immediately solicited twelve sets of measuring apparatus (each set including an andrometer, a spirometer, dynamometer, a goniometer, a platform balance, calipers, and a measuring tape). He consulted with leading medical and anthropological professionals for their guidance, including Louis Agassiz, one of the leading proponents of ethnology and polygenesis at the time.[57] Under their advice, he revised the printed form used by earlier investigators with new kinds of measurements he and his advisors thought appropriate to the Black body (figure 3.1), and he hired and trained inspectors to conduct exacting measurements and questioning, as well as additional clerks to tabulate the results.[58] Twenty-two of the thirty-eight items on the form required measurements of feet, arms, legs, head, waist, and chest; respirations had to be counted, mechanical readings recorded, facial angles ascertained, distance between nipples and around heels measured, and girth of neck noted. About half of the Black soldiers were measured unclothed; less than a tenth of the white soldiers were.[59] Soldiers were also asked about their ancestry, the current state of their health, their marital status, whether they were accustomed to athletic activities, their occupation, and if they knew the place of birth of their parents and grandparents. Inspectors were also instructed

[Form EE.]

SANITARY COMMISSION.

INDIVIDUAL INSPECTION.

1. Number of soldier in order of examination? — *1*
2. Name of soldier: — *Alfred Richards*
   rank? — *Private*
3. Regiment? — *New Recruit*
4. Entire height (in stockings—inches and tenths)? — *62.0*
4½. Distance from tip of middle finger to level of upper margin of patella, (in 'attitude of the soldier')? — *7 - 6*
5. Height from ground to lower part of neck (spine of the prominent, i.e. 7th cervical vertebra)? — *54 - 3*
6. Height to perinæum? — *28 - 8   R. 18 - 3*
6½. Height to most prominent part of pubes? — *3 - 8*
7. Breadth of neck? — *12 - 7*
7½. Girth of neck? — *15 - 2*
8. Breadth of shoulders between acromion processes? — *11 5*
9. Breadth of pelvis between crests of ilia? —
10. Circumference of chest across the nipples full inspiration? — *35*
    after expiration? — *32 - 3*
10½. Distance between nipples? — *8 - 4*
11. Circumference of waist above hips? — *30 6*
11½. Circumference around hips on level with trochanters? — *33 - 6*
12 a. Length of arm—from tip of acromion to tip of middle finger? — *29 6*
    b. Distance from middle of top of sternum to tip of middle finger, arm extended? — *33 6*
    c. Distance from tip of acromion to extremity of elbow? — *13 4*
13. Capacity of chest in cubic inches, (i. e. amount exhaled after full inhalation)? — *15 0*
14. Weight (lbs. and half lbs.) without coat, hat, arms or accoutrements? — *120 ½*
14½. Weight (from memory) at enlistment? — *116*
15. Dynamometer? — *25 5*
16. In the opinion of the Inspector, from appearance and statements of subject, is he of American stock of three or more generations? (In cases where this question cannot be answered with confidence, affirmatively or negatively, it will be best not to pursue the examination.) — *Full Blood Negro*
17. If so, period of immigration of ancestry? (Detail of both sides desirable.) — *Can't tell*
18. Where born — country or state? — *Louisiana*
    county? — *N. Orleans*
    parish or town? — *"*
19. If foreign born, year of arrival in this country?
    Supposed about?
20. Country of birth — of father? — *La,*
    " of mother? — *"*
    " of grandparents? — *"*

21. Enlisted—wh
    " wh
    " for
22. Conjugal rela widower?
23. Age (last birth
24. Former occup
25. Hair—color?
    amount
    texture
    if bald,
    becom
26. Eyes—color?
    " distance
    " prominen
27. Complexion?
28. Pulse (regular)
29. Respiration (p minute, whe
30. Muscular deve
31. Is he in usual
    if reduced
32. Is he, when o and more vi entered the
33. Condition of te
34. Head—a. circ occiput?
    b. distan proce
    c. distance osses
    d. distance cesses o
    e. distance protu
    f. width b
    g. "
35 Facial angle?
36 Foot—a. length extremity of
    b. length fr above h
    c. thickness
    d. circumfere tensor lig
51. Was he, before recreations, &
55. Education.
    Lan
    Good
    High
    Colle
    Profe

Signature of Exa
Place and date of

FIGURE 3.1 Commission Examiner William S. Baker's notes on the measurement of Alfred Richards, conducted at Elmira, New York, on November 12, 1864, and recorded in Form EE. Courtesy of the New York Public Library.

to record their observation of the subject's intelligence (with the average white man's intelligence as their norm), the color of their complexion (thus confirming or rejecting the subject's own report of their ancestry), along with descriptions of the texture and amount of their hair.[60]

The examiners—a dozen men, supported by more than a dozen clerks—enthusiastically set about "obtaining the length & breadth & thickness of a few specimens of Ethiopians" as they traveled to encampments in both the eastern and western theaters of war.[61] (One also pursued measurements of several of the human spectacles hired by P. T. Barnum for his museum, including giants, dwarves, "three huge fat women, some albinos, one Circassian girl and 10 Indians," as well as some "wild Australian children"; he also argued that measurements should be obtained from Chinese men in California.)[62] As one examiner noted, "I like the work much—very much—To me—it is a Science of studying man as I never before have studied him I have almost a passion for measuring naked men."[63] Another described peering, self-consciously, at hundreds of naked bathing soldiers in the waters of the James River in his efforts to assess patterns of pilosity, understood at the time as a racial marker: greater pilosity among white men, especially fuller beards, was thought to indicate their fuller manliness.[64]

Among their many requests for clarification about proper and accurate methods of measurement, the examiners especially puzzled over the slippery logic involved in determining soldiers' racial classification: "Is there no name for any grade between Full Black and Mulatto? He is a Mulatto if he is 1/8 white and the same if he is 1/2 white."[65] Gould himself occasionally expressed his excitement with the project's goals. Writing to a field agent, Gould exclaimed, "My results on the relative length of arms will do very well to go by the side of yours on the brain, though of course less new & interesting. —In another month I hope to have some *heel* results!"[66]

The investigation's objectification of the soldiers and their bodies met resistance from some soldiers. Several examiners inadvertently acknowledged how research subjects both asserted their humanity and shaped the course of the investigation. Black soldiers at Camp Nelson resolutely refused to report for measurement on Saturdays, which they regarded as their holiday from work.[67] Some men refused measurement, fearing it was a prank, or an effort to select the best men for a standing army, or to prevent desertions, or some other suspect scheme. Some refused to give their names; others thought better of it after being measured and tried to steal or destroy the records.[68] Many refused to remove their clothing for the inspectors, and others submitted only when ordered to do so by their officers.[69] Some would yield to measurement only if they were paid.[70]

Men who had been enslaved would have been familiar with the practices of whites in the slave markets and slave trade of the South, who prodded, inspected, and assessed the worth of enslaved men. Soldiers who resisted the investigators' examinations may well have been defending their bodily dignity, their privacy, and their self-worth by rejecting the dehumanizing inspections that might have linked their experience of the slave market to the USSC's inspections. Yet in the City Point, Virginia, contraband camp, freedwomen apparently wondered why their capacities were not being measured. Over the course of two weeks, eighty women presented themselves to be tested with the spirometer, and half also tried their hand at the dynamometer, to the alarm of the inspector.[71] Did they view the equipment as a source of entertainment, something sorely lacking in the lives of people in refugee camps? Were they pursuing what might be an opportunity to earn some small pay? Were they insisting on their inclusion in a project that excluded women from the conception of Black bodies?

Gould's project and the pressure to gather as many measurements of Black and Native troops as possible before the regiments were mustered out reached an anxious pace in the late summer and fall of 1865. Harris wrote repeatedly to Gould about his specific desire to have the soldiers of the 20th and 81st U.S. Colored Troops measured. (Organized in New York City, the 20th was "the pet of our N.Y. Loyal League—made up of negroes of northern birth"; the 81st U.S. Colored Troops "notwithstanding they were plantation boys that regiment is the pride of all Cold. Troops.")[72]

The examiners struggled with time pressures, the conditions of their work, hostile army officers, and Gould's criticisms of the inaccuracies that inevitably and persistently crept into the project.[73] Working in a surgeon's busy office was not ideal, noted William Baker, due to the lack of space and the apparent unhappiness of the men who appeared there for sick call.[74] Others complained of crowded and unheated huts and tents.[75] There were frequent delays as equipment failed to arrive or arrived damaged. "I have had constant vexations delays and disappointments since I landed," wrote one exasperated agent.[76] One agent noted that "it takes rather more time to measure a negro than a white man."[77] George W. Avery insisted, "It is not a work that I feel disposed to trifle with or hurry," and he expressed deep concern that his work on the project be recognized "as having been accurate and reliable."[78] Productivity varied greatly; one agent completed seventy-two measurements in one week and 100 the next.[79] Supervisors harangued the agents when they slept late or when their productivity slipped.[80]

For these reasons as well as others, the body of measurements collected by the USSC Statistical Bureau varied a great deal in their consistency and exactness. Agents used the apparatus differently; some positioned the calipers incorrectly, and some missed measurements. Wide variations in the work amassed by each of the agents pointed to worrisome deviations from the instructions provided by commission supervisors.[81] Gould worked hard to develop correctional computations to account for these variations, but he conceded that their findings suffered from human error.

Yet the USSC regarded the work as a success. The commission gathered measurements of nearly 16,000 soldiers; 10,876 of white soldiers, 517 of Native Americans, and 2,883 of "full-blooded Negroes and Mulattoes."[82] Gould's assembly and publication of the bodily measurements presented each set of measurements, first discussing white soldiers then Black, with considerable attention to variations among whites by nativity and among African Americans who were residents of free or slave states. His reports on the measurements of Black soldiers consistently referred to how much variance occurred from parallel measurements of whites. His reports of averages frequently referred to whether there was any indication of what Gould described as "ethnological significance." Gould repeatedly referred to his own minimal qualifications to assess the physiological and ethnological meaning of the measurements, yet he was confident that ethnological value was there.[83] Gould asserted that the measurements of Black soldiers were subjected to "strenuous endeavors" "using various bases of classification." He observed that "three or more distinct races of negroes are to be found in the Southern States," without comment on the Northern Black soldiers his agents encountered. He hoped that future researchers could investigate the effect of climate and soil "upon the blacks."[84] Gould concluded, "The most marked characteristics of the races, here manifested, appear to be—for the whites, the length of head and neck and short fore-arms; for the reds, the long fore-arms and the large lateral dimensions, excepting at the shoulders; for the blacks, the wide shoulders, long feet, and protruding heels."[85] Gould's project, focused on collecting and circulating raw data and statistical averages but not interpretations of that data, helped lay the foundation for the ripening of anthropometry and craniometry, for the development of scientific and medical theories of racial difference and racial inequality, and for the development of both a technical language, as well as data sets, to support these assertions.

Within this project, investigators only infrequently acknowledged the impact of structural racism and discrimination within the army on Black troops. Elisha Harris, supervising the investigations in New Orleans in the summer and fall of 1865, predicted that the commission would ultimately report "some startling truths to the people." Army officials were ignoring the influence of "overwork, exercise drilling, and . . . absolute neglect of the colored soldiers' health" on the high rates of mortality among Black troops. Harris concluded that mortality rate "pleases too many" of the army "regulars, the professionals who predated the war."[86] The commission's (and Harris's) dedication to anthropometric research and the embodiment of race did not necessarily blind individuals to the impact of military racism on the health of Black soldiers.

The cultural power and scientific authority of the USSC investigations drew not only on the large constituency of people involved as observers and investigators but also on circulation of their data and findings in the marketplace of war-related scientific literature. Gould's *Investigations in the Military and Anthropological Statistics of American Soldiers*, published in 1869 as part of the Sanitary Commission's monographic series, *The Sanitary Memoirs of the War of the Rebellion*, offered 650 pages of tables relating circumferences, weights, lengths, statures, complexions, dimensions, and proportions. It was also the largest anthropometric study yet conducted. The prevailing rhetoric of statistics allowed Gould to assert that the volume's measurements and computations were pre-evaluative and noninterpretive; they also held the rhetorical advantage of claiming both disinterest and objectivity.[87] Gould insisted that he would leave the work of interpretation to his readers and the experts in anthropology and ethnology, but he was confident that the work would permit a reliable comparison and determination of the position of the races.

Although the Sanitary Commission's records of the distribution of Gould's volume are not extant, the distribution list for another commission publication, also compiled by Gould (*Ages of U. S. Volunteer Soldiery*), suggests how the commission viewed its network of influence as well as its audience.[88] Of the first 481 copies, most were distributed domestically, although seventy-eight were distributed to foreign recipients. The domestic distribution list included learned and political clubs and organizations (the Union League, the Century Club); learned societies and organizations (historical, genealogical, philosophical, and ethnological as well as the American Academy of Arts & Sciences, the National Academy of Science, the Essex Institute, the Smithsonian Institution, and the American Philosophical Association); college and university libraries; municipal, state, and national public offices; and numerous life insurance companies. The long list of individuals included legislators, army officials, medical practitioners, lawyers, professors, civilian and military engineers, a wide range of elected and appointed public officials, bankers, and men associated with the commission (one woman was included on the list). The foreign distribution list was similar, including learned societies, college professors, medical practitioners, and public health officials in England, Scotland, Ireland, Germany, Denmark, France, and Switzerland. Nationally and internationally, fifty-two physicians were slated to receive free copies of the work.[89]

Commission president Henry Bellows was not content to await notice and review for commission volumes. He contacted potential reviewers and men associated with both national and regional publications, offering payment for reviews which, as Bellows stated it, should offer "thorough and complete" notices, the "attention and scrutiny" that would invite not only readers but also purchasers.[90] Whether because or in spite of Bellows's efforts, these USSC publications were widely reviewed in the state, regional, and national medical and popular press.[91]

Importantly to Gould and the USSC, *Investigations in the Military and Anthropological Statistics of American Soldiers* made it into print and circulation before the surgeon general's multivolume *Medical and Surgical History of the War of the Rebellion* began to appear. A sharp competition had developed toward the end of the war between the USSC and Surgeon General Joseph Barnes over who would provide the most authoritative medical and quantitative assessment of American soldiers. Using the army's enlistment records, muster rolls, records of sickness and mortality, and questionnaires forwarded to surgeons, the commission's Bureau of Vital Statistics engaged in wide-ranging research in search of "natural laws" that shaped the effectiveness and health of the army. Initially, the commission envisioned a number of publications to emerge from this research, including a medical history of the war, but in June 1865 Barnes blocked the commission's access to army information; by October of that year the adjutant general's office closed off all further access to the army's voluminous records. The commission's persistent critique of the army's Medical Department had come home to roost, and the commission's research for its medical history of the war ended.[92] However, the research for Gould's volume had already been completed, and when it was published in 1869 it would be the last volume printed by the commission.[93]

Woodward would never author a report based on his surveys, but commission inspector and physician Sanford B. Hunt summarized the responses to Woodward's circular in his twenty-five-page article "The Negro as a Soldier." The article poses and answers the question of Black men's capacity for military service. Hunt's report was not published by the commission as he originally intended (for reasons unknown); instead, it first appeared in 1867 in the *Quarterly Journal of Psychological Medicine*, and was reprinted two years later in the *Anthropological Review*, London's premier venue for the advancement of racialized science.[94] Hunt wrote his article after the war, when the military service of Black soldiers offered a profound rebuke to anti-Black racism. But Hunt, arguing that African Americans played only a passive role in the war, instead relied on white authorities—that is, the surveys collected by Woodward along with racist anthropological and ethnographic research, including the work of Samuel Morton. He invested anthropological research with the weight of what he called "natural law," but also suggested that education and environment might impact brain size and brain weight, key indices in racist arguments about Black inferior intellectual capacity.

Although he endorsed the ability of Black men to serve as soldiers, Hunt also offered a catalogue of the "physical facts" of racial characteristics in African Americans. These, he posited, included brain size and weight (as a "measure of intellectuality"), pulmonary capacity ("he has a tropical, or smaller, lung"), and liability to disease. He also pointed to their response to medical treatment: Black men's suspicious and mistrusting responses to white medical providers "are not intrinsic to his race, but are to a great extent educational, and may be expected to disappear." He also included their powers of digestion: Hunt describes African Americans as "heavy feeders" whose "instinctive fondness for fat bacon, opossum, and coon" could be attributed to their tropical origins. He offered conflicting assessments of Black men's ability to endure fatigue and of the impact of his "large, flat, inelastic" feet, "large joints," and "projecting apophyses of bone" on his ability to endure long marches. Hunt's acknowledgment of Black military abilities and consideration that environmental factors might impact enduring racial characteristics might lead us to view him as a more moderate voice on racial hierarchies at the time, but his endorsement of the most radical advocates of racist science undermines that impression.

TOGETHER, THESE INVESTIGATIONS did far more than simply document the deep interest of Sanitary Commission agents and military medical practitioners in (what they helped define as) the problem of race in the post-emancipation nation. The commission's investigations seized from abolitionists and slavery's advocates, as well as African Americans themselves, the power and authority to represent the social body of Black Americans to the nation. Together with other powerful organizations (including the army, the Smithsonian, and the American Freedmen's Inquiry Commission), the USSC work helped advance the relationship between modern governance and race-based medicine and science, and helped elevate the authority of state-sponsored knowledge in wartime and Reconstruction era debates about the future of American race relations and racial ideologies. Even the U.S. census was drawn into the endeavor. Although 1860 census enumerators were instructed that it was "very desirable" that each individual's race be "carefully observed," by 1870 enumerators were more forcefully advised that "important scientific results depend upon the correct determination" of color.[95]

Sanitary Commission members used the conditions of war to confirm the meanings and consequences of race thinking when they rejected African Americans as their peers and relegated them instead to the status of clients and specimens, and when they reserved for themselves, as white men and women, the expertise, authority, and social power to observe and interpret the meaning of race. Natural law, they argued, rather than presidential proclamations and constitutional amendments, would be the ultimate arbiter of the parameters of Black freedom.

CHAPTER FOUR

Anatomizing Race

It was not only the living Black body that Northern white medical men appropriated in their wartime pursuit of racial knowledge. The war's violence—as a military conflict, as a medical catastrophe, as an armed assault on a slaveholding republic—yielded a bounty of corpses. White medical personnel eager to take advantage of the wartime bounty of cadavers would claim, dissect, and disassemble thousands of Black war dead, both soldiers and civilian refugees from slavery. Regimental and contract surgeons, hospital stewards, and other medical employees performed tens of thousands of postmortem examinations on soldiers and civilians, Black and white, who died from wounds and disease. The war abruptly expanded access to hands-on anatomical knowledge, regarded as the hallmark of medical professionalism.[1] During the war as before it, surgeons and hospital workers made ample and focused use of the human remains of African Americans.

Prior to the war, dissection was central to the best medical training.[2] As historians of medicine have noted, the medical autopsy was critical to the advance of medical knowledge, especially knowledge about anatomy and the disease process. By the time of the war, both autopsy and dissection were key research tools, not only for the anatomical knowledge and the experience gained in the technical disassembling of a cadaver, but also for the insight it allowed into pathological processes.[3] For this reason, before the war many aspiring American physicians traveled to Europe for training, where clinics and hospitals were both more numerous and offered freer access to cadavers. In the nineteenth-century United States, cadavers were in short supply and therefore a commodified resource. They were typically secured, usually illicitly, from among marginalized populations who could not demand the dignity of respectful repose in death—executed criminals, paupers, individuals buried in Black cemeteries, and the impoverished and unfortunate who were unable to afford proper burial.

Southern anatomists relied primarily on cadavers of the enslaved, which were also trafficked to Northern medical schools.[4] Historian Daina Ramey Berry, more than any other scholar, has revealed the commodification of enslaved people's human remains, the "ghost value" that slave owners and white medical practitioners extorted from the bodies of the formerly enslaved.[5] Michael Sappol has similarly noted a commercial trade in Black cadavers shipped South from Northern cities.[6] Antebellum whites, who viewed the desecration of white burial yards and human remains with horror, turned a blind eye toward the targeted exploitation of Black human remains and cemeteries by body-snatchers and medical colleges.

The war's abundance of death tragically and dramatically transformed access to the single commodity that marked the authority and experience of the penultimate medical professional. However, the wartime and postwar drive to explore the bodies of deceased African American soldiers and refugees from slavery was about something more complicated. Before the war, comparative anatomy typically focused on the exterior surface and appearance of the human body (with the exception of craniology). As the independent scholar Molly Rogers noted in her study of Louis Agassiz and his collection of "ethnological photographs" of African-born enslaved South Carolinians, "Looking, . . . was more important than cutting" when it came to the antebellum science of race.[7] The war changed this. Some white medical practitioners appropriated and exploited African American bodies in pursuit of racial knowledge; others were motivated by opportunism — the availability of cadavers that whites deemed undeserving of dignity was an exploitable and valuable resource. However motivated (and motivations are rarely preserved in the archive), the disregard for Black human dignity was predicated on long-standing and popular practices of whites exploiting, objectifying, exhibiting, commodifying, and displaying Black bodies, particularly as ethnological specimens.

The display of living people and human remains was popular in the nineteenth-century United States and in Europe, and a means by which white audiences—professional and lay—could imagine themselves as astute observers of human difference.[8] It was also a source of spectacle, of white pleasure and entertainment that was popular and widely practiced in print, on the stage, at learned talks, and in museums, circuses, and other venues.[9] Britt Rusert argued that the visual archive of racial science was historically critical to its popularity. In the 1830s and 1840s, that archive was largely found in popular culture rather than in scientific texts: it appeared in joke books, broadsides, illustrated print forms, and ephemera emerging from the culture of minstrelsy.[10] Rusert also has argued that shows—such as the freak show and the minstrel show—were "staging grounds for exhibiting human difference and making the supposedly deep and essential differences of African American bodies hypervisible on the antebellum stage." This complemented the popular anatomical lecture, the hospital operating theater dissections, and the display of specimens at fairs, museums, and zoos.[11]

Non-white people were used as objects of display. So, too, were people of any race perceived as "freaks": the diseased, disabled, or disfigured.[12] Black women—African and African American—were particularly fascinating to the white gaze, whether veiled in scientific authority or not. Joyce Heth, only one of P. T. Barnum's many acts that exhibited Africans and African Americans as curiosities, was displayed by Barnum both as an unusually aged living person but also after her death. Like Saartjie Baartman, Heth would be dissected and anatomized, her human dignity rendered insignificant in light of the entertainment value that could be extracted from her human remains, at the crossroads of racist science and racial spectacle.[13] According to historian Benjamin Reiss, 1,500 people paid fifty cents each to attend the autopsy performed on Heth, an audience that included medical students, newspaper editors, and clergymen, among others.[14] The display of living people and their human remains was popular in the nineteenth-century United States and in Europe as a means by which white audiences—professional and civilian—trained themselves as astute observers of human difference and the racist ideologies that transformed difference into ranking and hierarchy.

The antebellum commodification of medical specimens, created without consent and used for personal or professional profit, played a role here as well.[15] By the eve of the war, the visual representation of what whites viewed as racialized bodies began to serve not only a white visual culture of amusement, repulsion, and entertainment, but also as a scientific endeavor that was increasingly comparative and dedicated to validating the role of science in defining race and illuminating racial hierarchy.[16] The bodies of the enslaved had long been commodified, whether alive or dead; we cannot expect white medical practitioners to have divorced themselves from the practices they had participated in and been accustomed to once the war began.[17]

These practices fueled the wartime developments explored in this chapter. In his Circular No. 2, issued in 1862, Surgeon General William Hammond encouraged all Union surgeons to forward specimens for the newly created Army Medical Museum in an endeavor to document the medical history of the war and advance medical knowledge in the nation. Autopsy reports, specimens, and artifacts were all encouraged with the surgeon general's assurances that the donor would be publically acknowledged both in museum displays and the museum's printed catalogues. Just as survey respondents gained authority as experts in pursuit of racial knowledge, so did those who contributed to the museum's collections.

In this context of racialized spectacle, vulnerability, and the commodification of Black bodies, this chapter considers military body-snatching, the anatomization of Black soldiers and civilians during and immediately after the war, and the different purposes associated with the dissection and anatomization of Black human remains.

Race and the Exploitation of the War Dead: Soldiers

The wartime interest in and commodification of the human remains of Black soldiers suggests a blurring of the distinction between autopsies (performed on subjects to ascertain cause of death) and dissection (performed on objects to gain anatomical knowledge).[18] It also set apart the interests of the U.S. Sanitary Commission (USSC) (concerned with the living bodies of Black soldiers) from those of the army (which quickly became as interested in the dead as in the living). The surgeon general requested careful case notes from military surgeons detailing medical treatments as well as postmortem reports from autopsies in the effort to document the unique medical history of the war — especially the carnage created by modern weaponry. Historian Shauna Devine has argued that the war's creation of unprecedented opportunities for postmortem examinations represented "the apex of wartime medical science." It helped launch the centrality of research, new knowledge, and refined practices in American medicine.[19] Military medical practitioners understood that their unprecedented access to the war dead not only could increase their knowledge and expertise but also, through their contributions to the surgeon general, could enhance their professional authority and standing.[20]

What the surgeon general could not have predicted was the way in which his order and the creation of the Army Medical Museum emboldened military surgeons to pursue opportunities for anatomical dissection. Union nurse Cornelia Hancock described surgeons practicing on amputated limbs they retained from postmortems and embalming cadavers to keep them for consultation purposes.[21] Burt Green Wilder (a comparative anatomist who would eventually serve as surgeon of the African American regiment, the 55th Massachusetts Infantry), while a medical cadet at Judiciary Square Hospital in Washington, D.C., spent hours in the hospital's dead house studying arterial systems to aid his familiarity with surgical anatomy and his goal of qualifying as a contract surgeon.[22]

The war may have launched American medicine toward scientific models in the pursuit of medical knowledge, but it also drew deeply on long-established white practices of dismembering and commodifying Black bodies. Wartime medical research authorized and incentivized the dismemberment of the remains of fallen soldiers, but it also empowered some white practitioners to particularly target the remains of Black soldiers and civilians—either as cadavers that could be dissected without the same social costs associated with similar treatments of the white dead or because the remains were available in abundance.

In 1864, William Chester Minor—an 1863 graduate of Yale Medical School with an interest in comparative anatomy—privately published a pamphlet containing thirty-five autopsy case reports from postmortem examinations he conducted as an acting assistant (contract) surgeon in the U.S. Army at New Haven's Knight U.S. General Hospital.[23] More than 23,000 patients were admitted to Knight Hospital over the course of the war, some of them members of the two Black regiments organized in Connecticut. Just over 200 deaths were recorded at the hospital.[24] The significant number of deaths among soldiers, even as they mustered into their regiments, enhanced Minor's medical education. Minor is best remembered for his postwar life: his mental illness, the murder he committed, his incarceration in insane asylums, and his contributions to the *Oxford English Dictionary* while an asylum inmate.[25] But during the war at Knight Hospital, he exemplified the young physician on the make. His wartime supervisors—well-known military surgeons—took great interest in his professional development, one describing him as "a skillful physician, an excellent operator, and an efficient scholar."[26] In 1865, one of his former professors described him as having "thorough knowledge" of human anatomy as well as a thorough acquaintance with comparative anatomy. He gained the latter "not from books alone, but also from extensive personal research."[27] During his time in Washington, D.C., hospitals, he prepared several specimens from dissections of Black soldiers and civilians, which he submitted to the Army Medical Museum. Minor's decision to publish his autopsy reports from Knight Hospital suggests a medical man with an eye to professional reputation and esteem. Assembling and publishing these case reports indicates that Minor understood there was an audience for such publications and that authorship was of value to his career and reputation.[28]

Minor's autopsy reports are technical, detailed, precise, and reflect in one particular way his interest in comparative anatomy. Of thirty-five case reports, twenty-four cases involved Black soldiers, and eleven involved whites—a disproportionate ratio that did not reflect the balance between Black and white patients at Knight Hospital. In five of his reports on Black soldiers and only one on whites, Minor commented on the subject's genitals. In the instance of the white soldier, he commented on a discoloration. In his reports on Black soldiers, he noted large size, color, evidence of a sexually transmitted disease, and a scrotal hernia. Minor's attention to disease, color, and size of genitals was unusual among published autopsy case reports, including those he would later write while posted at L'Ouverture and Slough General Hospitals, both in Alexandria, Virginia, where he conducted many more autopsies on Black soldiers, and from their remains, donated some sixty specimens to the Army Medical Museum.[29] Minor's observations suggest that a sexualization of Black men may have been part of the allure of securing cadavers to examine.

Ira Russell, who earned his medical degree from the University of New York in 1844, was already a well-respected physician when he enlisted in August 1861 as a Union surgeon.[30] By the spring of 1862, his military medical career accelerated as he began a series of postings at Union army hospitals. In addition to his work organizing and directing Union hospitals, Russell maintained a very active research program throughout the war. In his own words, he conducted a host of "pathological investigations," "in the wards and . . . in the dead house." He published widely, in USSC and surgeon general volumes, in Austin Flint's 1876 *Textbook of Human Physiology*, and he also wrote "Observations and Post-Mortem Results in Cerebro-Spinal Meningitis" as well as two other articles for the *St. Louis Medical and Surgical Journal*.[31] These investigations drew on several hundred dissections he conducted or supervised, the majority of them on the bodies of Black soldiers.[32] Russell kept detailed case summaries and tabular assessments of the progress of disease; he also anatomized, measured, and weighed the brains, lungs, livers, bowels, and other internal organs of the men whose bodies he opened.

An abolitionist, Russell supported the Emancipation Proclamation, gladly employed refugees from slavery in the hospitals he directed, and fought for the timely payment of their wages. He was a strong and public critic of the discrimination and maltreatment that African American soldiers experienced, and he was very interested in the status, health, and physiology of Black troops.[33] Several Black regiments organized and trained at Benton Barracks while he was posted there, which was also a refuge for the formerly enslaved as well as white civilians fleeing the Confederacy and the violence of war. Tens of thousands came under his care and supervision while he was on duty in Missouri. Experiencing an upward career trajectory thanks to the war, Russell did not hesitate to create and extract personal professional value out of the multitude of deaths that occurred under his charge.

Russell was an iconoclast when it came to the beliefs about race, susceptibility to disease, and ideas about the biology of race that were held by most white medical workers. He emphasized context when reporting his findings about the higher rates of infection and mortality in pulmonary infections in Black troops. He noted the exhaustion and exposure experienced by enlisted men when they first fled slavery, the severe winter conditions in 1863–1864; the denial of adequate shelter, heat sources, and hospital provisions for ill Black soldiers; and the arrival of white troops infected with measles, smallpox, and other diseases which then quickly spread to the Black troops. Slavery, severe weather, the conditions of war, and discriminatory treatment by white medical directors and surgeons ranked highest in Russell's accounting for Black illness and death.[34]

Yet among his findings, Russell also focused on what he understood to be physiological differences between Black and white bodies. He did not find Black troops more vulnerable to tuberculosis than whites, "a fact differing I believe from the commonly received opinion upon that subject," he noted. Russell did assert what he believed was evidence of a greater vulnerability to inflammatory pulmonary disease among African Americans. He found a greater occurrence of scarring on the lungs of the cadavers of Black men than among whites, and also that the lungs of African American men were on average four ounces lighter than those of whites. Russell wondered if this might explain what he described as the proven inability of Black soldiers to endure forced marches as well as whites. Even with his insistent attention to the material impact of slavery, racism, and discrimination on the health and survival of Black troops, Russell was nonetheless willing to seek out and accept the common argument that race was embodied, a biological fact, rather than an ideological justification for race-based slavery.[35]

We will return to Russell's medical investigations in the following chapter's attention to the care and disposal of the dead, but one additional point should be noted. Knowledge of Russell's extensive practice of postmortem examinations and dismemberment of the Black war dead must surely have circulated among the Black troops stationed at Benton Barracks. This raises important questions: how did the soldiers and civilians at Benton Barracks respond to Russell's disassembling of the dead? Former slaves and Northern Blacks alike must have been well aware of their unique vulnerability to white medical interest. Did this likely knowledge affect the willingness of Black soldiers to seek medical care or hospitalization? There is evidence that white officers of Black regiments felt that the practice of dissecting Black bodies had to be hidden from Black soldiers to prevent unrest and erosion of discipline among the troops.[36] Again, current sources only allow us to raise these questions, not answer them.

IN MARCH 1865, Surgeon George J. Potts, serving with the 23rd U.S.C.I., was court-martialed and dishonorably discharged for "unjustifiably mutilating the body of a deceased soldier in the presence of enlisted men of that command."[37] Because of the extant court-martial record, we have a much fuller record of the complex attitudes and motivations concerning the army's and Pott's individual views on the autopsy and dismemberment of Black soldiers. In this instance, the deceased soldier, Private Benjamin Anderson, had escaped slavery and enlisted in the 23rd U.S.C.I. during the war. He had much to live for, including his wife Sarah and his toddler son, James.[38] Anderson's unit saw a great deal of action in the eastern theater, including the Battle of the Crater, yet Anderson survived until an unknown illness struck him down as his regiment approached Richmond in March 1865. When he became ill, the regiment's assistant surgeons diagnosed at least three different illnesses and prescribed a number of different treatments. Nothing seemed to help; Anderson could not perform his duty for several days. He died very suddenly, collapsing outside his tent and dying within an hour.

Bennett Bethel, the acting assistant surgeon who had last treated Anderson, asked Potts whether a postmortem should be made because the cause of death was unclear. Potts went to Anderson's quarters, conducted a brief physical examination, and read his case files, quickly confirming that there was no clear diagnosis. Anderson's was the third sudden and similarly inexplicable death in the regiment; in consultation with the regiment's commanding officer, Lt. Col. Dempsey, Potts decided that an autopsy was necessary. He ordered the hospital steward to bring the body to the dispensary, an improvised log hut and tent shelter to the rear of the regiment's encampment, where Potts conducted the postmortem later that evening by candlelight. Helping Potts was Private Leonard Gant, a Black soldier who served as an aid to the hospital steward and who had assisted with two other postmortems.[39]

At that point, Potts directed Acting Assistant Surgeon Bethel to perform the autopsy, but Bethel refused, insisting that he had never performed one himself and, in fact, had never even seen a corpse opened — despite the fact that he had completed a medical degree at the University of Pennsylvania. Bethel remained, however, as an observer. Dempsey, the commanding officer of the regiment, had expressed a desire to observe—according to Potts, he "had never seen a man opened and was anxious to see the case," but Dempsey did not appear when Potts sent for him. Potts—who had before the war conducted over 100 postmortem examinations as a coroner—therefore conducted the autopsy. According to his narrative account of the procedure, it was thorough and typical—the opening incision, the removal and examination of organs, of arteries, of swollen glands. There is no suggestion in the surviving records that Potts was in pursuit of anatomical evidence of racial characteristics. However, it soon became clear that Potts's interest was not limited to understanding the cause of Anderson's death but also in securing medical specimens that he could forward to the Army Medical Museum. Potts remarked to Bethel he considered the case "of the *greatest importance*," so he intended to "send all the *viscera*, including the *Brain* to the *Surgeon General* at Washington D.C. either . . . for *microscopic examination* or to be placed in the *Medical Museum*." Potts insisted he was guided purely by "the *elevation* of our *science*," to which he was sure he could make an important contribution (while also gaining professional recognition) from Anderson's anatomized human remains.[40]

Almost five hours into the dissection, the dispensary was besieged by rain coming in through the roof and flooding the floor, and Potts felt "perfectly exhausted" but still wanted to dissect Anderson's brain. He sewed up the torso and then removed Anderson's head from his torso with the brain intact. Aware that the body now had an "unsightly appearance," Potts inserted a quart bottle and some canvas in place of the removed head. He decided that the body was now of sufficiently "normal" appearance that Anderson's remains could be readied for interment. With the removed organs stored in the dispensary, Potts offered Private Gant a dollar to sleep in the hut and guard the remains while Potts retired to his quarters. During the night Potts grew anxious that the valuable specimens might be discovered by the dogs that ran through the camp and so he returned, retrieved the sack of organs, and brought them to his own quarters for safe keeping.[41]

But Acting Assistant Surgeon Bethel was shocked by what he had observed during the examination. What Potts insisted as a "creditable autopsy" was represented by Bethel, in the court-martial that followed, as something very different—a "horrible mutilation" that left Anderson's corpse in "a bloody and shameful condition." Bethel testified that Potts had removed Anderson's organs without properly ligating the blood vessels, so blood flowed freely over the scene.[42] Bethel had complained immediately after the autopsy and dissection to the lieutenant colonel, who went to Potts's quarters and demanded the return of the organs and the head, which Potts reluctantly agreed to. Anderson was finally interred.[43]

Bethel's complaint made its way up the chain of command, and it was agreed that rather than an autopsy Potts had conducted a dissection "for the purposes of practice rather than scientific information," which threatened the army's Medical Department with disrepute. At the court-martial, Bethel alleged that the "dissection" was improperly conducted in the presence of "several" enlisted men from the regiment (in fact, only the hospital steward and Private Gant observed the procedure). Bethel and the commanding officer of the regiment further asserted that "such actions as these upon being known to enlisted men of such a superstitious cast of mind as colored soldiers, will utterly demoralize and destroy all confidence and discipline among them." No testimony was offered by enlisted men to support that allegation, but certainly word had spread about the treatment of Anderson's remains throughout the regiment.[44]

Potts accused his critics of describing his work in the "the very worst light" and asserted that "non-medical men, especially illiterate men cannot understand these things." The "ordinary horror with which a simple Post-Mortem is looked at by the vulgar" had led to exaggerated accounts. Potts was nonetheless convicted and dishonorably discharged from the service in April 1865. He appealed to the adjutant general, and the secretary of war approved a reversal of the charges and Potts returned to his position a month later.[45] Lurking behind Potts's story as it emerged in the documentary evidence is a harder-to-reach story of race, military medicine, and designs on professional advancement. As noted earlier in this chapter, surgeon general William Hammond had issued a call for medical officers to forward specimens for study and display at the new Army Medical Museum in Washington, D.C. Hammond also announced that the name of each contributor would be appended to specimens. This would have been regarded at the time as a mark of professional achievement, and it certainly helped account for the flood of specimens to arrive in Washington over the course of the war and after.

Potts's desire to participate in this form of personal and professional advancement was viewed skeptically by his fellow white officers. The charges they leveled against him portrayed the anatomization of Anderson as a personal indulgence rather than a professional exercise. Neither Potts nor his accusers spoke to the fact that Anderson was African American, and Potts offered no commentary that he was motivated by any desire to document racial characteristics. But his accusers were incensed that the dissection was carried out in front of Black soldiers, who might have responded by creating disarray and discontent in the regiment—not because Pott's actions would be understood as yet another racially motivated indignity to which Black soldiers were subjected, but because African Americans were "by nature" "superstitious."

White officers' concerns with regimental discipline were probably shaped by the June 1864 execution of Private William Johnson, one of the regiment's members, for his alleged attempted rape of a white woman at Cold Harbor, Virginia, and for desertion.[46] Performative executions of Black soldiers were, according to historian Jonathan Lande, often motivated by white officers' presumption that Black soldiers who violated or witnessed violations of military discipline required severe reminders of their obligations to the army.[47] The white officers of the 23rd U.S.C.I. may have feared that Anderson's mutilation would inspire mutinous protest; certainly Anderson's comrades, Henry Bush and Franklin Weaver, would attest to their knowledge of his postmortem two years later when Anderson's wife applied for pension benefits.[48] We cannot document the thoughts or feelings of his comrades or his widow about Benjamin Anderson's anatomization, and neither can we track how or if ideas about race motivated Potts. The recorded history of the event tracks only the bitter exchange of arguments between white officers, men whom Potts had belittled and challenged on more than one occasion and who had grown to dislike him. Anderson, his widow, and the men of the 23rd U.S.C.I. fall away from the record. But Benjamin Anderson was among tens of thousands of African American soldiers and civilians whose cadavers came under the investigatory and intrusive eyes of white medical authorities.

MINOR, RUSSELL, AND POTTS were unique figures in Civil War medicine, yet all three shared an investment in dissection as a key element of professional performance. Historian Michael Sappol has described the medical anatomist as a charismatic figure, uniquely positioned to transgress rigid cultural boundaries "between life and death, purity and contamination . . . and the sacred and profane." In focusing their work on the remains of Black soldiers, white surgeons avoided the opprobrium and wrath of white communities and survivors who would have challenged and decried similar use and abuse of their deceased racial kin.[49] At the same time, their use of Black soldiers' human remains was part of a larger pattern of racism in wartime military medicine.

Black Refugees as Medical Commodities

In December 1864, a white man passed over for appointment as superintendent of the Green Heights contraband camp at Arlington, Virginia, attempted to undermine his competitor by sending fraudulent complaints to President Lincoln. Writing two letters that purported to be from refugees from slavery, he accused his competitor of tolerating abuse and mistreatment of the camp's Black residents. Prominent among the charges he made in the voice of "Sally Brown" was that the residents "are sadly treated by the Doctors who sell us after we are dead they put us into barrels and send us to the north for the New York and Philadelphia Docts to cut us up."[50]

Although the letter was fraudulent, the charge gives us reason to pause. After all, refugees from slavery died by the thousands in Washington, D.C., and neighboring Virginia both during and after the war. Human remains overwhelmed the hospitals, camps, and streets of the capitol city, but also provided medical practitioners with an abundance of a valued commodity: fresh cadavers, the source of essential professional experience and knowledge. Importantly, the made-up complaint had grounding in fact, according to Julia Wilbur, who volunteered among the refugee camps and hospitals in Washington, D.C., and Alexandria and kept a diary of her experience. In April 1864 she wrote, "There are deeds done at that Hos. that I think would not bear the light. In the Hos. here the dead were laid out decently. Now they are rolled up in the clothes they [died] in taken out at once & that is the last that is seen or known of them. I presume every woman that has died in the new Hospital has been dissected. It is not certain that all have been buried. One coffin was taken to the graveyard with nothing but a little dirt in it & it was brought back again!"[51] In the nation's capital, no less than in St. Louis, New Haven, Baltimore, as in Union army camps and hospitals across the South, army surgeons, medical college faculty and students, hospital staff, and other medical practitioners found in the carnage of war a particular benefit: the unprecedented availability of fresh cadavers—male and female, civilian and soldier—on which they could perform postmortem examinations and dissections.

It was the human remains of Black soldiers that white surgeons like Minor, Potts, and Russell eagerly exploited in their pursuit of professional knowledge, skill, and standing. However, in Washington, D.C., the surgeons, hospital stewards, and health care workers also found in the quickly expanding population of civilian refugees from slavery a ready source of human remains to sharpen their skills on. The inclusion of so many civilian postmortem examinations in the autopsy records of the Army Medical Museum contradicts the surgeon general's assertion that the museum's goal was to document the war's impact on soldiers.[52]

The war and its uncertain destruction of slavery created a vulnerable population, and medical employees and military officers were not above exploiting their access to the African Americans who fell victim to the war. Many of the 35,000 to 40,000 men, women, and children who came into Washington, D.C., during the war were voluntary refugees from slavery, seeking a place of safety (Congress ended slavery in the city in April 1862). The armies operating in the eastern theater of the war brought many more to Washington; for example, the army recruited refugees from Fortress Monroe, Virginia, and New Bern, North Carolina, to meet the army's ever-increasing need for laborers on Washington's fortifications.[53] As historian Katherine Chilton has noted, fortifying the nation's capital against Confederate assault created an extraordinary demand for labor.[54] One historian estimates that 10,000 were employed in this effort.[55] By the end of the war, sixty-eight forts surrounded Washington, D.C., and their construction and maintenance relied very heavily on the labor of refugees from slavery. The more than two dozen military hospitals in the city also relied on their labor; as many as a third of Washington's hospital workers consisted of Black civilian employees who waited on surgeons and other officers, carried water and cleaned clothing, buried night soil and scrubbed privies, sawed wood and kept fires going in laundries and kitchens, cooked, and dug graves for the human and equine dead.[56] Their labor was essential, as one surgeon explained: "Some of these duties require strong, vigorous men, and others are so repugnant to the soldiers, that they will not even imperfectly, perform them, except under the fear of punishment."[57] The city itself was also a significant employer of refugees from slavery, for everything from the most demeaning labor of cleaning cesspools to building and maintaining the roads that were necessary for both commerce and military defense.[58]

The formerly enslaved coming into Washington faced tremendous obstacles in their struggle to secure basic shelter, food, clothing, and fuel. As desperate as the city and the army were for laborers, they made few preparations to house or care for the workers they relied on, especially the exhausted, ill, malnourished people whose bodies bore the scars and injuries of abuse and torture at the hands of former masters and mistresses. After temporarily housing refugees in the Old Capitol Prison, the city established its first camp for refugees from slavery early in 1862 in a group of tenements on Capitol Hill known as Duff Green's Row.[59] This and eventually all the area's contraband camps—including those established across the Potomac in nearby Alexandria and Arlington—were created to serve dual purposes: as employment depots as well as housing for the homeless.[60] Overcrowding and epidemic smallpox led to the army's June 1862 relocation of healthier refugees to Camp Barker, while they left the smallpox patients at Duff Green's Row, which became a smallpox hospital. Although situated in a dismal and unhealthy location, Camp Barker—formerly a cemetery and brickyard—had the advantage of military-style barracks, including forty-eight small huts and two sex-segregated hospital buildings. It served largely as an employment depot, with nearly half the residents employed as military or city laborers.[61] Another camp, Mason's Island, was established in 1864, also as an employment depot.[62]

Camp Barker was quickly overcrowded and became the site of a deadly cholera outbreak; mortality among camp and hospital residents was severe—700 out of about 5,000 people died between June 1862 and June 1864.[63] In December 1863 the army shut down Camp Barker's barracks, and the residents were forcibly relocated to Freedmen's Village at Arlington; many, however, rejected the move and made their way deeper into the city to fend for themselves.[64] In neighboring northern Virginia, two buildings in Alexandria were dedicated to sheltering refugees, and soon after the construction of Alexandria's L'Ouverture General Hospital (exclusively for Black soldiers and civilians), the army developed a contraband camp alongside. Five temporary camps were created in Fairfax and Arlington (in addition to Freedman's Village).[65]

Horrible mortality rates were the result of the arrival of an impoverished population of refugees in a city that relied on their labor but offered inadequate shelter and support. Persistent delays in paying wages that were desperately needed for food and shelter contributed to the precarity of life among refugees. Washington and neighboring northern Virginia were awash in death throughout the war, as evidenced by the flood of daily requests during and after the war to the city's quartermaster for the removal and internment of corpses from contraband camps, hospitals, and the homes, streets, and alleys of the nation's capital.[66]

Daniel S. Lamb, Samuel S. Bond, and Adolphe J. Schafhirt exemplified the city's white hospital workers who saw in this deadly consequence of war the opportunity to advance their personal and professional knowledge and standing. To a significant extent, they did so using the bodies of Black refugees who fell victim to the violence of war, to slavery's violent collapse, or to the severe circumstances of refugee life and labor in Washington,

D.C., and nearby Virginia communities. Like many enlisted or contract medical workers during the war, they were influenced by wartime developments: an unprecedented access to human remains (freed from the encumbrance of legal or ethical restrictions) and the creation of the Army Medical Museum, with its call for specimens and its promise of professionally advantageous acknowledgment of those who contributed case histories and specimens. All three men shared employment ties to the museum as well. Their shared professional ambitions help us understand how and why they and so many others chose the anatomization of Black civilian human remains as a professional opportunity not to be missed.

Samuel S. Bond was born in 1835 in Pennsylvania; he joined a regiment of Pennsylvania cavalry in 1861 and served three years as a hospital steward. When his term of service ended in 1864, he requested and received appointment as hospital steward in Washington and worked at Harewood Hospital.[67] A city directory from 1865 lists him as a clerk, but that year he completed his courses and earned his medical degree from Georgetown College. In 1866 he operated a private medical practice. By 1870 his practice had already secured him considerable financial success, and he continued working as a physician until his death in 1900. Bond anticipated that his wartime experience would be pivotal to his successful career as a physician. In 1867 he had established his medical practice in Washington, and he sought to increase his professional success with an advertisement in the *Weekly Monitor* (a Washington newspaper) announcing that he had served as a "late pathologist in the United States Army Medical Museum" and had "dissected and mounted most of the medical and pathological specimens" and "contributed a greater number of specimens to the museum than any one person." He added that a "long experience in the army in postmortem examinations has given him superior advantages in that specialty."[68]

Daniel S. Lamb also came from Philadelphia to Washington. Lamb, who would become a central figure in the Army Medical Museum in later decades, started as an enlisted hospital steward, working from 1862 to 1865 in an Alexandria military hospital. There he observed autopsies and dissections conducted by a former Barbadian planter and slave-owner Thomas Bowen as well as by William Chester Minor (noted earlier in this chapter).[69] Lamb was encouraged by his supervising surgeon to pursue his college degree. He began working at the Army Medical Museum after the war, organizing and collecting medical specimens, including postmortem work. He worked as an acting assistant surgeon at the museum from 1868 to 1892, when he was promoted to chief pathologist. In addition, he was on the medical college faculty at Howard University and on the staff at Freedmen's Hospital. An esteemed physician, Lamb was regarded as one of the city's most skilled autopsy pathologists. From 1883 until 1917 he was crucial to the work of the museum, contributing over 1,500 specimens, and Lamb served as the chair of the anatomy department at Howard University from 1877 to 1923.[70] He was regarded by some as an advocate for Black and female physicians in the District, but Lamb did not always act to support Black physicians: he failed to leave the white Medical Society of the District of Columbia when they rejected Black applicants for membership—who, in protest, formed the interracial National Medical Society. Furthermore, in 1877 Lamb supplanted Dr. Alexander Augusta—the highest-ranking Black physician during the war and one of the founders of Howard's medical school—as head of anatomy at Howard University's medical school. Augusta protested his replacement and left the faculty as a result.[71]

Adolph J. Schafhirt, who had emigrated as a child to Philadelphia from Germany, served as an enlisted hospital steward—as did his brother Ernst and his father Frederic. All three served in Washington, D.C.: Adolph and Ernst as hospital stewards, their father Frederic at the Army Medical Museum from its very beginning. During and for a time after the war Adolph and his brother assisted their father in his work as the leading anatomist at the museum. Adolph worked as an artist, preparing battlefield paintings as backdrops to the specimens, as well as a "bone connoisseur."[72] Following his December 1865 discharge, Adolph pursued a career as a druggist, owning and operating his own pharmacy into the 1890s. Ernst would continue his work as an anatomist and clerk with the museum, and he made plaster and clay models for exhibits into the 1880s.[73] Their father Frederic, a German-trained anatomist who was opposed to slavery but also had an established pedigree in racist science, brought Adolph and his brother into the museum work.[74]

Frederic Schafhirt had worked with two of the world's leading racial theorists. In Europe, he worked with Johann Blumenbach, acknowledged now as a founder of race-focused craniometry; after emigrating to Philadelphia, Frederic worked with the father of the racist "American school" of ethnography and advocate of polygenesis, Samuel Morton, assisting Morton in preparing *Crania Americana*, the 1839 text widely regarded as foundational to the development of scientific racism in the United States. Frederic also worked at the University of Pennsylvania under the renowned paleontologist Dr. Joseph Leidy, who was committed to the notion of biodeterministic racial difference and was a close correspondent with the foremost advocate of polygenesis, Josiah Nott.[75] Fredric moved to Washington intending to assume a position at Columbian College but found the medical faculty there so divided by their Civil War politics that he began to look elsewhere; he asked his former associate Professor Leidy to secure him a position with Louis Agassiz, another prominent public intellectual, naturalist, and advocate of racist science. In Washington, Fredric found a new path: he became a central figure in the early development of the collections at the Army Medical Museum. He was the museum's first hospital steward, and he remained employed with the museum from 1862 until his death in 1880. His museum colleagues described Fredric as an admirable bone-cleaner and anatomist, and they admired his skill in preparing and organizing the display of specimens.[76] He also lectured at the National Medical College and worked with the Smithsonian Institute.[77] In addition, he created a personal collection of human specimens, which he willed, with its glass cases, to Adolphe's son.[78]

Lamb, Bond, and Adolphe Schafhirt, like many other white surgeons and hospital workers, found that the harvest of death among refugees from slavery offered the perfect opportunity to hone their professional skills. They consumed the war's windfall—a grim abundance of corpses—to advance their study of human anatomy, yet another example of the contradictory logic of medical racism that posited Black bodies as simultaneously racially different and neutrally human. In 1865 and 1866, Freedmen's Hospital—established in 1863 near the site of former Camp Barker—permitted the three hospital steward employees of the museum to perform autopsies on and dismember the hospital's deceased patients.[79] They gained invaluable anatomical experience, and their employer, the museum, gained 150 specimens that the three created from the autopsies.[80] Although Schafhirt and Bond listed themselves as the authors of the manuscript casebook they had prepared for the museum documenting the postmortem examinations, Schafhirt conducted only nine of the 100 autopsies. Bond and Lamb conducted the vast majority.

It was more than fifty years later before Lamb acknowledged in print that their exploitation of freed people's remains would not meet the ethical standards of the twentieth century. Lamb would recall, "The time was that, at least in the hospitals, if we wanted a post mortem examination we simply made it without asking leave of anybody. That time has passed. The consent of relatives or friends must now be first obtained, and this consent is often refused."[81] If we are to judge by the narrative case histories prepared by Bond, Schafhirt, and Lamb, Freedmen's Hospital patients were not merely the anonymous poor that medical professionals had exploited. Some of the postmortem reports included case histories, presumably obtained from the patient by the attending physician; these antemortem histories some-times included considerable personal detail (such as names, ages, history of ailments, etc.). They also often indicated that a patient had been brought into the hospital by friends or family. Among them was Cinta Howard, aged about eighteen years old, who was very emaciated. Her friends had ex-plained her symptoms to the attending physician: they had brought her to the hospital after she lost the ability to speak and fell into a comatose state. After she died, Adolph Schafhirt autopsied and anatomized her, forward-ing a number of specimens from her remains. Like so many Black women autopsied for the museum, the specimens prepared from Howard's remains included several made from her reproductive organs.[82] This, too, was con-sistent with white ethnological fascination with the genitalia and reproduc-tive organs of African and African American women.[83] The logbooks that noted the arrival of specimens during and after the war and the accompany-ing case histories reveal that Black female deceased patients frequently had their internal reproductive organs removed and turned into specimens.[84]

Although the case histories offer a heartbreaking record of the physical trauma of slavery, war, and wartime labor on Black people, for the most part they do not reflect a systematic attempt to invent or document imagined ra-cial characteristics (with the exception of the attention to women's sexual organs already noted). Instead, the postmortem reports simply record the operator's observations during his disassembly of cadavers, including a narrative and tabular record of the weight of fourteen major internal or-gans. This suggests that most white medical workers were not performing autopsies and dissections on African American human remains in the ex-plicit pursuit of racial science; rather, they regarded the remains of African Americans as exploitable objects, not people entitled to a dignified burial. The combined effect of poverty and race, from the perspective of white sur-geons, hospital, and museum employees, made the Black civilian war dead dispensable.

The records of the Army Medical Museum reveal that Bond, Lamb and Schafhirt were joined by dozens of additional surgeons and hospital stew-ards in using the human remains of refugees from slavery and, of course, Black soldiers to practice their skills at autopsy, dissection, and anatomy. The hospitals of Washington, D.C., were prominent among the contributors—due to the very large and concentrated population of former slaves as well as the ease of transferring records and specimens to the museum—but post-mortem records and specimens came in from across the nation. The army's medical officers and employees eagerly seized on their access to the war dead to enhance their knowledge and authority in the profession.[85] This included some of the few Black physicians enlisted and employed by the army. Alexander Augusta, his pupil Anderson Abbott, Jerome Riley, William Powell, Charles Purvis, John Rapier, Willis Revels, and Alpheus Tucker all served during or after the war at Freedman's Hospital or the city's various contraband hospitals — the strictures of segregation meant they could not serve at hospitals for white soldiers.[86] They also conducted postmortem examinations, but if they prepared and submitted specimens to the museum, the surgeon general chose not to include them in the *Medical and Surgical History of the War of the Rebellion*.[87]

Making Specimens, Making the Army Medical Museum

Beyond the opportunity to practice dissection, white medical workers disassembled the human remains of Black soldiers and civilians to create specimens for the growing collections held and displayed at the Army Medical Museum. Surgeon general Hammond's 1862 Circular No. 2, establishing the Army Medical Museum to illustrate "the injuries and diseases that produce death or disability during war," providing the opportunity to study and develop methods for alleviating the medical challenges of war.[88] Hammond envisioned the museum as a place where knowledge would be created and where a new kind of medical and scientific learning could take place.[89] By collecting and exhibiting specimens that exemplified battlefield medicine and the human damage of war, the museum would become the first nationally funded institution for medical research. Surgeon John Brinton, named by Hammond as the museum's first curator, would clarify in later months the exact procedures for preparing and forwarding specimens. They should only be roughly prepared, tagged, and submersed in a keg of whiskey, allowing the museum's staff to do the precision work of preparing specimens. The museum also solicited detailed case reports to accompany each specimen as well as the name of the contributor, who would be acknowledged both at the museum and in future publications.[90] The museum covered the transportation costs.

The immediate flow of donations from surgeons and hospital stewards bore witness to the professional aspirations of medical officers and employees as well as their interest in contributing to wartime knowledge production. By the end of the museum's first year, curator Brinton reported that the museum had already collected 1,349 objects, including 985 surgical specimens, 106 medical specimens, and 133 missiles mostly extracted from the body, including bullets, shot, canisters, shell fragments, and arrows.[91] Some of those specimens Brinton had collected himself from the aftermath of the battle at Fredericksburg. Brinton was quick to point out that the museum easily surpassed the size and significance of similar collections in Britain and France, and he insisted it was not "a mere museum of curiosities" but rather "a collection which teaches."[92]

The United States could finally claim international prestige in medical research. By the end of 1864, the museum's collection had grown to include 3,500 surgical specimens, 500 medical specimens, 150 plaster casts and models, 100 drawings and paintings, and 1,100 microscopical preparations.[93] Like the respondents to surveys described in chapter 3, the contributors understood that their participation in these nation-building and professionalizing efforts would bring individual acknowledgment and recognition. Many would have already been familiar with the "gift economy" that enhanced both private medical and anatomical collections as well as public museums wherein specimens were exchanged or donated with a view toward future reciprocation.[94] And some, like surgeon Reed B. Bontecou (among many others), had already begun building private collections when they began forwarding specimens to the museum.

Bontecou was a well-known natural scientist, medical researcher, and physician when he enlisted in 1861 as a surgeon. Early in the war he had charge of Hygeia Hospital at Fort Monroe. From October 1863 to June 1866 he was the surgeon in charge of Harewood Hospital at Washington, D.C., one of the largest hospitals of the war with a capacity of 3,000 beds. He became known as one of the most prolific contributors to the Army Medical Museum and as a pioneering medical photographer, capturing preoperative and postoperative views of wounded soldiers. Before as well as during the war Bontecou was also an avid collector of natural history specimens— whether flora and fauna from his antebellum trip up the Amazon River, or specimens taken from the hospitals and battlefields of the war. While he was posted in charge of Hygeia Hospital, Bontecou collected human heads (not crania)—whether these came from deceased refugees from slavery or from soldiers is unclear, but it seems unlikely he would have risked opprobrium by mutilating the remains of white soldiers. Bontecou was one of several military surgeons called upon by the curators of the museum to deliver to the museum the privately held specimens they had collected during their military service. Bontecou had made a gift of the human heads to another physician, but curator Brinton demanded them as property of the army.[95]

Hammond's vision, the work of the museum's curators and employees, and the enthusiastic responses of contributors accelerated the development of American medical science but did so as part of the development of scientific racism and the medical objectification of non-white people. It is impossible to imagine that the museum's work was isolated from the increasingly popular scientific racism that was central to American medical science and practices at the time, especially in light of Frederic Schafhirt's central role at the museum. Popular anatomical museums had already been established in several leading cities by midcentury, and they participated in practices of commodifying, appropriating, and displaying Black and especially enslaved human remains—along with those of paupers, criminals, and other marginalized people.[96] Historians Stephen Kenny, Michael Sappol, Ann Fabian, and Samuel Redman agree that anatomy museums lent legitimacy and popular support to evolving notions about the biological determinism of race and racial hierarchies.[97]

However, the racial project of the Army Medical Museum was inconsistent. The published catalogues of the museum's collection of specimens clearly demonstrate less interest (either on the part of donors or museum curators) in Black bodies as exemplifying the human cost of war. Alfred Woodhull's *Catalogue of Surgical Section of the U.S. Army Medical Museum* (1866) included only 223 specimens from African Americans out of more than 4,700. Edward Curtis's *Catalogue of the Microscopial Section of the United States Army Medical Museum* (1867) referred to only ten specimens from African Americans out of 149; George Otis's *Catalogue of the Anatomical Section* of *the United States Army Medical Museum* (1880) included only fourteen specimens from African Americans out of almost 7,000.[98] Although the museum received hundreds of reports on postmortems and dissections conducted on African Americans, it would seem that most contributors to the museum's collections were either not interested in taking specimens from African American bodies or assumed such specimens were not as useful or welcome as those taken from whites. Certainly white soldiers suffered battlefield wounds more frequently than African Americans, whose regiments were less likely to be deployed on the battlefield. Perhaps surgeons simply had greater access to white cadavers. Or, alternately, the curators may have preferred to display specimens from white soldiers in representing the human body; they could see Black bodies only as evidence of embodied race, not as examples of racially neutral consequences of war's injuries and disease. Whatever the cause and motivation, the donation and creation of specimens underrepresented the cost of warfare on Black soldiers and civilians.

When and how the Army Medical Museum became more openly complicit in explicit scientific racism is part of the story of the wartime production of medical and scientific racism, particularly the rooting of race in biology. While neither the surgeon general nor the museum's curators appear to have explicitly solicited specimens for the purposes of documenting "racial characteristics" in Black bodies during the war, at war's end the museum charted a new path and purpose: What kinds of collections would they pursue? What would be the postwar future of a museum founded to document and commemorate the medical crisis of warfare? The answer, as Ann Fabian explained in her study of museums and collectors and their pursuit of scientific foundations for racial difference, was to turn to the army's war on Native people in the western plains and collect Indian skeletons, crania, and other "objects of ethnological or archaeological interest."[99]

Military expeditions in the west and genocide against Native Americans generated a substantial wave of collecting, as did the looting of sacred mounds and burial sites. After the war and until the end of the nineteenth century, the museum's central work focused on ethnology and comparative anatomy, fueling the museum's then-explicit investment in scientific and medical racism. This endeavor was complemented by an 1869 exchange with the Smithsonian Institution in which the museum transferred "objects illustrating the manners and customs of the Indians" in exchange for the "entire collection of crania" at the Smithsonian.[100] It is less well known that the museum's postwar curators also continued to collect African American crania—both actively soliciting donations and purchasing individual crania as well as crania collections from medical colleges, from Southern physicians, and from individual collectors.[101] A circular issued to the medical officers of the Freedman's Bureau in 1868 directed them to participate in the collection of specimens for the museum, further evidence that African American remains were an important target of the museum's postbellum collecting.[102]

Samuel Morton's influence—as the great popularizer of the notion that race had a biological basis—continued to shape the museum in the decades to come.[103] In 1869, curator George Otis was excited at the prospect of having created a collection of crania that "will rival the famous Mortonian cabinet," and by the mid-1870s the museum's "Craniological Cabinet," situated just off the main entrance, was arranged just as Morton arranged his, in an imagined hierarchical order.[104] By 1871 the museum had collected over 900 skulls.[105] Morton's influence also played out in the methods used to measure crania, volume being (incorrectly) associated with intellectual ability.

After the war, many specimens were donated or purchased from nearby faculty and students at Washington-area hospitals and college dissecting rooms, including Columbia College, Georgetown College, and Howard University.[106] Washington-area physicians were similarly interested in contributing specimens that would advance the museum's ethnological interests. An ophthalmologist, Dr. S. M. Burnett, donated twenty-three specimens of eyes from Black patients, asserting that these specimens, too, could help the museum ascertain "how far this change in their condition has influenced their susceptibility to and immunity from certain diseases," referring to the race work of Josiah Nott and George Glidden.[107] Some contributions were accidental. Construction at the Washington, D.C., Soldiers Home apparently disturbed a Black burial ground there, from which another U.S. officer extracted and donated crania to the museum. Large numbers of specimens also continued to be taken from deceased patients at Freedmen's Hospital.

Autopsies by Bond, Schafhirt, and Lamb from 1866 to 1867 generated some 150 specimens, but hundreds more were secured in the decades to follow.[108] The museum continued to capitalize on the abundance of Black illness, injury, and death in postwar Washington. Late in the 1880s, even as the museum's ethnological interest focused on Native Americans, the museum curator kept up a substantial correspondence with medical researchers and medical school professors in the South who were anxious to offer their various specimen collections of Black crania and skeletal remains that, they and the curator both believed, revealed anatomical racial characteristics.[109]

The Army Medical Museum had a profound impact on American medicine. Beyond the authority offered to contributors and the great popularity of its collections with the American public as well as medical researchers, the museum collections (both material and textual) became an important source for the surgeon general's second major project about medicine and the war. The 1862 circular that announced the formation of the museum also indicated the surgeon general's intent to publish an official medical history of the war, the *Medical and Surgical History of the War of the Rebellion*. Composed of six volumes published between 1870 and 1888, the series offered a comprehensive account of military medicine and surgery, including thousands of case histories and autopsy reports. Like the volumes published by the U.S. Sanitary Commission, the surgeon general's volumes would ultimately catalog and describe, rather than analyze, the tens of thousands of cases describing treatments of disease, wounds, autopsy results, and specimens that fueled the unprecedented number of dissections performed by medical practitioners at all ranks during and immediately after the war.

Like the work of the museum, the assembling of materials for the six-volume work would reveal the tensions inherent in a project where race held both definitive and precarious meaning in the production of medical knowledge. The first volume opens by noting the "scientific and historical" "propriety" of arranging medical data by race, so obvious a service to humanity that it needed no further explanation—silently affirming the centrality of whiteness to the project and the relegation of Black bodies to peripheral studies of "race."[110] The surgeon general announced that the volumes would contribute "to our knowledge of the influence of race-peculiarities on disease," but that influence proved difficult to determine. As noted in chapter 2, the results did not always conform to existing assumptions about racial difference.

The surgeon general found it even harder to locate the meaning of race in the case reports assembled for the surgical volumes. Reports of surgery performed on Black patients are scattered throughout, but there were no conclusions suggesting "race peculiarities" in surgical outcomes.[111] This mirrored the Army Medical Museum's catalogs of presurgical and postsurgical specimens and case reports. In both catalogs and Baxter's medical history, Army Medical Museum curator Otis solicited additional case information in several instances of surgeries performed on Black soldiers and civilians, but his aim was to gather complete information on particular procedures rather than grist for the field of comparative anatomy.[112] In other words, case reports and specimens from Black bodies were simultaneously used as evidence of racial difference that suffused anatomy and physiology, yet also they were also used interchangeably with specimens and case reports from white bodies.[113]

Historian Katherine Cober has noted that on the eve of the Civil War anatomical illustration and modeling offered and created the Caucasian male as the universal body.[114] To the extent that anatomical illustrations and representations included non-whites, they were most often used to exemplify deviation from the universal white norm. Yet medical students and physicians, even the strongest advocates of biological racism, did not give a second thought to their reliance on the cadavers of non-whites in gaining anatomical expertise. This core contradiction in the logic and science of race that should have troubled scientists and medical practitioners went unexamined, whether in the treatment of the ill and injured or, as we see in the next chapter, in the treatment of the dead.

CHAPTER FIVE
The Afterlife of Race

After white medical staff had their fill of observing, assessing, measuring, probing, disarticulating, and anatomizing the bodies of African American soldiers and civilians who came to the army's medical practitioners for care and healing, they treated the human remains of the Black war dead without dignity or respect. Some were sent to segregated cemeteries, at best. Others were sent to unmarked or mass graves, and some to anonymous medical waste pits. For African Americans, wartime death was often met with continued acts of discrimination and injustice. Many whites viewed the bodies of Black soldiers and civilians as both more exploitable than those of whites and less deserving of the dignified burial that white soldiers and their survivors hoped for. The wartime culture of "A Good Death" pursued by so many white Unionists was distantly removed from the experiences and possibilities that followed the passing and postmortem exploitation of Black soldiers and civilians, who had offered their lives (or whose lives were taken) in a war to end slavery.[1]

The war's abundance of death came to soldiers and civilians, white and African American, but Black soldiers (and likely Black civilians) died at a far greater rate than did whites. Although it is the dramatic number of fallen soldiers on Civil War battlefields that drew the attention of the nation and most modern scholars today, we should remember that the majority of wartime mortality occurred ingloriously in camps and in hospitals from disease. Not only did disease take the life of most soldiers who died during the war, but also notably a much higher proportion of Black than white soldiers. Of the estimated 37,000 Black soldiers who died during the war, 30,000 died from disease in hospitals and camps. Black troops were almost ten times as likely to die from disease as from combat; among white troops, death from disease was only twice as likely as death from combat injuries.[2] Once sick, Black troops died about five times more frequently than white troops. Black soldiers were more likely to die than whites from diarrheal diseases, pneumonia, scurvy, tuberculosis, smallpox, and malaria.[3] In other words, the mortality *"rate"* among the United States Colored Troops in the Civil War was 35 percent greater than that among other troops.[4] This unprecedented mortality (although not the racial disparity), led historian Drew Gilpin Faust to describe the Civil War as creating a new national relationship to death.[5] For African Americans—those who died and those who survived to mourn—wartime death extended the impact of slavery as well as state racism in significant ways, as this chapter will reveal.

Additionally, African Americans were disproportionately numbered among the unknown dead. More than 40 percent of all military war dead were never identified, but among African American soldiers that proportion grew to 66 percent.[6] Some of that difference might be accounted for by the Confederate practice of killing Black prisoners or refusing to allow the Union army to retrieve and bury its dead after battles had concluded. However, considering that the great majority of Black deaths occurred in Union hospitals and in camps rather than in battle, it would seem that the circumstances of Black soldiers' deaths were *more likely* to allow their proper identification. The commanding officer of the 62nd U.S.C.I., in his farewell speech to the regiment at the conclusion of their service, noted that "Death held high carnival day after day for months. The four hundred graves—many of them nameless"—were witness to that fact.[7] But why were so many nameless? How and why so many died unnamed and unacknowledged demands explanation.

The chaos of war—especially on the battlefield—often forced the Union army to ignore its own regulations dictating ritual honoring and burial of the dead and instead to dispose of human remains in improvised ways. White soldiers were also left in unmarked and mass graves or never buried at all. However, for Black soldiers and civilians, white scientific and medical investigations further diminished the extent and meaning of their wartime sacrifice, adding a final degradation to the wartime indignities visited on them.[8] As Black bodies were removed from camps, from segregated hospitals and hospital wards, from where they collapsed and died while at work on fortifications or in streets and alleyways, they were often allotted a segregated and inferior resting place. In undercounting the extent and aftermath of Black mortality and by failing to expose the legacy of racist mortuary practices, historians have underestimated the extent to which racism shaped and permeated the institutions of war and death.

Certainly, we can point to instances of dignified and notable burial practices claimed for some African American servicemen. Captain Andre Cailloux of the First Louisiana Native Guard was buried with full military and Catholic honors in New Orleans, witnessed by thousands of city residents who turned out to honor their native son.[9] For many uncounted African Americans, however, wartime burial occurred without ceremony, in improvised and anonymous burial grounds. Even worse, particularly for comrades, their kin and friends, wartime burial practices could not ensure that the integrity of the corpse was preserved. This was sometimes the result of wartime conditions, but it was also the result of decisions by military surgeons and hospital workers to dissect, anatomize, and reduce soldiers' remains to medical specimens. At contraband hospitals across the South, Black civilians met similar fates in death.

Whites' wartime pursuit of embodied race in living and recently deceased Black soldiers and civilians revealed their unwillingness and perhaps incapacity to recognize the full personhood of people of African descent. Using the bodies of Black soldiers for dissection and anatomization, often in search of biological justifications for social hierarchies and race-based privileges, turned people into objects—objects that had no claim on funeral rites, a military burial, notification of next of kin, or official registration. Even those whose remains were not exploited by medical investigators faced inequities. The medical and military context in which death occurred was steeped in racist practices that preceded the war, as well as the wartime context noted here. The story of the war dead, as historians have long emphasized, was central to the experience, meaning, and memory of the war, for soldiers and noncombatants alike. Historians have far to go toward understanding how the disparaging treatment of Black war dead shaped the meaning of the war for whites and for African Americans.

Death outside the Reach of War

Outside the reach of the war, African Americans met the death of loved ones as their status (enslaved or free), spiritual practices, cultural expectations, and resources demanded or allowed.[10] On May 1, 1862, anyone who happened to be at the Arch Street Wharf in Philadelphia would have witnessed the large funeral procession for Mrs. Elizabeth A. Schureman, wife of an African Methodist Episcopal (AME) pastor. Before the procession, Mrs. Schureman's remains had been laid out "beautifully and appropriately" by Mrs. Sarah Williams, a Philadelphia shroudress. Her body had been carried on a bier from her home to the wharf, in a procession that included the brothers and sisters of her fraternal order, her congregation's officiants, her church women's society members, her family, and friends. The procession departed Philadelphia for Burlington, New Jersey, where they entered the AME church. There, the choir sang, the congregants offered hymns, and the pastor spoke from the book of Revelation. After the benediction, her remains were escorted to the cemetery, where her pastor and the male and female officers of her fraternal society performed final rituals. It was, by report, the largest funeral ever witnessed in Burlington.[11]

Elizabeth Schureman's funeral rites were those of an elite member of her community, enmeshed in the religious, fraternal, and business life of her social circle. It was, in many respects, a privileged passage and not typical of what the mostly working-class, military-aged Black men and their families in the North would have encountered or experienced. The example of Schureman's rites points to the layered meanings of a dignified death for the deceased, their family, and their community. It highlights the important social context of death and funeral rituals. However wealthy or poor, African Americans in the North would have hoped and expected that on their death (during peacetime), a family member or a close friend would bathe their body, place it on a cooling board, drape it in a shroud or dress, in a new or at least clean suit of clothes, and that friends would join the family in sitting up with the corpse while sharing food, hymns, and stories. A friend or a local carpenter would build a coffin, and the next day—if possible—the deceased would be carried to their church for a funeral service and then taken by wagon or pallbearers to a cemetery for final burial rites. At the very least, one hoped for close attendance to the body by loved ones and a dignified (and undisturbed) burial, even if in a potter's field.[12]

Prior to the Civil War, the nineteenth-century politics of race had material consequences—dictating, for example, which burial grounds were open to African Americans. In the context of segregation (whites frequently excluding African Americans from public, denominational, or municipal cemeteries, or relegating them to inferior sections), Northern African American congregations and communities established their own burial grounds and celebrated the successful founding of Black cemeteries. The Black press covered these as especially noteworthy events. In reporting on the establishment of a Black cemetery in Cincinnati, a reporter in Frederick Douglass's paper, *The North Star*, described it as a "splendid acquisition," "a most useful institution," equivalent to the importance of public halls and meeting places to the Black community.[13] Similarly, the dedication of Olive Cemetery in Philadelphia was attended by over 400 local African Americans, who understood it to be "an extraordinary occasion . . . calculated to do us imperishable honor—for, amongst all civilized communities, an interest is always manifested for the proper sepulture of the dead."[14] From the pages of the *Christian Recorder*, the organ of the AME church, congregations that purchased cemetery lots announced the achievement as a great blessing.[15] The

Recorder asserted that these developments placed Black citizens on an equal footing with whites, but more importantly ensured dignity and respect in death.[16]

When "resurrectionists" targeted Black burial grounds (as they frequently did), Black communities expressed outrage and trauma. In both the North and the South, Black Americans, free and enslaved, often experienced insult to the burial places of their friends and family. Grave robbers, in their endless pursuit of cadavers for anatomy instruction and practice, had a long history of violating and commodifying African Americans in death. Resurrectionists profited handily by exhuming and selling fresh corpses to medical schools and museums, and they haunted Northern Black cemeteries and slave cemeteries in the South to obtain "fresh" bodies for medical schools. African Americans in the North and South petitioned local authorities for protection of Black burial grounds against resurrectionists to no avail.[17]

Historians Daina Ramey Berry and Stephen Kenny have revealed the antebellum traffic in the corpses of enslaved people to be modeled on the slave trade itself, one that solicited and supplied both the dying and the deceased to Southern and Northern medical professionals, collectors, and museums. The violation and stolen dignity associated with exhuming human remains and commodifying the corpses enlarged the scope and impact of racism to include the bodies of the dead as well as those who mourned them.[18] On the eve of the Civil War, white supremacy was often manifested in denying a dignified death and burial to African Americans, exemplifying the profound disregard with which so many white Americans viewed the personhood of Black people, alive and dead.

This was especially the case in the antebellum South, where death was not only a commonplace feature of the torture and exploitation of the enslaved but also a promise for final liberation. In the enslaved communities of the 1850s, community-based death rituals were constrained by the demands of slave owners on the time, mobility, and cultural practices of the enslaved. Funerals were widely regarded by slave owners as events too easily adapted to organizing resistance and rebellion, which prompted white surveillance and efforts to prevent or curtail them. During the years and generations of American slavery, legislatures and municipalities strove to police and repress the funerals and burial ceremonies of enslaved communities — documented as early as 1680 in Virginia.[19] Enslaved and free Blacks in Richmond protested a law passed in the aftermath of the 1831 Nat Turner rebellion that prohibited religious assemblies because it prevented them from conducting

dignified burial services.[20] Whites often followed the execution of enslaved participants in rebellions by refusing a proper burial for human remains, intended as a further punishment and as a warning to the community
of enslaved people. Other executed rebels had their remains mutilated.[21]

Some former slaves reported hasty burials, sometimes in crude coffins,
sometimes in no more than the clothes in which people died. The brusque and
dishonoring treatment of the enslaved dead typically meant that if there were
funeral services offered, they occurred days, weeks, even months later.[22]
Historian David Roediger has pointed to evidence, in both slave narratives
and the Works Progress Administration (WPA) interviews, that enslaved
people deeply resented the callous disregard of slave owners for the dignified funerals and burials of the enslaved. Enslaved people defied their owners'
disregard and pursued their own rituals around death. Some survivors of
slavery described tender rituals of bathing the deceased, dressing the corpse
in either a suit of clothes (men) or a clean winding sheet (women), and carefully tending the deceased until a well-fit coffin was built. The deceased would
then be carried to the burial site, and a church service would be held the next
Sunday.[23] Drumming and singing were key in some enslaved communities;
ring shouts accompanied burial rites in others. One former slave recalled the
"big time" that occurred at a service, where survivors witnessed to the life
of the deceased. Most who had experienced slavery, however, reported long
delays before services were held for the deceased, a delay imposed by
the endless work demands of slavery.[24] Yet funeral rites were also part of the
geography of resistance among the enslaved, especially in the plantation regions of the South: vitally important, deeply sacred, and, when possible,
hidden from white observation.[25]

Burial practices and burial grounds among enslaved communities varied
widely, but Lynn Rainville's important study of African American cemeteries in Virginia explains that the frequent use of uninscribed fieldstones as
markers likely reflected the context of proscribed illiteracy, inaccessible resources, and reliance on oral history to identify gravesites, and practices that
emphasized family rather than individual burial sites. Yet she also found a
tremendous variety of inscribed markers and decorative practices at burial
sites.[26] The burial places that free and enslaved Black Southerners used were
always vulnerable to the authority and power of whites. In a typical example,
white municipal authorities deemed a Black burial ground in Augusta, Georgia, less important than the expansion of a city wharf.[27] Part of the campus
of the University of Richmond was built over a burial ground of enslaved

people.[28] Several Black cemeteries and burial grounds in Washington, D.C. fell victim to changing city ordinances and city growth as well.[29]

Rites Worth Fighting For

Black Civil War troops brought their own ideas about and experiences with death to their wartime service. They also understood that their access to the honor of a military burial, the same ritual that white soldiers received in death, was worth fighting for and one of the ways in which the war accelerated their claims to racial equality and citizenship rights.[30] Historian J. T. Roane reminds us that historically, burial grounds, like plantation provision grounds, were sites of Black insurgency, challenging white social control both during and after slavery. As such, they were also sites of white assault.[31] What historian Vincent Brown names as "mortuary politics"—the power struggles reflected and revealed in contested treatments of the dead—were also clearly evident in the disposal of Black bodies by white military and medical men during the war.[32]

Some white commanders fully embraced equitable burial rites as one of the earned privileges of Black military service. A "regular military burial" was described by Thomas W. Higginson, commander of Black troops, including a military escort bearing a flag-draped coffin to an appropriate burial place "and three volleys fired over the grave."[33] Colonel Samuel Armstrong described the funeral of another Black soldier, formerly a slave: his coffin was draped in the U.S. flag, the procession included a dirge-playing brass band and a group of comrades who bore arms reversed, and the rite was attended by three commissioned officers.[34] In coastal South Carolina, Black and white soldiers under the command of Major General Rufus R. Saxton were buried together in the Soldiers Cemetery near Beaufort.[35] Saxton, military governor over the South Carolina coastal islands, instituted what Corporal James Henry Gooding of the 54th Massachusetts proudly described as a "very important and humane arrangement" that the brave soldier who died from disease or wound must be *decently* buried." Citing orders from the provost marshal's office (pertaining to the death of white soldiers), Saxton required that each corpse be provided with a "good, substantial" coffin, clean garments, and a white-painted board to identify his name, regiment, and age. Furthermore, Gooding noted, "The relatives and friends of the deceased are to receive an official notice of the facts, detailing the manner of death, or sickness before death, and every item so far as known of the conduct of the deceased in the field." This, he noted, was an improvement on the "old order of things," with no report of what those previous practices had been.[36] Gooding, an advocate for Black enlistment, may have appreciated that detailing the formerly egregious practices of burying Black soldiers in segregated burial spots or in unmarked graves would not endear Northern Blacks to military service.

Some army chaplains were dedicated to providing honorable services and burial for the Black soldiers with whom they served; the fourteen African Americans among the 133 chaplains who served during the war were among them.[37] Chaplain James Peet, stationed at Vicksburg with his regiment (the 50th U.S.C.I.), in September 1864 noted, "The burial of the dead is properly attended with Religious Services and Military Escort."[38] At Knight Hospital in New Haven, Chaplain James Crane reported accompanying to the grave and performing services for Black soldiers who died in the hospital, services that included an "address in each case."[39] Chauncey Leonard, assigned to L'Ouverture Hospital in Alexandria that served Black soldiers and civilians, reported committing Black soldiers to the grave with "appropriate religious services."[40] Many more may have acted similarly; the extant record, however, is very thin.

When Private John Cooley died in May 1864, his coffin received an escort to the cemetery and a graveside service led by the Reverend Albert Gladwin (a Black Baptist minister and the government-appointed superintendent of contrabands at Alexandria).[41] However, Gladwin made no mention of the war or of the Black soldiers defending the nation, and he included no military honors. This was one of several indignities that prompted Black soldiers to protest.[42] In December 1864, 443 Black soldiers in L'Ouverture Hospital petitioned Major Edwin Bentley, director over the area's hospitals, to end Gladwin's practice of burying Black soldiers with Alexandria's civilian refugees from slavery. For the last year, the "soldiers burying ground" (now Arlington National Cemetery) had been undergoing major improvements, but the burial ground for the refugees from slavery was essentially a potter's field where the bodies were "packed away," three or four to a grave.[43] The soldiers were furious: "We . . . [feel] deeply interested in a matter of so great importance."

> As American citizens, we have a right to fight for the protection of her flag, that right is granted, and we are now sharing equally the dangers and hardships in this mighty contest, and should shair [sic] the same privileges and rights of burial in every way with our fellow soldiers

who only differ from us in color. To crush this rebellion, and establish civil, religious & political freedom for our children, is the height of our ambition. To this end we suffer, for this we fight, yea and mingle our blood with yours, to wash away a stain so black, and destroy a Plot so destructive to the interest and property of this nation, as soldiers in the U.S. Army.

They demanded "our bodies may find a resting place in the ground designated for the brave defenders of our countries flag."[44] Their carefully written petition did not express any disdain for burial with Black civilians but rather directly protested the army's refusal to recognize them as soldiers, due a soldier's honor. Relief workers Harriet Jacobs and Julia Wilbur joined in the protests and outcry, and by the end of the month the quartermaster general's orders finally instructed that Black soldiers had earned the right to burial in the military cemetery along with white soldiers.[45]

Military racism continued to shape burial practices throughout and after the war. In March 1864, at Helena, Arkansas, the commander of the 56th U.S.C.I. noted that since "the dead of this Regiment having not been buried according to army regulations the following order will be observed—A commissioned officer will be required to be present at any funeral connected with their respective companies and see that the graves are dug at least four feet deep and that the noncommissioned officers are properly instructed in the duties and forms connected with military funerals."[46] In July 1865, white abolitionist, journalist, and author James Redpath wrote to the *National Anti-Slavery Standard* and reported the burial of Black soldiers and civilians in the Charleston area in a potters' field. In Tennessee, their interment occurred in "sloppy and slimy ground at the bottom of a hill," away from white Union and Confederate burials. In Savannah, he reported, the commanding officer refused to bury Black and white soldiers in the same cemetery, despite protests from one of the chaplains assigned there.[47] At Camp William Penn, on the outskirts of Philadelphia, the men of the 32nd U.S.C.I. protested the mistreatment of a fallen comrade, when, in the spring of 1864, the regimental surgeon failed to attend to a soldier whose remains were left, unburied, in the warm barracks.[48]

The Right to Know and to Mourn

There was no official procedure in place to notify families of a soldier's death during the war. Newspapers often printed casualty lists from battles, but they commonly included inaccurate or incomplete information. The *Christian Recorder* occasionally received and published reports of the dead from Black regiments. Comrades or sympathetic commanding officers or chaplains sometimes took it on themselves to notify survivors with reassuring notes about how a soldier had met his end. On the eve of battle, the soldiers who served in the 28th U.S.C.I. asked their (Black) chaplain Garland H. White to notify their loved ones if they were killed and to report they had died like men.[49] They wanted the honor of their sacrifice recognized and acknowledged.

For Black families, information about a loved soldier's death was often hard to come by. The many letters of inquiry sent by worried family members and survivors to the army for information about whether a loved soldier was living, injured, or dead tells us how difficult it was to access accurate and timely information.[50] The efforts of the U.S. Sanitary Commission (USSC) and the Christian Commission to assist families who sought confirmation of the status of their loved ones helped some. But the majority of Black soldiers were enlisted in the slave South and were formerly enslaved; it would have been exceedingly difficult to get word to loved ones, many of them illiterate and still held as slaves. In addition, hundreds of thousands of women, children, and the elderly accompanied men when they fled slavery for Union lines with the intent to enlist. Those family members would have faced uncertain destinations and destinies as refugees from slavery. Complicating the likelihood of kin notification was the fact that regimental records of death sometimes noted not the names of survivors but the names of the slave owners who had claimed the soldiers as their property—Unionist slave owners who were entitled to compensation for the loss of their human property during the war.[51]

When the widows of fallen Black soldiers applied for veteran's pension benefits, they were required to provide evidence of their husband's death, and we therefore might expect their applications to include some insight into how families learned of the death of a loved one or how their regiment acknowledged the death. The USSC's Army and Navy Claim Agency, established in 1864 to assist soldiers, their widows, and surviving family members apply for back pay, bounty, and pension benefits, registered a large number of pension applications that failed because the widows and survivors could not provide proof of death.[52]

The pension records confirm that the widows and survivors of African American soldiers were infrequently provided with official notice, let alone thoughtful correspondence, relaying the death of their loved ones. In a sample of 240 pension applications from the widows of Black soldiers, only twenty-five of the widows had anything besides the official service record that documented their husband's death and burial.[53] Widows appear to have only rarely received comforting words initiated by regimental chaplains, commanding officers (company captains or regimental commanders), or USSC or Christian Commission agents; only three of the 240 applications included this kind of communication (none from commission agents). Another three commanders responded only when prompted by a widow's inquiry about the details of her husband's death. In eleven of those pension applications, the widow included informal testimony she had received from friends and comrades. They described attending or assisting in their comrade's burial. Some of these also witnessed their comrade's death, noting that they held his hand as he died, or had administered his last dose of medicine, or had been assigned to nursing duty, which included preparing his body for burial and assisting with the burial detail.

Only four of 240 applications included testimony by comrades describing a funeral service. Willis Johnston's commanding officer reported that he was buried "by a platoon of his company in as respectable a way and place as circumstances would permit. All of his near friends were with him and know the spot he was buried," he reported. Elijah Cannon's commanding officer reported he was "present at his funeral and can assure you that he was buried as a soldier and a patriot should be, with all the honors of war and with appropriate religious service." Jane Tobia Purnell received word that her son was buried in the shade of a large elm tree and that "a very large number of the boys testified their respects to the memory of your son by accompanying him to the grave." These communications were comforting but apparently all too rare for the families of African American war dead.[54]

Many of the white war dead had families who worked to bring fallen soldiers' bodies home. For Black families, this was far less likely, even among those in the North. They rarely received timely notification and they lacked the resources to pay for the significant embalming and shipping costs involved with reclaiming their dear ones.[55] Augustus Wells, of the 28th U.S.C.I., probably died in the post hospital at Brownsville, Texas, but his grieving mother, Martha Wells, sought assurance and the opportunity to bring his body home to West Virginia for reburial. Writing to the commander at Brownsville, she explained that she was unsure if the reported death actually referred to her son, having heard from comrades that he was still alive. She urged that a careful search of the records as to the deceased's color, age, height, and other characteristics (which she assumed the army kept careful and accurate records of) could yield an affirmative identification and "gratify a poor distressed mother." She would write to the hospital director if necessary. If an affirmative identification could be made, she explained,

> I will go to texas & Bring him Home: . . . and let me know if I can get him[.] please let me know the distance to Texas and what it would cost[.] now dear Sir I hope you will not consider me putting you too much trouble in making these inquiries about my son when you consider that I am a fond mother and now a distressed mother being in doubts about the death of my son[.] as I have said there may be *one* of the same name in the same Regiment who has *died* at that time[,] if so you can soon find out and let me know. the Doctor of the Hospital I suppose can give full information[.] I will be under many obligations for any further information from you and this will relieve a fond but distressed mothers mind[.] please let me know if he died with a wound or natural sickness.[56]

Although Mrs. Wells was unsuccessful in her effort to bring her son's body home, there were apparently a few, rare, exceptions. Sergeant John Bird of the 55th Massachusetts died in January 1864, and his Black Masonic brothers honored his last wish—to be sent home for burial—by paying for his body's return home to Michigan for burial with Masonic honors.[57] When Sergeant Major Robert Bridges Forten of the 43rd U.S.C.T., son of Philadelphia's wealthiest and most prominent Black couple, James and Charlotte Forten, died in Maryland, his remains were shipped home to Philadelphia. He was the first African American to receive the full honors of a military funeral in the city—although 11,000 Black soldiers passed through Camp William Penn and nearly 1,000 of them died there.[58]

Whose Death Counts?

Early in the war, the War Department recognized the importance of careful and accurate death records. The unexpected number of battlefield deaths at Antietam, and the slow and haphazard process of burials, put tremendous external and internal pressure on the army to establish clear procedures and regulations for registering and burying the dead.[59] The chaos that met the disposal of the dead at Antietam appalled the public, and the army could not hope to sustain success at enlistment if families and likely enlistees believed their mortal sacrifice would go unnamed and unacknowledged. In addition, strategic planning required the War Department to have up-to-date and accurate records of manpower and human resources.

Nonetheless, the wartime registration and regulation of death was unsystematic, and battlefield chaos was not always to blame.[60] The assignment of responsibilities—for moving bodies from the battlefield, hospital or camp to a burial site; for securing coffins, conducting rites, and preparing graves; for informing next of kin; for the registration of the dead and marking of burial sites—all relied on old, new, and piecemeal regulations and orders. The unanticipated scale of war causalities stressed all efforts to regularize this process. On September 11, 1861, General Orders No. 75 assigned to the Quartermaster Department the responsibility for ensuring an accurate "mortuary record" by issuing the necessary forms for registering those who died in hospitals and camps and providing materials for grave markers (but not burial locations). In the spring of 1862, those orders were extended to battlefield deaths, stipulating that remains of the dead be interred.[61] At the urging of the USSC, the War Department adopted new, triplicate reports to be filled out registering each soldier's death and burial, with copies retained at the hospital, the cemetery, and at the adjutant general's office at Washington, D.C. This greatly improved the War Department's record keeping.[62] The Christian Commission also kept records, and printed and distributed identification tags to soldiers, listing family contact information to avoid an anonymous death.[63] Commanding officers in charge of hospitals and posts bore the ultimate authority for the execution and retention of the requisite forms.[64] Yet the names of Black soldiers, who succumbed to wounds, or infectious disease, or workplace injuries, were far too often lost, misplaced, or forgotten. The names of the members of the 56th Massachusetts Infantry (African Descent) who succumbed to cholera and were buried on Quarantine Island (near St. Louis) were recorded, but when their remains were reinterred at nearby Jefferson National Cemetery, they were placed in a mass grave without markers or a record of their names.[65] At what became Virginia's City Point National Cemetery, 29 percent of white soldiers' burials were unknown, compared to 75 percent of Black soldiers' burials.[66]

In April 1863, general orders dictated the procedures for burial at the battlefield: marking off suitable locations for burial, interment, marking graves with wooden headboards and registering the interments, conducted by fatigue parties.[67] As historian Drew Gilpin Faust has noted, the Union Army had "no regular burial details, no graves registration units, and until

1864 no comprehensive ambulance service."[68] The scale of battlefield as well as hospital causalities required improvised responses rather than well-organized rituals and procedures.[69]

The volunteers of the Sanitary and the Christian Commission also became involved in recording deaths and assisting survivors in locating and recovering fallen soldiers. In an elaborate but highly effective "hospital directory" system, the USSC both compiled information on hospital patients and pursued family inquiries about the status of individual soldiers through their network of agents and associates in Union hospitals.[70] Through USSC agents in the North, wives and kin sought information about a soldier's death. Word might reach a family of a death, or a battlefield wound, or a hospital admittance, but without detailed information (hospital, chaplain, surgeon, cause). Others heard about specific regiments being involved in deadly actions (Petersburg, Olustee, etc.) and wrote to know if their kin had survived. Although the system was designed in 1862 prior to Black enlistment, and therefore with white soldiers and their families in mind, some agents assisted Black family members in their search for information. Both commissions also assisted families who could afford it in locating and shipping bodies home for burial, in conveying descriptions of the soldier's death, and in forwarding the effects of the dead.[71] They widely publicized these efforts, to increase white public support and successful wartime fundraising.[72] The Union army reported its battlefield success and failures in Northern newspapers and frequently noted the number of fallen enemy they took the time to inter before leaving a battlefield, as if to claim their civilized conduct in war—and affirming the social significance of a decent burial.

Unrecorded burials and a failure to provide funeral rites and a recognized burial place shaped the experience of Black soldiering. Despite military and civilian efforts to enumerate the dead, a large proportion of Black soldiers went to their death without a record made. Some reasons for a high proportion of unknown war dead affected white and Black war dead similarly. The vast majority of gravesite headboards quickly deteriorated under the weather and other environmental conditions, and this was all the more the case in some places, like the Atlanta burial grounds, where fifteen hundred headboards had paper cards attached with identifying information—cards that were entirely obliterated before the war was over.[73] In addition, some of the Black soldiers buried at Quarantine Island (across from Benton Barracks) were lost to flooding.[74]

At St. Louis, where several Black regiments were organized, mustered in, and hospitalized, the recorded number of soldier deaths tell us that their burials went unmarked and unregistered. A U.S. Sanitary Commission relief agent writing to USSC headquarters described the great mortality associated with the initial organization of the 62nd, 65th, and 67th USCT at St. Louis. By the winter of 1863/64, with a year and a half of war to go, 1310 newly enlisted soldiers in these regiments had died—more than the total number of burial sites in the St. Louis area registered for fallen Black troops at the end of the war.[75]

Surgeon Ira Russell, noted in chapter four for conducting an estimated 800 autopsies and dissections on Black soldiers and refugees from slavery, failed to register the death of more than half of the soldiers whom he autopsied, dissected, and anatomized (in a sample of ninety-one named autopsies, only 48 percent of their deaths were properly recorded in military service records).[76] Many were anonymously disposed of. Commanding officers of men stationed or hospitalized under Russell's care at Benton Barracks complained of Russell's failure to register the names of the deceased.[77]

Yet Russell, for all his concern with the discriminatory mistreatment of Black soldiers, failed to secure a proper burial for the Black men he autopsied and anatomized.[78] He kept meticulous records of their names, companies and regiments as he and his subordinate surgeons tracked the postmortem examinations they carried out; but there is no record that the human remains they handled were transferred to registered graves at city cemeteries or the neighboring Jefferson National Cemetery. Incomplete mortuary records for the adjoining national cemetery list many Black soldiers, unknown, buried in numbered graves, but certainly not the number we would expect to see at a depot through which so many Black soldiers traveled.[79] Of the nineteen white soldiers Russell autopsied, however, all but three were properly identified and buried.[80]

It is possible, in the case of the human remains generated by Russell's dissections, that many were not buried in cemeteries but rather were consigned to medical waste pits. Waste pits would have been necessarily a part of wartime hospital complexes like that at St. Louis, and they rarely appear on maps or sketches, including those of Benton Barracks.[81] They certainly were never designated in death registers as "burial" places for soldiers. But the greater likelihood that Black, rather than white, soldiers were subjected to dissection and anatomization suggests this as one of the many reasons why Black soldiers who died at Benton Barracks cannot be traced to marked burial sites.[82]

Burial Places: Soldiers

When it came to the mortality of Black soldiers, the considerable military bureaucracy that focused on an accurate record and registration of death and the location of internment, often failed. Across the national cemetery system, a disproportionate number of African American troops are among the "unknown," interred in unmarked and mass graves, despite orders from the War Department instructing both the Quartermaster Department and hospital and regimental surgeons to see to properly marked and recorded burials. Records of hospitals at Baltimore; City Point, Virginia; Camp Nelson, Kentucky; and Nashville also reveal apparent disregard for standard burial registration practices when it came to the remains of Black soldiers, anatomized or not.[83]

Where the army was much more successful, however, was in ensuring that the remains of Black soldiers who were interred (or after the war, reinterred), were buried in segregated sections of cemeteries. Early in the war, private undertakers were often engaged to remove and bury the dead, often in local, civilian cemeteries.[84] By the time African Americans were permitted to enlist, the War Department had adapted to the demands of the war and established military rules and procedures for interring the dead. Fourteen Union military cemeteries had been established by the end of 1862, and more would follow before the end of the war.[85] The national cemetery system that resulted maintained the practices of segregation that shaped every feature of military life and death during the Civil War.[86] Both the maps and plans for new cemeteries and the extant records of interments document segregation both within and between cemeteries. Arlington National Cemetery is perhaps the best known, segregated from its beginning.[87] Lebanon Cemetery outside Philadelphia was established for Black soldiers only; as of 1875, Woodlands, Glenwood, Odd Fellows, Bristol, Mechanics, Chester, Lafayette, and Mount Moriah—the other Philadelphia cemeteries—admitted only white soldiers for burial. Whitehall held one Black soldier of sixty total.[88] In Nashville, the record of Union burials in 1864 and 1865 indicated the careful segregation of burial sites.[89] At Jefferson National Cemetery, African Americans were buried in a separate section, and as was typical, adjacent to Confederate prisoners of war—widely regarded by Union veterans and their families as the least favorable location in any national cemetery.[90]

Quartermaster General Montgomery Meigs, when queried after the war about the reasons for past and continued segregation in national cemeteries like Arlington, was both duplicitous and evasive, refusing to concede that segregation was practiced for the benefit of whites, rather than African Americans.[91] According to historian Micki McElya, when the massive postwar reburial program concluded in 1871, 30,000 of 300,000 Union soldiers reinterred in national cemeteries were Black, and all buried in segregated sections.[92] Despite overwhelming evidence to the contrary, even today some representatives currently associated with the national cemeteries assert they were "never segregated."[93] Yet we know that even record keeping was segregated. The Quartermaster General's office used printed forms to keep track of deaths, interments and reinternments, and at least as late as 1875, those printed forms listed white and Black soldiers separately.[94] In their design, construction, and function, these military cemeteries — eventually national cemeteries — reinforced the segregation and exclusion of Black America from the Union's national vision.[95]

Civilian Burials and Burying Grounds

Deep in the winter of 1864, a mother and refugee from slavery approached a white captain at his office in the Quartermaster Department in Washington, D.C.[96] Her baby had died, and she asked for help in securing a decent burial. The white officer in turn sent a note to the quartermaster in charge of burials in the city. The captain noted that she "represented herself" as contraband but also noted that she was "not in our employ" — that is, not one of the hundreds then employed by the quartermaster office to labor on defense works, or wharfs, or streets, or in hospitals. He seemed ambivalent about her eligibility for assistance but referred the case to his commanding officer and included the address where the mother and child resided. In this and more than 1,600 similar requests that survive in the archives today, local quartermasters' depots took up what they probably understood to be a significant public health concern and arranged for the dead to be picked up by ambulance or hearse, provided a coffin, and interred. As tens of thousands of refugees from slavery made their way to Washington, a new wave of misery hit that already burdened population as disease, hardship, and the lingering consequences of slavery's deep violence took their lives by the thousands. The April 1862 abolition of slavery in the capitol increased the pull of the city to refugees. The accounting of their deaths was scattered and incomplete. In February 1863, one official estimated that twelve to fifteen refugees from slavery died each day; in December of that year, the estimate was twenty-five per week. By contrast, for one six-month period in 1864, fourteen white paupers died who were buried by the city.[97]

Importantly, the mothers, fathers, godparents, siblings, aunts, uncles, spouses, and friends who showed up at quartermasters' depots (or at a military hospital, at the East Capital Street Barracks, at the city's police station, or after the war at a Freedman's Bureau office) refused to allow their loved ones to be reduced to an abstract count of the dead. Their requests might have been made in desperation, or because they believed the federal government had extended its protective arm over them, or because they believed that in laboring on behalf of the Union war effort they were entitled to the most basic decencies of life and death. Through their actions, these survivors of the brutality of slavery and wartime emancipation testified to the significance of a decent final resting place for their loved ones. The bodies of the deceased mattered. They were beloved, even in death. To the extent that they could, their survivors rejected the commodification and objectification that so many of the enslaved had experienced at the hands of their owners and that the Black war dead experienced at the hands of some white Unionists.

These requests, filed as "Unknown Contraband Negroes Also Known" in the quartermaster records, tell us a number of important things. Many of the dead needing burial were not, in fact, "unknown." Hundreds of requests were the result of a spouse or family member or friend appealing to the quartermaster office for help in securing a decent burial for their loved ones. Their requests frequently included the age of the deceased, the name of the deceased and their survivors, the location from which they had come to secure safety in Washington, and the cause of death. In many instances where no name of the deceased was recorded, the age was, and this suggests that someone who knew and cared about the deceased had a hand in making the request, and the clerk simply did not bother noting their name. Disturbingly, some refugee families without resources or shelter were forced to simply leave their loved ones' remains on the street to be collected and interred by the army while other refugees were left in the streets and alleyways by white employers. Some appear to have simply died, exposed, where they walked or lay. Others died on the job from injury.[98]

In response to the requests, coffins were dispatched (some requests specified the length of the coffin required).[99] Very rarely, requests indicated the time set for funeral rituals so that the coffin could be provided in a timely manner. But often the request for removal referred to an "unknown contraband." Many of the requests were for infants and children (and children's ages were most consistently reported); some were for the elderly. Most rare were indications of where the deceased would be interred. One of those exceptions occurred with the report of the death of 104-year-old Esther Young, who succumbed to smallpox and was buried by the quartermaster at Black-owned Harmony Cemetery.[100] After the war, the quartermaster reported that his department had conducted 20,727 burials, 5,726 of them African Americans.[101]

The requests also tell us that different officers varied in their response to the requests. Some—notably, African American physicians who worked in Washington-area military hospitals, such as Anderson Ruffin Abbott, Alexander T. Augusta, William B. Powell Jr., Charles Purvis, John Rapier Jr., and Alpheus W. Tucker—offered detailed notes, including names, ages, and cause of death. Others—from Kalorama Hospital (for smallpox patients) in particular—made the briefest of requests, often omitting names and cause of death but carefully indicating the length of the coffin needed. Notably, the requests that were made at hospitals were not always about patients. Survivors appear to have approached whichever office or institution was closest to their residence when making their requests, and sometimes that was a hospital. Finally, nomenclature also varied. Many of the white officers continued describing the deceased as "contraband" in the years after the war, and one contract surgeon referred even to infants and children as "freedmen."[102]

The quartermaster office in Washington, D.C., was the heaviest employer of refugees from slavery; by 1863, they not only were organizing refugee labor, but they had also been charged with responsibility for the removal and burial of refugees who died in the city and neighboring northern Virginia—whether the deceased labored for the Union army or not.[103] City authorities provided interment for white paupers, but passed the cost and responsibility for removing and interring deceased refugees to the army, which during the course of the war brought hundreds if not thousands of Black men, women, and children from Fort Monroe, New Berne, North Carolina, and other points in the eastern theater of war, to Washington, where the labor of the able-bodied was urgently needed.[104]

These refugees, along with thousands more who made their own way to the city, became critical laborers. They worked as stevedores, teamsters, laundresses, and servants; they built and maintained the ring of defense works that protected the city; they loaded and unloaded the Commissary Department cargo carried by the many ships plying the Potomac River; they maintained the streets and avenues that permitted both commercial and military traffic; they also "policed" the city—that is, shoveled up and carted away animal carcasses, night soil, manure, and other offal that private citizens, businesses, and the army tossed out onto the street. They also became a third of the hospital workforce.[105] Yielding to the advice of Chief Quartermaster Elias Greene, the War Department agreed that the laborers should be taxed from their wages for the support of unemployed refugees. These funds, argued Greene, went toward sheltering, feeding, and clothing the refugees—but they also went toward the cost of removing and interring the formerly enslaved people who died in the city.[106]

The occurrence of death among Black refugees in the city met the illogical and contradictory impulses of racism. In all of the hospitals of the city—especially in what became Freedmen's Hospital and Alexandria's L'Ouverture Hospital (which served Black soldiers and civilians)—deceased Black patients were considered exploitable resources on which white medical workers practiced their dissection and anatomical skills. As noted in chapter 3, this was not necessarily in pursuit of identifying anatomical racial characteristics but rather because white medical practitioners did not approach the Black war dead as they did whites. No medical investigators set up shop in a hospital serving white soldiers or civilians to conduct hundreds or thousands of dissections—the white public would not have tolerated it. Race mattered in how the dead were treated. Race mattered so much that the racially demarcated responsibilities for Washington's civilian burials led to a standoff when authorities could not determine the race of the deceased. Neighbors were forced to bear the odor and threat of infection when the race of a woman's corpse, a smallpox victim, could not be firmly identified and therefore was left for several days.[107]

With the exception of the contraband camp at Mason's Island, none of the requests that made their way to the quartermaster office came from the city's contraband camps—they apparently had their own means of burying the dead because we know refugees themselves were employed as gravediggers by the army and assigned to hospitals and contraband camps.[108] The camps had their own procedures, however crude, for gathering the dead in anticipation of removal and interment. Harriet Jacobs, in a letter written for publication in the *Liberator*, described the room at Duff Green's Row reserved for the dead, a small room on the ground floor: "This room was covered with lime. Here I would learn how many deaths had occurred in the last twenty-four hours. Men, women and children lie here together, without a shadow of those rites which we give our poorest dead. There they lie, in the filthy rags they wore from the plantation. Nobody seems to give it a thought. It is an every-day occurrence, and the scenes have become familiar. One morning, as I looked in, I saw lying there five children."[109]

Jacobs's eyewitness accounts of the mistreatment and exploitation of refugees from slavery draws a through-line from the treatment of the living to the treatment of the dead. Presumably, all of the area contraband camps had similar "dead rooms," where survivors could bring their deceased family members and friends, to await collection and burial by fellow refugees employed as grave diggers. When any of those camps closed—as Camp Barker did in early 1864—the refugees from slavery faced greater obstacles in their efforts to secure the burial of kin. Relief worker Cornelia Hancock noted that Camp Barker's closure meant that refugees had "no place to go to get themselves coffins for their friends," and "sometimes they lay unburied for a week because there is no one to hunt up an order for them."[110]

EARLY IN THE WAR the bodies of refugees from slavery might have been interred at the city's potter's field, on the grounds of the Old Soldiers' Home, at one of the city's five Black-owned cemeteries (Columbian Harmony, Payne's, Mount Olivet, Mount Zion, and Mount Pleasant), or, in Alexandria, at the city's potter's field (Penny Hill), or at burial grounds associated with the military hospitals (Claremont, L'Ouverture, and Contraband Hospital). In January 1864, the depot quartermaster at Alexandria took charge of an acre and a half of abandoned land to establish a cemetery near L'Ouverture Hospital. The quartermaster there authorized the employment of gravediggers and provided for a hearse and driver; had extra coffins stored at the hospital; and established routine hours and days when burials, requested by the local superintendent of contraband, could take place.[111] Beginning in July 1864, with the creation of Arlington Cemetery, and its segregated Section 27 (which became known as Contraband Cemetery), more than 3,600 Black civilians would be buried there.[112] Only 20 percent of them were brought from hospitals; 76 percent came from contraband camps and city streets and alleyways. Four percent came from barracks, likely employees laboring for the army. Fifty-eight percent were men, and 42 percent women.[113] Freedman's Village, established on the Union-confiscated Lee-Custis estate in Arlington, had its own burial ground at Arlington.[114]

Wherever their final resting place, interment meant the deceased were laid in coffins, carried by a hearse or ambulance to a cemetery, and buried in marked graves. This stood in sharp contrast to other wartime locations where refugees from slavery gathered. As relief worker Maria Mann observed at Helena, Arkansas, deceased contraband were buried in pits with dead mules and horses.[115] John Williams, a North Carolina Black soldier at New Berne, wrote to both military and medical authorities to declaim the practice where Black smallpox victims who died "have A hole dug and put them in without a coffin." "I think this is A most horrible treatment," he wrote, and demanded better treatment.[116]

The uncounted Black war dead—men and women whose remains were exploited, scavenged by white medical practitioners, and discarded in waste pits, mass graves, or the least desirable acreage of burial grounds— became part of the material afterlife of an idea that people of African descent were immutably, biologically, and sociologically fixed in a subordinate relationship to whites. Although American anti-Black racism was firmly rooted in the effort to justify slavery's extortion of human lives and labor for the benefit of one group over the lives of another, early in the nation's life the ideology of race had become useful and fundamental to an entire nation, well beyond the borders of a slave-owning South. White Northerners may have fought and won a war against Southern slaveholders, but the modern nation to which they aspired emphatically embraced a scientific and medical empiricism that advanced white authority and depended on the continued subordination and objectification of Black bodies, the living as well as the dead.

Conclusion

After the Civil War, the measurements, medical cases, autopsy reports, and observations whites generated from their study of African American soldiers and civilians were used by white medical professionals, anthropologists, educators, statisticians, and insurance companies to support a wide range of flawed and fallacious conclusions. They were used to endorse the idea of race and also the notion of a racial hierarchy—and, most explicitly, the biologically determined inferiority of "the negro." Out of these conclusions came a profoundly injurious health legacy: the rationale for dangerous public health policies, unsound medical theories and practices, harmful medical research and experimentation, and discriminatory insurance company practices. All would have long-term consequences for the health and well-being of people of African descent well into the next century.[1]

The data collected and published by the U.S. Sanitary Commission (USSC) and the army would enjoy a long life in the scientific and medical literature published decades after the war. Notoriously self-promoting, the USSC circulated, free of cost, thousands of pamphlets and booklets among army physicians during the war, creating an eager audience for their ongoing publication concern. (As Benjamin Gould noted, those circulated works directed "public attention in some degree to the fact that the Comm. is doing scientific work as well as charitable."[2]) The commission's publications also paved the way for future military studies.[3] Its wartime investments in the search for "racial anatomical peculiarities" added legitimacy, authority, and prestige to a wide array of racist research that deeply shaped medical and scientific culture. Journals as wide ranging as the *American Journal of Dental Science*, the *Medical Examiner and General Practitioner: A Journal Devoted to Physical Diagnosis*, and *Popular Science* published this research. It reached both professional and lay audiences, elevated the authority of the authors, and in turn sustained the centrality of race in medical and scientific education, as well as to the culture of professionalization in these fields of endeavor.[4]

Whether they sought racial difference in the hyoid bones or in the varying degrees of convexity in the external condyloid surface of the tibia, in the volume of the crania or the breadth of the heel, white researchers continued their pursuit of physical manifestations of race, the necessary foundation for a racial ideology that ranked the value of people of African descent below whites. Although the project of bringing scientific authority to the "'ordinary' social fact" of racial difference had its origins well before the Civil War, the war was pivotal in accelerating the pace of that research, its legitimacy, and the investment of the state in supporting and circulating the conclusion that humans could be categorized and reduced to biologically distinct, ranked races.[5]

The question that began this book's research—why the Civil War ended slavery but failed to more substantially undermine anti-Black racism—might better be framed as a question about what happened during the war to reinforce white supremacy with the tools and legitimacy of medical and scientific research. The wartime modernization of the American race project was made both necessary and possible by the destruction of slavery (in the minds of many white Northerners, emancipation meant an unimaginable new status for Black Americans), as well as the unprecedented availability of an abundance of African American bodies. Wars and armies produce vulnerable populations, and, both before and after the Civil War, nations used armies and military conflict to pursue race science and race medicine. Regimental surgeons studied race medicine among Black soldiers in the nineteenth century West India regiments. European, African, and Asian prisoners held by Germans during World War I were exploited for anthropometric study.[6] The U.S. Army conducted race studies on Japanese American, African American, white, and Puerto Rican soldiers as test subjects for mustard gas experiments in World War II.[7]

As important and powerful as these long-term consequences were in sustaining the respectability and authority of medical and science-based arguments about the meaning of race and the inferiority of African Americans and other people of color, we should not overlook the immediate impact of this work on the experience and meaning of the war itself. The Union war effort—among both armies and civilians—was not only about waging a war to defeat the Confederacy and the destruction of slavery. The Union war effort was also turned into a race-making project, ultimately assuring Northern whites that the nation's racial hierarchies and, specifically, the subordination of African Americans, would continue in the aftermath of the war.

As military officers and surgeons commanding or attending to Black troops, white men were conferred a new source of authority and identity: as astute observers of "race," their government solicited their views to assess the manifestation of racial inferiority in the bodies of Black soldiers, whom they were empowered to observe, measure, prod, and objectify as something "other." Whatever their motivations for joining the army and serving in the war, their government invited whites to participate in a process of race-making, and many entered into the endeavor with confidence, revealing in the process the many popular sources of their race knowledge. For many, it was not prior contact with people of African descent, but commonplace white assumptions masquerading as "well known facts" and widely circulated historical or biblical sources. "Universal opinion," too, stood in for empirical grounding.

The officers who assigned Black soldiers the dangerous and difficult fatigue labor of building defense works and fortifications under constant enemy shelling expressed a confident assessment of a wide range of racial characteristics that confirmed the suitability of these particular and inferior soldiers not for fighting but for hard labor. The military surgeons assigned to Black regiments or to hospitals serving Black soldiers and civilians viewed the injured, diseased, and deceased that they encountered as useful objects upon which they could freely practice their surgical, medical, and anatomical skills. Particularly in locations where surgeons and other hospital workers had unprecedented access to Black cadavers, the opportunity to dissect and anatomize without regard to popular opprobrium was priceless. And, for a few whites, the Black ill, injured, and dead they encountered in their practice became the raw material for building their professional authority on the distinct features of the Black body. These commitments to racial ways of thinking—their own unearned privilege and the objectification of others as inferior—are shown here as widespread and substantial, regardless of their attitudes toward slavery.

The civilian men and women of the USSC also played an important role in the war's racial project. As advocates of medical and social modernization through the work of the commission, the white women and men of the USSC envisioned the modern nation's midwives as white. They rejected nearly all the Black organizations formed to assist with soldiers' relief, and they stumbled over the commission's obligations to assist the nation's most needy population during the war—the refugees from slavery. White women who found themselves capable leaders and effective managers were unwilling to risk learning that Black women, too, shared those skills, and many were unwilling to share public recognition with the Black women who also organized and led patriotic relief efforts. They were unwilling and unable to embrace an integrated democracy.

Furthermore, the men of the commission understood that relief was after all "women's work" — not the kind of work or accomplishment that would establish commission men as "men of mark." That achievement would lay in medical and scientific advancements that modernized the organization and delivery of wartime medical care, and in exploiting their access to Black soldiers to conduct the nation's first large-scale, government-authorized racial research. Even the white soldiers who were measured, their lung capacity tested, their lifting power assessed, likely understood this as a competition they were ordained to win.

For Black Americans, their encounters with the race project of white Unionists magnified the devastating impact of military conflict and the tenuous and fitful wartime destruction of slavery. Called to military service by their own dedication to freedom and by the expanded rights that many imagined would follow, many Black soldiers faced military command and medical treatment that made the war far more dangerous for them than their white comrades in arms. The experience of joining an army that they believed was committed to Black emancipation, only to encounter officers and a bureaucracy that viewed them as objects of study, animal-like, and beasts of burden, must also have shaken their hopes for survival, let alone expanded citizenship after the war. As Margaret Humphreys noted in her study of Black soldiers, the policies and actions of white officers and health care workers showed them to be "poor stewards of the men in their care. Their decisions, great and small, careless and deliberate, doomed these soldiers to early graves."[8]

For Black civilians, especially refugees from slavery, the human cost of the war remains uncounted. No historian has yet been able to estimate with any reliability the mortality among Black civilians in the South. Certainly recent works on life in refugee camps, by Chandra Manning and Amy Murrell Taylor, have documented the inadequacies of army-supervised refugee camps. Jim Downs, in his study of illness and suffering among freed people in the postwar South, has shown the continued loss of life that followed the failures of the Freedmen's Bureau Medical Division and federal policy in providing for the health care needs of Southern Blacks after the war.[9] But Civil War historians have long focused on death rates to easily convey the significance of the war; as long as the civilian dead remain uncounted, so too their experience of the war remains outside the more easily recited "facts" of the war.

As historian Rana Hogarth has noted in her study of medical ideas about Blackness in the Atlantic world, the pursuit of medical theories of race and the practice of race-based medicine has a long and storied past.[10] *Medicine, Science, and Making Race in Civil War America* helps historicize race-making. It demonstrates how this race project accelerated during wartime emancipation—at the moment when race-based slavery was undermined by the actions of enslaved people, Union military victories, and federal policy. Northern white commitments to the constitution and to the abolition of slavery were accompanied by their commitments to racial ideologies that sustained white supremacy, which attempted to root the subordination of Black Americans in nature rather than the institution of slavery. The result was and continues to be catastrophic for people of African descent, weaving a dedication to racial essentialism into the practice and professionalization of medicine in the United States.

It is a matter of grave concern that medical racism and the ideology of biological race continue to deprive Black Americans of health and life in the twenty-first century. As historians Deirdre Cooper Owens and Sharla Fett have recently highlighted in the *American Journal of Public Health*, institutional racism and racial bias in health care provision are distressingly evident in the three to four times higher pregnancy-related mortality rate Black women experience compared with whites in the United States.[11] As they note in reference to the practice of medicine, "Black people have a right to be suspicious of an institution that has historically victimized their ancestors for centuries."[12] This centuries-old practice of dismissing Black ill health, devaluing Black life, and regarding Black patients through a lens uninformed by a critical consideration of the long legacy of medical racism has life-and-death consequences. Medical science and medical care continue to replicate ideas and practices that not only fail to heal but also perpetuate the lethal consequences of American investments in anti-Black racism.

Medical historian Lundy Braun has conclusively illuminated the persisting impact of medical and scientific racism in the "race correction" that continues to be used with spirometers, a practice that draws uncritically on centuries of assertions that lung function varies by race. More pointedly, people of African descent are considered to have biologically determined pulmonary dysfunction. As Braun notes, the spirometer, a tool that is essential to the diagnosis of respiratory disease and to the assessment of eligibility for compensation for workplace hazards, regularly dismisses lower lung function of Black Americans as a product of biological race rather than as evidence of disease or impairment. "Race correction" infiltrates a wide range of medical algorithms and has a daily effect on the diagnosis and treatment of African Americans.[13] Similarly, scholar Dorothy E. Roberts has pointedly argued that the routine use of "race-based adjustments" in diagnostic algorithms "shows a failure to understand the meaning of race and its connection to racism."[14]

My intention in *Medicine, Science, and Making Race in Civil War America* is to encourage readers to grapple with the historical, in order to be better equipped to challenge and change one of the many ways in which racism, so substantially a part of Civil War medicine and science, shapes our present.

Acknowledgments

I owe a deep debt of gratitude to the generous and inspiring support of friends, scholars, archive and library professionals, and funding agencies for the many ways in which they encouraged and assisted my work on this project. Historians are lost without archives and knowledgeable archivists, and I have benefitted from the knowledge and expertise of exceptional professionals. Archivists and reference librarians at the National Archives and Records Administration, the National Museum of Health and Medicine, and the Manuscript and Archives Division of the New York Public Library all played a crucial role in my research. DeeAnn Blanton, retired senior archivist for military records at the National Archives, kindly and expertly guided me through collections as I looked for answers about wartime burial practices. Laura Cutter, chief archivist at the National Museum of Health and Medicine, generously helped me navigate the archives of what was once the Army Medical Museum. I am especially indebted to Susan Waide, reference archivist at the Manuscripts and Archives Division of the New York Public Library Manuscript Division, for her tremendously important work reorganizing the papers of the U.S. Sanitary Commission and also for guiding me through those voluminous collections. Her generosity in sharing her knowledge was crucial to my efforts to navigate this still under-explored resource.

Funding for this project came from several sources. I wish to acknowledge the support of the National Endowment for the Humanities; the New York Public Library Short-Term Research Fellowship Program; the University of Iowa's Arts and Humanities Initiative; the University of Iowa College of Liberal Arts and Sciences DSHB Faculty Scholar award; the University of Iowa's Office of the Provost; and the University of Iowa's Obermann Center for Advanced Study, the latter providing the necessary respite and lovely office where I finally began writing chapters.

I am indebted to several scholars who organized conferences, gave feedback on papers and presentations, provided insightful comments on article drafts and the book manuscript, and helped me make this book better than it would have been without them. Susan Lynn Smith, professor emeritus at the University of Alberta, invited me to participate in a conference on "Health Legacies: Militarization, Health, and Society" in 2009, and in preparing that presentation I began my work on this project. I am deeply indebted to her for helping me think about my work in the context of the history of medicine. Kathleen Diffley, professor emerita at the University of Iowa invited me to present my work at the 2013 Midwestern Modern Language Association Civil War history group, where fellow panelists and commenters gave me much to think about. I am also grateful to have been invited to participate in the 2015 University of Maryland conference honoring the work of Ira Berlin, "Slavery, Freedom, and the Remaking of American History," where a number of people offered helpful guidance and suggestions. Christopher Willoughby and Sean Smith organized an important conference on "Medicine and Healing in the Age of Slavery" at Rice University in 2018, which provided rich and fertile ground for the ideas I was struggling with. The anonymous readers for the chapter I subsequently submitted to the volume they co-edited were also very helpful.

Judith Giesberg and three anonymous readers at the *Journal of the Civil War Era* offered enormously insightful critiques that helped me sharpen that article and the larger project as well.

At the University of Iowa, the graduate students and faculty of the History Department responded with probing questions and generous support as I struggled to make sense of the project. Also at Iowa, the History of Medicine Society invited me to present a part of this project, and the questions and feedback from that audience provided important guidance in my work finishing the manuscript. The historians Noralee Frankel and Jane Schultz offered critical feedback and support that were deeply helpful. Of course, even with the blessing of all this careful thought and comment from other historians, I take all responsibility for any errors that managed to slip through.

I wish also to acknowledge a long-term debt to the scholars and activists who pushed and pulled me into history, women's history, and African American history. As an undergraduate working in women's studies, I was fortunate to work with Margo Culley, Elizabeth Petroff, and Joyce Berkman at the University of Massachusetts at Amherst, all brilliant feminist scholars who drew me into the magical world of archives and research on the history of women and gender. A conversation among women's studies students and teachers at the University of Massachusetts with Barbara Smith (of the Combahee River Collective) and Gloria Joseph (professor emerita at Hampshire College) compelled me to think carefully about the importance and necessity of studying African American women, and Gloria Joseph gifted me with the critical opportunity to read, learn, and organize my thinking about Black women's history.

By some lucky star, I made my way to the first class of PhD students in the Women's History Program at the University of Wisconsin, where I developed lasting friendships and deep intellectual ties with an amazing group of fellow graduate students who went on to become prominent feminist activists, historians, and archivists, and I consider myself lucky indeed to have learned with them and survived graduate school because of them. My teachers at Wisconsin, Linda Gordon, Gerda Lerner, Judy Leavitt, Jeanne Boydston, Vanessa Northington Gamble, Nellie McKay, and Tom Shick, shaped me into the historian I became. I learned so much from all of them, all excellent scholars and teachers in their own way. They trained me and supported me as I struggled to succeed as a historian. Steve Engle also supported my graduate work by providing me with a decade's worth of training and employment as a house painter, for which I am eternally grateful.

My colleagues in Gender, Women's and Sexuality Studies at the University of Iowa kept my head on straight and proved through their activism and their feminist commitments in the university, in the classroom, in their scholarship, and through the best department meetings ever, that the academy can be a place of compassion, justice, and devilish humor. This wonderful group included Rachel Williams, Teresa Mangum, Laura Kastens, Naomi Greyser, Lina Murillo, Brady G'Sell, Marie Kruger, Janette Taylor, Pat Dolan, Corey Creekmur, Christopher Rasheem McMillan, Meena

Khandelwal, Meenakshi Gigi Durham, Aniruddha Dutta, Natalie Fixmer-Oraiz, David Gooblar, E. Cram, Kristy Nabhan-Warren, Hyaeweol Choi, Lisa Heineman, Linda Kroon, Maurine Neiman, Anna Bostwick Flaming, Mary Ann Rasmussen, Ellen Lewin, Miriam Thaggert, and Susan Birrell.

The solace, nourishment, and laughter provided by friends and family sustained me through the years it took me to complete this book. The Schwalms—Ray and Doris, Bruce, Kim, Olivia, Victor, and Pearl, of course—asked when the book would be done, hosted and distracted me on many a research trip, and helped me keep perspective. Meredith Alexander and Kim Marra fed me, sustained my spirit, walked and hiked with me, and said all the right things to keep me at it when writing a book seemed like a fruitless ordeal. Kathy Janz and Nancy Reincke frequently reminded me that friends, the woods, the pond, and, of course, the animals we share our lives with are the icing on the cake in our daily lives. Booker, Beecher, Otis, Tolliver, Lucy, Mitchell, and Grayson, thanks for all your assistance. Most of all, I want to thank Doris Stormoen, "Dr. D.," my spouse and life partner, for your engagement in this project, as well as for the laughter, the dances, the songs, the projects, the food, the travels, and your enduring love.

Notes

Preface

1. The reference here to "libidinous investments" draws from Saidiya Hartman, "Venus in Two Acts," *Small Axe* 26, no. 2 (June 2008): 1–14: "The libidinal investment in violence is everywhere apparent in the documents, statements and institutions that decide our knowledge of the past" (5).

2. Christina Sharpe, *In the Wake: On Blackness and Being* (Durham, NC: Duke University Press, 2016), 43.

3. Quoting here from Marisa J. Fuentes, "A Violent and Violating Archive: Black Life and the Slave Trade," *Black Perspectives*, March 7, 2017, https://www.aaihs.org/a-violent-and-violating-archive-black-life-and-the-slave-trade/, part of an online roundtable devoted to Sowande Mustakeem's *Slavery at Sea*.

4. This is now a rich body of scholarship; see, for example, Daina Ramey Berry, *The Price for Their Pound of Flesh: The Value of the Enslaved, from Womb to Grace, in the Building of a Nation* (Boston: Beacon Press); Marisa J. Fuentes, *Dispossessed Lives: Enslaved Women, Violence, and the Archive* (Philadelphia: University of Pennsylvania Press, 2016); Brian Connolly and Marisa J. Fuentes, "Introduction: From Archives to Liberated Future of Slavery to Liberated Futures," *History of the Present* 6, no. 2 (2016): 105–116, an introduction to a special issue of that journal with many important essays devoted to the archives of slavery; Britt Rusert, "New World: The Impact of Digitization on the Study of Slavery," *American Literary History* 29, no. 2 (2017): 267–286; Sasha Turner, "The Nameless and the Forgotten: Maternal Grief, Sacred Protection, and the Archive of Slavery," *Slavery and Abolition* 38, no. 2 (2017): 232–250; and Laura Helton et al., "The Question of Recovery: Slavery, Freedom, and the Archive," *Social Text* 33, no. 4 (2015): 1–18.

5. Robert Penn Warren, *The Legacy of the Civil War* (1961; repr., Lincoln, NE: Bison Books, 1998).

6. Ruth Wilson Gilmore, "Fatal Couplings of Power and Difference: Notes on Racism and Geography," *Professional Geographer* 54, no. 1 (2002): 15–24, p. 16; Harriet A. Washington, *Medical Apartheid: The Dark History of Medical Experimentation on Black Americans from Colonial Times to the Present* (New York: Harlem Moon Broadway Books, 2006); Dorothy E. Roberts, *Fatal Invention: How Science, Politics, and Big Business Re-create Race in the Twenty-First Century* (New York: New Press, 2011).

Introduction

1. In his article, "'His Native, Hot Country': Racial Science and Environment in Antebellum American Medical Thought," Christopher D. Willoughby notes on the basis

of examining over 4,000 medical school examinations that racial medicine was a common theme in medical education, North and South. *Journal of the History of Medicine and Allied Sciences* 3 (2017): 328–351.

2. Sadiah Qureshi, *Peoples on Parade: Exhibitions, Empire, and Anthropology in Nineteenth-Century Britain* (Chicago: University of Chicago Press, 2011) brilliantly traces this development in Great Britain.

3. There is a rich literature on the rise of scientific racism and medicine. In addition to the previously cited Willoughby, see Owen Whooley, *Knowledge in the Time of Cholera: The Struggle over American Medicine in the Nineteenth Century* (Chicago: University of Chicago Press, 2012); Melissa N. Stein, *Measuring Manhood: Race the Science of Masculinity, 1830-1934* (Minneapolis: University of Minnesota Press, 2015); and Deirdre Cooper Owens, *Medical Bondage: Race, Gender, and the Origins of American Gynecology* (Athens: University of Georgia Press, 2017). On the popular appetite for scientific knowledge and literature, see Katherine Pandora, "Popular Science in National and Transnational Perspective: Suggestions from the American Context," *Isis* 100, no. 2 (2009): 346–358, especially 353–356, and Conevery Bolton Valencius et al., "Science in Early America: Print Culture and the Sciences of Territoriality," *Journal of the Early Republic* 36 (2016): 73–123, especially 83–84. On professional authority and popular science, see, among others, Hyman Kuritz, "The Popularization of Science in Nineteenth-Century America," *History of Education Quarterly* 21, no. 3 (1981): 259–274, especially 266–268.

4. Although never simply a matter of physiology, post-Enlightenment ideas about race were consistently obsessed with race as a "body-centered phenomenon," as noted by Geraldine Heng, *The Invention of Race in the European Middle Ages* (New York: Cambridge University Press, 2018), 26. Heng further offers a very useful working definition of race: "Race is one of the primary names we have—a name we retain for the strategic, epistemological, and political commitments it recognizes—attached to a repeating tendency, of the gravest import, to demarcate human beings through differences among humans that are selectively essentialized as absolute and fundamental, in order to distribute positions and powers differentially in human groups. . . . Race is a structural relationship for the articulation and management of human difference, rather than a substantive content" (27).

5. For parallel overlaps in disciplines that were not yet fully differentiated, see Andrew D. Evans, *Anthropology at War: World War I and the Science of Race in Germany* (Chicago: University of Chicago Press, 2010), chapter 1, and the introduction to Tim Lockley, *Military Medicine and the Making of Race: Life and Death in the West India Regiments, 1795-1874* (New York: Cambridge University Press, 2020).

6. Margaret Humphreys, *Intensely Human: The Health of the Black Soldier in the American Civil War* (Baltimore: Johns Hopkins University Press, 2008); Chandra Manning, *Troubled Refuge: Struggling for Freedom in the Civil War* (New York: Knopf, 2016); Amy Murrell Taylor, *Embattled Freedom: Journeys through the Civil War's Refugee Camps* (Chapel Hill: University of North Carolina Press, 2018); Jim Downs, *Sick from Freedom: African-American Illness and Suffering during the Civil War and Reconstruction* (New York: Oxford University Press, 2012).

7. Shauna Devine's authoritative history, *Learning from the Wounded: The Civil War and the Rise of American Medical Science* (Chapel Hill: University of North Carolina

Press, 2014), challenges the long-standing myth of wartime surgical butchery and argues instead that the war "prompted major developments in the life and work of northern physicians who doctored in the war and in the process transformed American medicine and research" (11). Humphreys, in *Marrow of Tragedy: The Health Crisis of the American Civil War* (Baltimore: Johns Hopkins University Press, 2013), emphasizes "the vast differences brought by the war" to the organization of health care delivery and to medical knowledge and research (7).

8. Gretchen Long, *Doctoring Freedom: The Politics of African American Medical Care in Slavery and Emancipation* (Chapel Hill: University of North Carolina Press, 2012); Humphreys, *Intensely Human*; Manning, *Troubled Refuge*; Taylor, *Embattled Freedom*; and Downs, *Sick from Freedom*. See also Gaines M. Foster, "The Limitations of Federal Health Care for Freedmen, 1862–1868," *Journal of Southern History* 48 (August 1982): 349–372; Randy Finley, "In War's Wake: Health Care and Arkansas Freedmen, 1863–1868," *Arkansas Historical Quarterly* 51 (Summer 1992): 135–163; and, on the long-term postwar impact of segregation and racism on health care of African Americans, see Washington, *Medical Apartheid*.

9. On anthropometry, phrenology, spirometry, and other aspects of nineteenth-century scientific racism as well as their lasting impact on ideas about race, see John S. Haller Jr., *Outcasts from Evolution: Scientific Attitudes of Racial Inferiority, 1859–1900* (Urbana-Champaign: University of Illinois Press, 1971); Lundy Braun, *Breathing Race into Science: The Surprising Career of the Spirometer from Plantation to Genetics* (Minneapolis: University of Minnesota Press, 2014); Ann Fabian, *The Skull Collectors: Race, Science, and America's Unburied Dead* (Chicago: University of Chicago Press, 2010); Samuel J. Redman, *Bone Rooms: From Scientific Racism to Human Prehistory in Museums* (Cambridge, MA: Harvard University Press, 2016); Paul H. D. Lawrie, "'Mortality as the Life Story of a People': Frederick L. Hoffman and Actuarial Narratives of African American Extinction, 1896–1915," *Canadian Review of American Studies* 43 (Winter 2013): 352–387; Bruce Dain, *A Hideous Monster of the Mind: American Race Theory in the Early Republic* (Cambridge, MA: Harvard University Press, 2002); Todd Savitt, *Medicine and Slavery: The Diseases and Health Care of Blacks in Antebellum Virginia* (Urbana-Champaign: University of Illinois Press, 1978), especially chapter 9; Washington, *Medical Apartheid*, especially chapters 4 and 5; and Stein, *Measuring Manhood*, chapter 1.

10. Daina Ramey Berry, *The Price for Their Pound of Flesh: The Value of the Enslaved, from Womb to Grave, in the Building of a Nation* (Boston: Beacon Press, 2017), chapter 6.

11. Sarah K. A. Pfatteicher, "Rebecca Lee Crumpler," in *African American Lives*, ed. Henry Louis Gates Jr. and Evelyn Brooks Higginbotham, 199–200 (New York: Oxford University Press, 2004).

12. Britt Rusert, *Fugitive Science: Empiricism and Freedom in Early African American Culture* (New York: New York University Press, 2017), chapter 5.

13. Robert J. C. Young, *Colonial Desire: Hybridity in Theory, Culture, and Race* (London: Routledge, 1995), 126–127; and James Hunt, "Introductory Address on the Study of Anthropology," *Anthropological Review* 1 (May 1863): 1–20.

14. Rusert, *Fugitive Science*, 200–201; Long, *Doctoring Freedom*, 32–33; Stein, *Measuring Manhood*, 60–62; Charles Richard Weld, "History of the Royal Society; with the

Memoirs of the Presidents," *British Quarterly Review* 39 (January–April 1864): 105–110, *Anti-Slavery Standard*, September 26, 1863; Mia Bay, *The White Image in the Black Mind: African-American Ideas about White People, 1830–1925* (Oxford: Oxford University Press, 2000), 58–63; Vanessa Northington Gamble, *Making a Place for Ourselves: The Black Hospital Movement, 1920–1945* (New York: Oxford University Press, 1995).

15. I am grateful to my colleague, the wonderful social and labor historian Shel Stromquist (professor emeritus, University of Iowa), for pushing me to think about this. Although I address this point as it becomes pertinent in the chapters that follow, this book points to the profound weight of medical and scientific racism against Black Americans at the time of the Civil War. For critical discussions of whiteness, see Barbara Fields, "Whiteness, Racism, and Identity," *International Labor and Working-Class History* 60 (Fall 2001): 48–56, p. 50; Sharrona Pearl, "White, with a Class-Based Blight: Drawing Irish Americans," *Eire-Ireland* 44, nos. 3 and 4 (2009): 171–199, pp. 182, 195; James R. Barrett and David Roediger, "Inbetween Peoples: Race, Nationality and the 'New Immigrant' Working Class," *Journal of American Ethnic History* 16, no. 3 (1997): 3–44. The latter essay offers persuasive arguments historicizing the increasingly debated concept of a "white" race in structuring workplaces and in naturalization law in post–Civil War America.

16. S. B. Buckley to B. A. Gould, October 12, 1865, Folder 11, Box 1, Part I: Administrative Records, Statistical Bureau Archives, MssCol 18780, United States Sanitary Commission Records (New York Public Library Manuscripts and Archives Division, New York).

17. In his summary of the mean dimensions of the body, Benjamin A. Gould asserts that while his work "discloses many curious and interesting facts, full of significance to the physiologist and ethnologist. . . . it seems more proper to leave the discussion to experts, trusting that the results may have been so elaborated and presented, as to be available to them in a convenient form" (317); *Investigations in the Military and Anthropological Statistics of American Soldiers* (Cambridge, MA: Riverside Press, 1869).

18. I am prompted to clarify this by the excellent work of Stein (*Measuring Manhood*) in linking the history of masculinity with the history of nineteenth-century race science.

19. I. A. Newby, *Jim Crow's Defense: Anti-Negro Thought in America, 1900–1930* (Baton Rouge: Louisiana State University Press, 1965), offers an exhaustive account of the popular and professional scientific literature of racism.

20. Haller, *Outcasts from Evolution*, 19–20. Lundy Braun traces the use of spirometry in race science after Gould's use of the technique in "Spirometry, Measurement, and Race in the Nineteenth Century," *Journal of the History of Medicine and Allied Sciences* 2 (April 2005): 135–169. See also Michael Yudell, *Race Unmasked: Biology and Race in the Twentieth Century* (Ithaca, NY: Cornell University Press, 2014), introduction and chapter 1.

21. Haller, *Outcasts from Evolution*, 86–87.

22. Haller, *Outcasts from Evolution*, 204; Joseph Alexander Tillinghast, "The Negro in Africa and America," *Publications of the American Economic Association* 3 (May 1902): 403–637. W. E. B. Du Bois wrote a review of the book-length article in *Political Science Quarterly* 18 (December 1903): 695–697. Cope was a member of the "American School"

of biology; his reliance on the Sanitary Commission work and his contributions to racial science are described in Haller, *Outcasts from Evolution*. Cope's biographer, Jane P. Davidson, noted that Cope's theories, in turn, were widely quoted "as scientific proof of the superiority of whites" (178); *The Bone Sharp: The Life of Edward Drinker Cope* (Philadelphia: Academy of Natural Sciences of Philadelphia, 1997).

23. Rudolph Matas, *The Surgical Peculiarities of the American Negro: A Statistical Inquiry Based upon the Records of the Charity Hospital of New Orleans, La., Decennium 1884-'94* (Philadelphia: [no identified publisher], 1896), 20.

24. Frederick L. Hoffman, *Race Traits and Tendencies of the American Negro* (New York: Macmillan Co., 1896).

25. William Z. Ripley, *The Races of Europe: A Sociological Study* (New York: D. Appleton, 1899), 85, 88, 95, 100, 107, 111, 139, 407.

26. The Sanitary Commission donated its measuring equipment to American colleges and universities to promote continued research in biometrics. Roberta J. Park traces the extensive postwar history of anthropometry among physical educators in "'Taking Their Measure in Play, Games, and Physical Training': The American Scene, 1870s to World War I," *Journal of Sports History* 33 (2006): 193–217; see especially pp. 195–201, focusing on the measure and creation of the ideal white body. Also see, for example, Jay W. Seaver, *Anthropometry and Physical Examination: A Book for Practical Use in Connection with Gymnastic Work and Physical Education* (New Haven, CT: Press of the O. A. Gorman Co., 1896); and Charles B. Davenport and Albert G. Love, *The Medical Department of the United States Army in the World War*, vol. 15 of *Statistics, Part One: Army Anthropology* (Washington, DC: U.S. Government Printing Office, 1921), 52–53.

27. Aleš Hrdlička, "Anthropology of the American Negro: Historical Notes," *American Journal of Physical Anthropology* 5 (April–June 1927): 205–221. Hrdlička was the first curator of physical anthropology at the Smithsonian Institution, founder of the *Journal of Physical Anthropology* and an early advocate for formation of the American Association of Physical Anthropologists. Adolphe H. Schultz, "Biographical Memoir of Aleš Hrdlička," *National Academy of Sciences of the United States of America Biographical Memoirs* 23 (1944): 305–338.

28. See Frank Spencer, "Anthropometry," in *History of Physical Anthropology: An Encyclopedia*, ed. Frank Spencer, 80–90 (New York: Garland, 1997), which firmly places Gould's work in a long-lasting and significant history of racial classification and study.

29. Paul A. Lombardo, "Anthropometry, Race, and Eugenic Research," in *The Uses of Humans in Experiment*, ed. Erika Dyck and Larry Stewart," 215–239 (Boston: Brill Rodopi, 2016).

30. Hoffman, *Race Traits*; and Kelly Miller, "A Review of Hoffman's *Race Traits and Tendencies of the American Negro*," in *American Negro Academy, Occasional Papers* (Washington, DC: The Academy, 1897), 20–22.

31. W. E. Burghardt Du Bois, ed., *The Health and Physique of the Negro American. Report of a Social Study Made under the Direction of Atlanta University; Together with the Proceedings of the Eleventh Conference for the Study of the Negro Problems, Held at Atlanta University, on May the 29th, 1906* (Atlanta, GA: Atlanta University Press, 1906). See Maria Farland, "W.E.B. DuBois, Anthropometric Science, and the Limits of Racial Uplift," *American Quarterly* 4 (December 2006): 1017–1044, especially 1021–1023. Du

Bois, of course, made a number of contributions to dismantling the notions of biological determinism and the supposed health inferiority of Black people, including *The Philadelphia Negro*. Kellee White offers an important overview of Du Bois's critique of race science and race medicine in "The Sustaining Relevance of W. E. B. Du Bois to Health Disparities Research," *DuBois Review* 8 (2011): 285–293.

32. Virginia Jeans Laas, ed., *Wartime Washington: The Civil War Letters of Elizabeth Blair Lee*. (Urbana: University of Illinois Press, 1999), 223.

33. Chandra Manning, *What This Cruel War Was Over: Soldiers, Slavery, and the Civil War* (New York: Vintage Civil War Library, 2008); Andrew J. DeRoche, "Freedom without Equality: Maine Civil War Soldiers' Attitudes about Slavery and African Americans," *UCLA Historical Journal* 16 (1996): 24–38.

34. See John Harley Warner, "The Fall and Rise of Professional Mystery: Epistemology, Authority, and the Emergence of Laboratory Medicine in Nineteenth-Century America," in *The Laboratory Revolution in Medicine*, ed. Andrew Cunningham and Perry Williams, 110–141 (Cambridge: Cambridge University Press, 1992); Whooley, *Knowledge in the Time of Cholera*.

35. The best history of social investigations in the nineteenth century is Oz Frankel's *States of Inquiry: Social Investigations and Print Culture in Nineteenth-Century Britain and the United States* (Baltimore: Johns Hopkins University Press, 2006). Much of that reportage consisted of large uninterpreted collections of data. See James H. Cassedy's *American Medicine and Statistical Thinking, 1800-1860* (Cambridge, MA: Harvard University Press, 1984), 230; and "Numbering the North's Medical Events: Humanitarianism and Science in Civil War Statistics," *Bulletin of the History of Medicine* 66 (1992): 210-233. Also Ian Hacking, "Biopower and the Avalanche of Printed Numbers," *Humanities in Society* 5 (1992): 279–295.

36. Berry, *Price for Their Pound of Flesh*, 148–193; see also Michael Sappol, *A Traffic in Dead Bodies: Anatomy and Embodied Social Identity in Nineteenth-Century America* (Princeton, NJ: Princeton University Press, 2002).

37. American Social History Project/Center for Media and Learning, "The What Is It? Exhibit," *The Lost Museum Archive*, City University of New York, 2015, https://lostmuseum.cuny.edu/archive/exhibit/what/. Barnum was a slave trader as well.

38. Carolyn Sorisio, *Fleshing Out America: Race, Gender, and the Politics of the Body in American Literature, 1833–1879* (Athens: University of Georgia Press, 2002); Jane Desmond, *Staging Tourism: Bodies on Display from Waikiki to Sea World* (Chicago: University of Chicago Press, 1999); Sharon Macdonald, ed., *The Politics of Display: Museums, Science, Culture* (New York: Routledge, 2010); Pamela Scully and Clifton Crais, "Race and Erasure: Sara Baartman and Hendrik Cesars in Cape Town and London," *Journal of British Studies* 47 (2008): 301–323; and Daphne A. Brookes, *Bodies in Dissent: Spectacular Performances of Race and Freedom, 1850-1910* (Durham, NC: Duke University Press, 2006).

Chapter One

1. Portions of this chapter first appeared in Leslie A. Schwalm, "'A Body of 'Truly Scientific Work': The U.S. Sanitary Commission and the Elaboration of Race in the Civil War Era," *Journal of the Civil War Era* 8 (2018): 647–676.

2. Ira Berlin, Joseph P. Reidy, and Leslie Rowland, eds., *The Black Military Experience*, series 2, book 1, of *Freedom: A Documentary History of Emancipation, 1861-1867, Selected from the Holdings of the National Archives of the United States* (New York: Cambridge University Press, 1982).

3. John David Smith, "Let Us All Be Grateful That We Have Colored Troops That Will Fight," in *Black Soldiers in Blue: African American Troops in the Civil War Era*, ed. John David Smith, 1–77 (Chapel Hill: University of North Carolina Press, 2002), 8–9.

4. See Brian M. Taylor, "'To Make the Union What It Ought to Be': African Americans, Civil War Military Service, and Citizenship" (PhD diss., Georgetown University, 2015), for an excellent study of Black political thought and community mobilization around military service during the war.

5. These practices extended to record keeping; the records of the 65th U.S.C.I. in RG 94 are filed under "65th Nigger Infantry," Box 42, Regimental Papers, U.S. Colored Troops, 61st-65th Colored Infantry, Record Group 94: Records of the Adjutant General's Office, 1780-1917, National Archives and Records Administration (NARA), Washington, DC.

6. Smith, "Let Us All Be Grateful," 40. See also Kelly D. Selby, "The 27th United States Colored Troops: Ohio Soldiers and Veterans" (PhD diss., Kent State University, 2008).

7. Benjamin Woodward, "Observations on Injuries, and Repair, etc.," Folder 4.7 Box 111, Section E: Medical Committee Archives, Part IV: Historical Bureau Records, New York, NY, Archives, MssCol 22263, New York Public Library Manuscripts and Archives Division, United States Sanitary Commission (USSC) Records.

8. The survey was circulated by J. H. Baxter, the Chief Medical Officer of the Provost Marshal-General's Bureau, and appeared in 1875 as part of a major postwar U.S. government publication: *Statistics, Medical and Anthropological, of the Provost-Marshal General's Bureau, Derived from Records of the Examination for Military Service in the Armies of the United States during the Late War of the Rebellion, of over a Million Recruits, Drafted Men, Substitutes, and Enrolled Men: Compiled under Direction of the Secretary of War* (Washington, DC: Government Printing Office, 1875).

9. The persistence of racist military medicine during peacetime as well as World War I is cogently discussed in Jennifer Keane, "A Comparative Study of White and Black American Soldiers during the First World War," *Annales de démographie historique* 103 (2002): 71–90.

10. Henry Boltwood to Dr. Blake, August 20, 1864, Box 2, Vol. 1, Part 1: Main Office, Department of the Gulf Archives, MssCol 18590, New York Public Library Manuscripts and Archives Division, USSC Records.

11. Observer Julia Wilbur quoted here by Chandra Manning, *Troubled Refuge: Struggling for Freedom in the Civil War* (New York: Knopf, 2016), 47; see also Richard Sears, *Camp Nelson, Kentucky: A Civil War History* (Lexington: University Press of Kentucky, 2002), 67.

12. Carlina de la Cova, "Army Health Care for Sable Soldiers during the American Civil War," in *Bioarchaeology of Women and Children in Times of War*, ed. Debra L. Martin and Caryn Tegmeyer, 129–148 (Basel, Switzerland: Springer International, 2017); *Daily National Republican* (Washington, DC), March 31, 1864.

13. Joseph T. Glatthaar, *Forged in Battle: The Civil War Alliance of Black Soldiers and White Officers* (New York: Free Press, 1990), 169–206. Racist ideas about disease were also circulated by non-medical officers: Assistant Inspector General Lt. Col. W. N. Thurston, of the Department of the Gulf, wrote to department headquarters in New Orleans affirming the assessment by the regiment's surgeons of the bad condition of the 65th U.S.C.I. ("morally and physically"), which they attributed in large part to their assumption that Black men "were full of the seed of disease" (Lt. Col. W. N. Thurston to Major George B. Drake, October 29, 1864, Regimental Papers, 61st–65th U.S.C.I., U.S. Colored Troops, Box 42, , Record Group 94: Records of the Adjutant General's Office, 1780–1917, NARA, Washington, DC).

14. Samuel Ferguson Jaynes to Charlie Jayne, July 12, 1864, Jayne Papers, James S. Schoff Civil War Collection, William L. Clements Library, University of Michigan, Ann Arbor.

15. Berlin et al., *Black Military Experience*, 640.

16. Tom Lowry and Jack Welsh, *Tarnished Scalpels: The Court-Martials of Fifty Union Surgeons* (Mechanicsburg, PA: Stackpole Books, 2000), 76–79. The regiment's commander, Robert Gould Shaw, brought charges against Briggs, but there was no court-martial against him.

17. Pension file of John Bates, IC 219374; pension file of John Bandy, IC 840217; pension file of Jerry [aka Henry] White, IC 92134; and pension file of Henry D. Brown, IC 660715, all in Record Group 15: Records of the Veterans Administration, NARA, Washington, DC.

18. *Medical and Surgical Reporter*, May 27, 1865.

19. Freeman J. Bumstead et al., *Report of a Committee of the Associate Medical Members of the United States Sanitary Commission, on the Subject of Venereal Diseases, with Special References to Practice in the Army and Navy* (Washington, DC: Printed for Circulation by the United States Sanitary Commission, 1863), 13.

20. *Wartime Letters from Seth Rogers, M.D., Surgeon of the First South Carolina . . . 1862–1863*, transcribed by University of North Florida, *Florida History Online*, https://www.unf.edu/floridahistoryonline/Projects/Rogers/index.html. Burt Wilder, an abolitionist surgeon in the 55th Massachusetts, voluntarily prepared anthropometric measurements of Black soldiers for the USSC out of his commitment to the project (see chapter 2). B. A. Gould to Harris, December 25, 1865, Box 119, Section E: Medical Committee Archives, Part IV: Historical Bureau Records, New York, NY, Archives, MssCol 22263, New York Public Library Manuscripts and Archives Division, USSC Records.

21. Emily Parsons, *Memoir of Emily Elizabeth Parsons, Published for the Benefit of Cambridge Hospital* (Boston: Little, Brown & Co., 1880), 133–139. Jane E. Schultz notes several similar examples in *Women at the Front: Hospital Workers in Civil War America* (Chapel Hill: University of North Carolina Press, 2004), 103.

22. Jill Newmark, "Face to Face with History," *Prologue* 41 (Fall 2009): 22–25. I add to Newark's list D. O. McCord, who was noted by Margaret Humphreys as associated with a Louisiana regiment in *Intensely Human: The Health of the Black Soldier in the American Civil War* (Baltimore: Johns Hopkins University Press, 2008), 64.

23. Berlin et al., *Black Military Experience*, 356–567; Daryl Keith Daniels, "African Americans at the Yale University School of Medicine, 1810–1960" (MD diss., Yale University School of Medicine, 1991), 38–39.

24. Jane E. Schultz, "African American Men in the Union Medical Service," *Mercy Street Revealed*, February 21, 2017, http://www.pbs.org/mercy-street/blogs/mercy -street-revealed/african-american-men-in-the-union-medical-service/.

25. Daniels, "African Americans at Yale," 31–36.

26. Daniels, "African Americans at Yale," 37.

27. According to historian Jane Schultz, "Benjamin Boseman Jr., a 'promising' young Black student, whom Medical Director Joseph K. Barnes was considering for a position as Assistant Surgeon in an African American regiment. Barnes, who would follow the ousted William Hammond as Union Surgeon General in 1864, explained that he was willing to appoint Boseman with special permission from Secretary of War Stanton, but only after he had completed his medical coursework in upstate New York. This correspondence suggests that there were others who aspired to join the surgical corps during the war, even if they did not ultimately win appointments" (Schultz, "African American Men").

28. Emily Jones Salmon, "J. D. Harris (ca. 1833–1884)," *Encyclopedia Virginia*, December 22, 2021, https://www.encyclopediavirginia.org/Harris_Joseph_D_c_1833–1884.

29. Newmark, "Face to Face with History."

30. Humphreys, *Intensely Human*, 66.

31. Schultz, *Women at the Front*, 22.

32. Schultz, *Women at the Front*, 92–93; Jane E. Schultz, "Seldom Thanked, Never Praised, and Scarcely Recognized: Gender and Racism in Civil War Hospitals," *Civil War History* 48 (2002): 220–221.

33. In places where Black refugees from slavery and from the military conflict gathered—Nashville, Memphis, St. Louis, Helena, Washington, DC—many former slaves gained employment as contract hospital workers (Schultz, "Seldom Thanked," 22). See, for example, the African American women on the employment roster of the hospital at Helena, Arkansas, December 30, 1864. Entry 57-F, Hospital Muster Rolls, Arkansas, Box 1, Record Group 94: Records of the Veterans Administration, NARA, Washington, DC. Consider Milly Coleman, who left slavery along with her husband—he enlisting, and she making her way to Washington, DC, and finding work at Carver Hospital. There, she lived in a tent in the hospital yard. Her primary responsibilities were keeping two wards clean—the floors, the spittoons, the bedding, and the patients' dressing and clothing—but she often left her tent in the evening to come back to the wards to clean up; when sick and wounded soldiers were brought to the hospital, she noted, "Day or night, I had to be there" (Milly Coleman, Affidavit, July 21, 1897, IC 919698). Although the pension examiners discounted Black women's claims to have worked as nurses, the pay records often supported their claims. The applicant in this case was clearly employed and paid as a hospital matron, despite the Pension Bureau's doubts. Similarly, Laura Frazer (aka Givens) worked at Freedman's Hospital in Washington, DC, under Dr. Augusta as a cook in a Special Diet kitchen for two years; despite the suspicions of the pension examiner, she earned her pension as a nurse (Louisa Frazer aka Givens, IC 918938).

34. Leslie A. Schwalm, "Surviving Wartime Emancipation: African Americans and the Cost of Civil War," *Journal of Law, Medicine and Ethics* 39 (Spring 2011): 21–27.

35. Ira Russell, "The Sanitary Report of Benton Barracks Near St. Louis, Missouri; to the United States Sanitary Commission," Item 194, Folder 3.4, Box 110, Section E: Medical Committee Archives, Part IV: Historical Bureau Records, New York, NY, Archives, MssCol 22263, New York Public Library Manuscripts and Archives Division, USSC Records.

36. Humphreys, *Intensely Human*, chapter 4.

37. Glatthaar, *Forged in Battle*, 189.

38. Glatthaar, *Forged in Battle*, 190.

39. Humphreys, *Intensely Human*, chapter 3.

40. Berlin et al., *Black Military Experience*, chapter 15, contains several documents reporting this reality of Black military service; see, for example, the 1864 report by a medical inspector in Memphis (639-640) as well as the 1864 complaint filed by an anonymous Black soldier stationed at Brazos Santiago, Texas (640-641). See also Humphreys, *Intensely Human*, chapter 4; Edwin S. Redkey, ed., *A Grand Army of Black Men: Letters from African-American Soldiers in the Union Army, 1861-1865* (Cambridge: Cambridge University Press, 1992), 256-561; Edward A. Miller Jr., "Angel of Light: Helen L. Gilson, Army Nurse," *Civil War History* 43 (March 1997): 33-35; N., "Honor to Whom Honor Is Due," *Liberator*, December 16, 1864; Schultz, *Women at the Front*, 136; Jim Downs, *Sick from Freedom: African-American Illness and Suffering during the Civil War and Reconstruction* (New York: Oxford University Press, 2012), especially 35-36; and Glatthaar, *Forged in Battle*, 191.

41. Ira Russell, "The Sanitary Report of Benton Barracks Near St. Louis, Missouri; to the United States Sanitary Commission," Item 194, Folder 3.4, Box 110, Section E: Medical Committee Archives, Part IV: Historical Bureau Records, New York, NY, Archives, MssCol 22263, New York Public Library Manuscripts and Archives Division, USSC Records.

42. Londa Schiebinger, *Secret Cures of Slaves: People, Plants, and Medicines in the Eighteenth-Century Atlantic World* (Stanford: Stanford University Press, 2017); Rana A. Hogarth, "A Case Study in Charleston: Impressions of the Early National Slave Hospital," in *Medicine and Healing in the Age of Slavery*, edited by Sean Morey Smith and Christopher D. E. Willoughby, 143-164 (Baton Rouge: Louisiana State University Press, 2021); Stephen C. Kenny, "'A Dictate of Both Interest and Mercy': Slave Hospitals in the Antebellum South," *Journal of the History of Medicine and Allied Sciences* 65 (2009): 1-47.

43. Soldier Nathaniel Adams noted that he preferred his home remedy for diarrhea of black pepper tea to anything the regimental medical staff could provide (pension file of Nathaniel Adams, IC 472578, Record Group 15: Records of the Veterans Administration, NARA, Washington, DC). See Sharla M. Fett, *Working Cures: Healing, Health, and Power on Southern Slave Plantations* (Chapel Hill: University of North Carolina Press, 2002). Of course, white soldiers, both North and South, also found their medical officers lacking; see David Williams, *A People's History of the Civil War* (New York: Free Press, 2005), 208-210.

44. Humphreys, *Intensely Human*, 95-98; Joseph T. Glatthaar, "The Costliness of Discrimination: Medical Care for Black Troops in the Civil War," in *Inside the Confederate*

Nation: Essays in Honor of Emory M. Thomas, ed. Leslie J. Gordon and John C. Inscoe, 251–271 (Baton Rouge: Louisiana State University Press, 2005), 262; Ira Berlin et al., eds., *The Wartime Genesis of Free Labor: The Upper South*, series 1, vol. 2 of *Freedom: A Documentary History of Emancipation, 1861–1867, Selected from the Holdings of the National Archives of the United States* (New York: Cambridge University Press, 1993) 326. Glatthaar notes that that rate of illness with the disease was 764 percent higher among Black troops and the death rate 692 percent higher. Smallpox vaccination and treatment in contraband camps was also inadequate; the superintendent of Camp Barker in Washington, DC, reported both a shortage of vaccine matter and ineffective vaccine matter in the fall and winter of 1863.

45. The infection was likely erysipelas; see Henry Allen Pension file, WC 834236, Record Group 15: Records of the Veterans Administration, NARA, Washington, DC.

46. George Kebo pension file, WC 919204, Record Group 15: Records of the Veterans Administration, NARA, Washington, DC. Infected soldiers would consequently infect the women with whom they were intimate, and the women would pass the infection to their children.

47. For a positive report, see Sergeant-Major Rufus Sibb Jones [8th USCI], "Letter from Sergeant-Major Rufus S. Jones, 8th U.S. Colored Troops," *Christian Recorder*, May 7, 1864. See also Gretchen Long, *Doctoring Freedom: The Politics of African American Medical Care in Slavery and Emancipation* (Chapel Hill: University of North Carolina Press, 2012), 78; James G. Mendez, "A Great Sacrifice: Northern Black Families and Their Civil War Experience" (PhD diss., University of Illinois at Chicago, 2011), 119.

Chapter Two

1. Charles Stillé, *History of the United States Sanitary Commission, Being the General Report of Its Work during the War of the Rebellion* (Philadelphia: J.B. Lippincott & Co., 1866), 490. The authoritative works include Judith Giesberg, *Civil War Sisterhood: The U.S. Sanitary Commission and Women's Politics in Transition* (Boston: Northeastern University Press, 2000); Robert H. Bremner, *The Public Good: Philanthropy and Welfare in the Civil War Era* (New York: Knopf, 1980); Jane Turner Censer, ed., *The Papers of Frederick Law Olmsted*, vol. 4, (Baltimore: Johns Hopkins University Press, 1986), introduction; William Quentin Maxwell, *Lincoln's Fifth Wheel: The Political History of the United States Sanitary Commission* (New York: Longmans, Green & Co., 1956); and Jeanie Attie, *Patriotic Toil: Northern Women and the American Civil War* (Ithaca, NY: Cornell University Press, 1998).

2. Benjamin A. Gould, *Investigations in the Military and Anthropological Statistics of American Soldiers* (Cambridge, MA: Riverside Press, 1869), 246.

3. Stillé, *History of the United States Sanitary Commission*, 527. The USSC wrote its own histories, seeking to shape public perception of the value and breadth of the commission's contributions to the worlds of medicine, philanthropy, and modern nationalism. The first of these was Katharine Prescott Wormeley, *The United States Sanitary Commission, A Sketch of Its Purposes and Its Work* (Boston: Little, Brown & Co., 1863).

4. In its 1864 history, the USSC portrays a public clamor for "a decisive, prompt, and rigid rule over the mob of civilian benevolence." L. P. Brockett, *The Philanthropic*

Results of the War Collected from Official and Authentic Sources (New York: Sheldon & Co., 1864), 6.

5. Bellows was joined by W. H. Van Buren, Elisha Harris, and Jacob Harsen, all physicians, representatives from the "Advisory Committee of the Board of Physicians and Surgeons of the hospitals of New York" and "The New York Medical Association for Furnishing Hospital Supplies in Aid of the Army" (Brockett, *Philanthropic Results of the War*, 34–35).

6. The clearest account is offered in Brockett, *Philanthropic Results of the War*, 34–42.

7. The best overview of this formative period is offered by Giesberg in her authoritative *Civil War Sisterhood*; see also Censer, *Papers of Frederick Law Olmsted*, vol. 4, introduction, and Suellen Hoy's brief but effective overview in *Chasing Dirt: The American Pursuit of Cleanliness* (New York: Oxford University Press, 1996), chapter 2. Kathryn Shively Meier provides an overview of the commission's impact on modernizing American medicine in her essay, "U.S. Sanitary Commission Physicians and the Transformation of American Health Care," in *So Conceived and So Dedicated: Intellectual Life in the Civil War-Era North*, ed. Lorien Foote and Kanisorn Wongsrichanalai, 19–40 (New York: Fordham University Press, 2015). Attie notes that the extant record makes it difficult to establish how voluntary or not the merger was (*Patriotic Toil*, 82–86); certainly, in its 1864 history the USSC completely elides the preparatory work among women and the WCAR.

8. Charles Stillé, *The Sanitary Commission of the United States Army: A Succinct Narrative of Its Works and Purposes* (New York: Published for the Benefit of the United States Sanitary Commission, 1864), 3–6.

9. Maxwell, *Lincoln's Fifth Wheel*, 9. Giesberg estimates the number of local societies at 7,000 (*Civil War Sisterhood*, 5–6); Attie estimates them at 10,000–12,000 (*Patriotic Toil*).

10. Again, Attie notes that the extant record makes it difficult to establish how voluntary the merger was (*Patriotic Toil*, 82–86).

11. Stillé, *Sanitary Commission of the United States Army*, 517.

12. Attie, *Patriotic Toil*, 3; Stillé, *Sanitary Commission of the United States Army*, 172, 488; Mary A. Livermore, *My Story of the War: A Woman's Narrative of Four Years Personal Experience as Nurse in the Union Army, and in Relief Work at Home, in Hospitals, Camps, and at the Front, during the War of the Rebellion. With Anecdotes, Pathetic Incidents, and Thrilling Reminiscences Portraying the Lights and Shadows of Hospital Life and the Sanitary Service of the War* (Hartford, CT: A.D. Worthington & Co., 1889), 475.

13. Bremner, *Public Good*, 54–55.

14. L. P. Brockett, *Heroines of the Rebellion: Or, Woman's Work in the Civil War: A Record of Heroism, Patriotism, and Patience* (Philadelphia: Edgewood, 1867), title page. Brockett further characterizes women's relief work: "Everywhere started up women acquainted with the order of public business; able to call, and preside over public meetings of their own sex; act as secretaries and committees, draft constitutions and bye-laws, open books, and keep accounts with adequate precision, appreciate system, and postpone private inclinations or preferences to general principles; enter into extensive correspondence with their own sex: co-operate in the largest and most rational

plans proposed by men who had studied carefully the subject of soldiers' relief, and adhere through good report and through evil report, to organizations which commended themselves to their judgment, in spite of local, sectarian, or personal jealousies and detraction" (57).

15. Giesberg, *Civil War Sisterhood*, 170–171.

16. Giesberg, *Civil War Sisterhood*, 59.

17. Brockett, *Heroines of the Rebellion*, 534–545; Stillé, *Sanitary Commission of the United States Army*, 178–179.

18. The records of four lodges where commission volunteers and agents found shelter (two in Washington, DC, one each in Annapolis and Alexandria) show no African American visitors although Black women were extensively involved in relief work in these locations. See Lodge Number 6 record book (1864 December 1–1865 July 15), Folder 1; Home for Soldiers' Wives and Mothers admission register (1863 Dec 26–1865 Sep 22), Folder 2; and Alexandria Lodge, Admission register (1863 August 14–1865 June 21), Folder 3, all in Box 204, Part II: Special Relief Department, Washington, DC, Archives, MssCol 22261, New York Public Library Manuscripts and Archives Division, United States Sanitary Commission (USSC) Records. See also Annapolis Home for Wives, Mothers, and Children of Soldiers, Register (1863 July 35–1864 May 31), Folder 8, Box 2, Part I: Annapolis Records, Maryland Archives, MssCol 18817, New York Public Library Manuscripts and Archives Division, USSC Records.

19. White abolitionist Julia Wilbur described the racist comments she encountered when visiting the Alexandria lodge in January 1864 in the company of African American and white aid workers. Jean Fagan Yellin, ed., *The Harriet Jacobs Family Papers* (Chapel Hill: University of North Carolina, 2008), 2:539.

20. See United States Sanitary Commission, Philadelphia Branch, *Report of the General Superintendent Report of the General Superintendent of the Philadelphia Branch of the U.S. Sanitary Commission to the Executive Committee, January 1st, 1866* (Philadelphia: King & Baird, Printers, 1866), on the exclusion of Black women from lists of Philadelphia officers. See also Women's Central Association of Relief, *Second Annual Report of the Women's Central Association of Relief, No. 10, Cooper Union, New York* (New York: William S. Dorr, Book and Job Printer, 1863), 5; and Andrew Dickson White, *The Annual Report of the Women's Pennsylvania Branch, U.S. Sanitary Commission, Present April 1, 1864* (Philadelphia: Henry B. Ashmead, Book and Job Printer, 1864), 4, 18–32; as well as Supplies Received (1861 December–1865 September, vols. 6–12, Box 12, Part III: Supplies, New England Women's Auxiliary Association Archives, New York Public Library Manuscripts and Archives Division, USSC Records.

21. See, for example, Charles Brandon Boynton, *The History of the Great Western Sanitary Fair* (Cincinnati: C.F. Vent & Co., 1864), 93–94, 108–109; H. G. Gladding and Frederick A. Farely, *History of the Brooklyn and Long Island Fair, February 22, 1864* (Brooklyn: Union Steam Press, 1864), 70–71 (on the "superiority" of Black waiters), 77 (on the performance by the Hutchinson family), and 149 (on cash donations by African Americans). New York City's Colored School No. 7 and Colored Grammar School No. 2 sponsored evening entertainments for the benefit of the Metropolitan Sanitary Fair, noting that the USSC provided aid for both Black and white soldiers (*Weekly Anglo-African*, March 5, 1864, and March 12, 1865).

22. Western Sanitary Commission, *Final Report of the Western Sanitary Commission, from May 9th, 1864, to December 31st, 1865* (St. Louis: R.F. Studley & Co., 1866), 16.

23. Judith Giesberg, ed., *Emilie Davis's Civil War: The Diaries of a Free Black Woman in Philadelphia, 1863–1865* (University Park: Pennsylvania State University Press, 2014), 137.

24. *Weekly Anglo-African*, May 7, 1864.

25. Described by many historians as an exercise in "meaningful national civic action," the fairs rarely envisioned racial democracy as a central tenet of that nation. See Melinda Lawson, *Patriotic Fires: Forging a New American Nationalism in the Civil War North* (Lawrence: University of Kansas Press, 2002), 27. Among the sanitary fairs that excluded African American women from organizing committees: Baltimore in 1864 (although Black regiments were invited to parade as part of the festivities), see Robert W. Schoeberlein, "A Fair to Remember: Maryland Women in Aid of the Union," *Maryland Historical Society* 90 (1995): 467–488; St. Louis in 1864 (as with Baltimore, Black regiments were invited to perform guard duty, but white female attendants initially refused to serve Black clergymen who attempted to dine at the fair), see Louis Gerteis, *Civil War St. Louis* (Lawrence: University Press of Kansas, 2001); and Philadelphia in 1864, see Richard S. Newman, "All's Fair: Philadelphia and the Sanitary Fair Movement during the Civil War," *Pennsylvania Heritage* (Summer 2013): 56–65, p. 62. The executive committee chairman of the Philadelphia fair, John Welsh, refused the request of William Forten and Ebenezer Bassett in April 1864 to permit African American women to sponsor and staff a table; African Americans were also excluded from attending the fair during its first week; see Elizabeth Milroy, "Avenue of Dreams: Patriotism and the Spectator at Philadelphia's Great Central Sanitary Fair," in *Making and Remaking Pennsylvania's Civil War*, ed. William Blair and William Pencak, 23–57 (University Park: Pennsylvania State University Press, 2001), 50.

26. Other examples include the sketches on display ("Bringing in Contrabands") at the Brooklyn and Long Island fair, performances by the Hutchinson family as well as Hooley's minstrel troupe, and a slave whip as well as cotton and sugar produced by free labor on abandoned plantations in the South (Gladding and Farely, *History of the Brooklyn and Long Island Fair*, 42, 147, 148, 155).

27. *Weekly Anglo-African*, January 9, 1864. Boynton in *History of the Great Western Sanitary Fair* (102–103) failed to note the racial politics documented in the *Weekly Anglo-African*.

28. *Weekly Anglo-African*, February 13, 1864.

29. *Weekly Anglo-African*, February 4, 1865. As the Detroit Black women began organizing their own fair, they were approached by white women who "possessed kindness of heart, and magnanimity enough to brave the taunts and jeers of the Black-hearted portion of our [the wider, white community in Detroit] community," who made a "request to be permitted" to take part (April 8, 1865). While clearly communicating their own leadership and the lesser "assistance" of white women, these Black organizers also conceded that it took a certain amount of courage for white women to follow the lead of Black women.

30. White Detroit reformer Isabella G. D. Stewart, who was a frequent correspondent with Ellen Collins, expressed apprehension about the expansion of USSC women's

organizing among the "red hot" amalgamationists of Ohio. Stewart, a member of a prominent Detroit family, was well known for her religious and charitable activities; she presided over the city's first soldier's aid society, was involved with the Detroit Home of the Friendless and the city's Thompson Home for Old Ladies, and helped author and publish recipe books in the 1870s intended as fundraisers for these institutions; and was a member of the Woman's Christian Temperance Union (WCTU). Stewart's recollections of teaching a Sunday school at a Black congregation conveys her apprehension and distaste for working with people of color. See Morse Stewart, "Memorial of Mrs. Morse Stewart (1889)," 32–33 and 87–95, and Isabella G. D. Stewart to Miss Collins, August 13, 1861, Folder 7, Box 1, Women's Central Association for Relief Records, MccCol 22266, New York Public Library Manuscripts and Archives Division, USSC Records.

31. Nonetheless, the white Ladies' Union Aid Society in St. Louis decreed it inappropriate to use funds for former slaves that had been donated to support white soldiers; they insisted instead on an entirely separate organization, which the city's African American women quickly took up (*Daily Missouri Democrat*, January 23, 1863). On the WSC, see William E. Parrish, "The Western Sanitary Commission," *Civil War History* 36 (March 1990): 28–29. An unsigned and very sympathetic review of two WSC publications in the *North American Review* made two subtle statements of the WSC's commitment to relief regardless of status or race but does not explicitly state the extent of its work among former slaves in the South (W. S. Rosecrans, "Art. VIII: Annual Report of the Western Sanitary Commission for the Years Ending July, 1862, and July, 1863; Circular of Mississippi Valley Sanitary Fair, to Be Held in St. Louis, May 17th, 1864," *North American Review* 98, no. 203 [April 1864]: 522, 529), nor does it include any reference to its letter to President Lincoln pleading for assistance in helping 50,000 former slaves in the Mississippi valley. See James Yeatman et al. to President Abraham Lincoln, November 6, 1863, printed copy at the Gilder Lehrman Institute of American History, "History Resources: The Western Sanitary Commission Reports on Suffering in the Mississippi Valley, 1863," http://www.gilderlehrman.org/history-by-era /african-americans-and-emancipation/resources/western-sanitary-commission -reports-suffering. The USSC's extensive network of western branches is described in J. S. Newberry, *The U.S. Sanitary Commission in the Valley of the Mississippi, during the War of the Rebellion, 1861–1866* (Cleveland: Fairbanks, Benedict & Co., 1871).

32. Carol Faulkner's *Women's Radical Reconstruction: The Freedmen's Aid Movement* (Philadelphia: University of Pennsylvania Press, 2006) remains the authoritative work on this subject.

33. Faulkner, *Women's Radical Reconstruction*, 123–125; 1860 census; Gunja SenGutpa, *From Slavery to Poverty: Racial Origins of Welfare in New York, 1840–1918* (New York: New York University Press, 2009), 211. Faulkner notes several other women, white and African American, who were either employed by the Freedmen's Bureau or worked independently as employment agents in the North; see also Stephen Kantrowitz, *More Than Freedom: Fighting for Black Citizenship in a White Republic, 1829–1889* (New York: Penguin, 2012), 289–280, 297.

34. Commission women were very diligent in their correspondence and in nurturing close ties between local societies and branch leaders; Giesberg makes this point in

Civil War Sisterhood. The impact of excluding Black women in later social movements is noted in Lisa Tetrault, *The Myth of Seneca Falls: Memory and the Women's Suffrage Movement, 1848–1898* (Chapel Hill: University of North Carolina Press, 2014); and Louise Michele Newman, *White Women's Rights: The Racial Origins of Feminism in the United States* (New York: Oxford University Press, 1999), especially chapter 2.

35. For an example of a history of USSC work that excludes mention of African American wartime organizing, see Brockett, *Philanthropic Results of the War*.

36. Faulkner, *Women's Radical Reconstruction*, 124.

37. Ella Forbes, in *African American Women during the Civil War* (New York: Garland, 1998), documents the wide range of activities. Two hundred and eighty-eight women are listed as members and officers of these organizations (not all listed members' names). For my count, I relied primarily on reports in the *Christian Recorder* and the *Weekly Anglo-African*, counting only those societies for which there was evidence of ongoing activities (rather than single events), only those societies in which women predominated and led (some societies included men as advisors or supporters), and only those that included soldier relief (Black and/or white) among their goals. This, then, excludes the many societies organized for the primary purpose of relief to former slaves.

38. White, *Annual Report of the Women's Pennsylvania Branch*, 23, 24. At the time of this report, over 300 societies were affiliated with the USSC in Pennsylvania, Delaware, and New Jersey (3).

39. *Weekly Anglo-African*, May 7, 1864.

40. Forbes, *African American Women*, 103; C. Peter Ripley, ed., *The Black Abolitionist Papers* (Chapel Hill: University of North Carolina Press, 1992), 5:311–313; *Weekly Anglo-African*, February 27, 1864, April 30, 1864, January 28, 1865, and February 4, 1865. J. S. Newberry, in his official history of USSC work in the Mississippi valley, discusses the commission's work in Cleveland but does not mention this auxiliary (or any other Black-led organization in the West). See Newberry, *U.S. Sanitary Commission*.

41. *Weekly Anglo-African*, July 2, 1864 (Baltimore), August 13, 1864 (Boston).

42. *Weekly Anglo-African*, October 8, 1864; *Christian Recorder* February 11 and February 25, 1865.

43. United States Sanitary Commission, Philadelphia Branch, *Report of the General Superintendent 1866*.

44. For example, the *Weekly Anglo-African*, April 1, 1865, reports that treasurer Elizabeth Thompson of the New York Ladies Committee for the Relief of Sick Soldiers attended Lincoln's inauguration and visited the hospitals, schools, and orphan asylum in Washington, DC, Arlington, and Alexandria. A "deputation" from the St. Thomas Sanitary Commission auxiliary traveled to City Point, Virginia, to visit hospitals and camps, and distribute donations (*Christian Recorder*, April 8, 1865). The (unaffiliated) Boston Colored Ladies Sanitary Commission claimed chapters in Chelsea and Malden, Massachusetts. The Utica, New York, Colored Soldiers' Aid Society forwarded donations to the Soldiers and Freedmen's Aid Society in Washington, DC (*Weekly Anglo-African*, May 20, 1865; see also February 27, 1864, and January 28, 1865).

45. Janette Thomas Greenwood, *First Fruits of Freedom: The Migration of Former Slaves and Their Search for Equality in Worcester, Massachusetts, 1862–1900* (Chapel Hill: University of North Carolina Press, 2009), 64.

46. Emily Parsons, *Memoir of Emily Elizabeth Parsons, Published for the Benefit of Cambridge Hospital* (Boston: Little, Brown & Co., 1880), 138–139.

47. See, for example, Ladies' Union Association of Philadelphia, *Report of the Ladies' Union Association of Philadelphia, Formed July 20th, 1863, for the Purpose of Administering Exclusively to the Wants of the Sick and Wounded Colored Soldiers* (Philadelphia: G.T. Stockdale, 1867); and Carla L. Peterson, *Black Gotham: A Family History of African Americans in Nineteenth-Century* (New Haven, CT: Yale University Press, 2011), 264.

48. *Weekly Anglo African*, December 28, 1861, for an example of "colored" schoolgirls' donation to white soldiers.

49. *Weekly Anglo-African*, February 11, 1865.

50. Forty women organized a Ladies' Committee for the Aid of Sick Soldiers in New York City, staffing a special diet kitchen for the Black soldiers hospitalized on Riker's Island (*Weekly Anglo-African*, January 30, 1864). See also Ladies' Union Association of Philadelphia, *Report of the Ladies' Union Association*, 3.

51. The Cleveland society sent donations to the Philadelphia fair for colored soldiers (*Weekly Anglo-African*, February 4, 1865); the St. Thomas commission sent donations to the hospitals serving Black soldiers in Alexandria, Virginia (see *Christian Recorder*, March 4, 1865). On the forwarding of donations to the Norfolk society, see *Weekly Anglo-African*, July 30, 1864, and December 24, 1864.

52. Ladies' Union Association of Philadelphia, *Report of the Ladies' Union*, 4–5. Of nearly 6,000 men and women housed at that lodge in 1865, 390 included Black troops (United States Sanitary Commission, Philadelphia Branch, *Report of the General Superintendent 1866*, 21–22).

53. *Weekly Anglo-African*, October 8, 1864; Ladies' Union Association of Philadelphia, *Report of the Ladies' Union*, 4–5. On Washington, DC, see Robert Harrison, *Washington during Civil War and Reconstruction: Race and Radicalism* (Cambridge: Cambridge University Press, 2011), 218.

54. A "large assemblage," "a good portion of which were ladies," met in Brooklyn's African Methodist Episcopal (AME) church in March 1863 (*Weekly Anglo-African*, March 10, 1863).

55. *Weekly Anglo-African*, December 7, 1861, February 1, 1862, February 15, 1862, and March 8, 1862; *Liberator*, September 15, 1865. The Colored Ladies' Sanitary Commission of Boston held a fair, October 18–22, 1864, for the benefit of disabled Black Massachusetts soldiers and their "poor, suffering and destitute wives and children" (*Liberator*, May 27, 1864 quoted; see also October 7, 14, and 21, 1864), and the women congregants of Philadelphia's St. Thomas Episcopal Church, an official auxiliary of the USSC, held their own fair as well.

56. In New York, efforts began October 5, 1863, according to articles in the *Weekly Anglo-African*, October 10, 17, and 24, 1863. Another organization planned a fair for Black soldiers in 1864 (*Weekly Anglo-African*, November 26, 1864). The Philadelphia fair was held in October 1864 (*Weekly Anglo-African*, October 29, 1864), and the Boston fair in October 1864 (on white women staffing tables, see *Weekly Anglo-African*, November 5, 1864). In New Bedford, events were held in October and November 1863 (*Weekly Anglo-African*, December 5, 1863).

57. For example, at least ninety African Americans in New York and from across the country worked together in 1865 to hold a fair benefiting the *Weekly Anglo-African* newspaper (January 21, 1865).

58. *Weekly Anglo-African*, October 3, 1863.

59. *Weekly Anglo-African*, January 2, 1864.

60. Lewis Steiner, "Report on the Operations of the Eastern Department," *Sanitary Commission Bulletin*, November 1, 1863, 7.

61. See, for example, the correspondence of Samuel Ferguson Jayne, who noted about the treatment of Black patients, "When we came here most of the men were without beds—now we have them upon, not only beds—but every man has also an iron bedstead, entirely covered by mosquito netting" (Samuel F. Jayne to Charlie, July 12, 1864). Later he also wrote, "There are many contrabands connected with our camp. They are very destitute of all of the necessities of life. We sometimes give them things for which they are very grateful. We found them lying upon the ground with no beds, no blankets, and almost naked. We have furnished beds and blankets for them, and Miss Gilson got a piece of flannel and distributed it as far as it would go" (Samuel F. Jayne to Charlie, July 26, 1864). Jayne Papers, 1864, in James S. Schoff Collection, William L. Clements Library, University of Michigan, Ann Arbor.

62. Not all respected her work; a white colleague complained, "She will kiss a negro boy, or do anything for a soldier—but she will hardly treat any stranger politely" (Samuel Ferguson Jayne to Charlie, August 1, 1864). Jayne Papers, 1864, in James S. Schoff Civil War Collection, William L. Clements Library, University of Michigan, Ann Arbor. Also see "Dr Douglass to the Agts. San. Com. —Sept. 24/62," Folder 6, Box 4, Frederick Newman Knapp Papers, Massachusetts Historical Society, Boston; Samuel F. Jayne to Hon. Frank B. Fay, Supt. Auxiliary Relief Corps, July 11, 1864, Folder 7, Box 1, Part I: Letters and Reports, Department of North Carolina, MssCol 18581, New York Public Library Manuscripts and Archives Division, USSC Records; and Brockett, *Heroines of the Rebellion*, 133–148. On race relations in hospitals, see Jane E. Schultz, *Women at the Front: Hospital Workers in Civil War America* (Chapel Hill: University of North Carolina Press, 2004), 98–99.

63. May 25, 1863: J. H. Douglas to Dr. Page, Folder 15, Box 2, Part I: Letters and Reports, Department of North Carolina, MssCol 18581, New York Public Library Manuscripts and Archives Division, USSC Records; and Vol. 3, Page's 1864 journal, Box 7, Part I: Letters and Reports, Department of North Carolina, MssCol 18581, New York Public Library Manuscripts and Archives Division, USSC Records.

64. Jaynes's wartime correspondence has been preserved in May S. Briggs, ed., *The Ferguson-Jayne Papers, 1826–1938*, 2 vols. (Davenport, NY: Davenport Historical Society, 1981), which includes the diary of Samuel Ferguson Jayne, 1864 (1834–1904, photo included in volume), and the Jayne Papers, 1864, in the James S. Schoff Civil War Collection, William L. Clements Library, University of Michigan, Ann Arbor. Some of his letters were also printed in the *Sanitary Commission Bulletin* (see September 1, 1864, for example).

65. United States Sanitary Commission, Philadelphia Branch, *Report of the General Superintendent 1866*, 3–6; Brockett, *Heroines of the Rebellion*, 650–658 (on the Women's Relief Association of Brooklyn and Long Island). The commission created a separate

department for this work, called the Special Relief Service, led by Frederick Knapp, with headquarters in Washington, DC, where the need for this work was first incorporated into commission practice. It became an aspect of commission work in all of the regional branches as well. "New Orleans Soldiers Home and Brashear City Soldiers Rest," Folder 1, Box 107, Section D: Special Relief Archives, Part IV: Historical Bureau Records, New York, NY, Archives, New York Public Library Manuscripts and Archives Division, USSC Records. A partial and draft history of the branch (never published) is located in the papers of Frederick Knapp, director of the special relief branch. According to his draft, the branch—which was organized in late 1862—had only three employees by the end of that year; it grew steadily in size until June 1865, with 15 employees. Also attached to this branch was the commission's work advising and assisting soldiers in recouping back pay and bounties and applying for pensions. "Concerning the records and system of the Special Relief Office," undated, 22-page, handwritten manuscript, Folder 2, Box 4, Frederick Newman Knapp Papers, Massachusetts Historical Society, Boston. See also United States Sanitary Commission, Boston Branch, *Report Concerning the Special Relief Service of the U.S. Sanitary Commission in Boston, Mass. for the Year Ending March 31, 1864* (Boston: Prentiss & Deland, 1864), especially 3–7.

66. "New Orleans Soldiers Home and Brashear City Soldiers Rest," Folder 1, Box 107, Section D: Special Relief Archives, Part IV: Historical Bureau Records, New York, NY, Archives, MssCol 22263, New York Public Library Manuscripts and Archives Division, USSC Records.

67. Attie, *Patriotic Toil*, chapter 4.

68. *Weekly Anglo-African*, January 30, 1864, February 6, 1864, February 20, 1864, March 26, 1864, April 2, 1864, April 23, 1864, November 15, 1864, and August 19, 1865; Union League Club, *Report of the Committee on Volunteering, Presented October 18th, 1864* (New York, Union League Club, 1864), 17, 24; Peterson, *Black Gotham*, 264; and Forbes, *African American Women*, 75.

69. *Christian Recorder*, December 12, 1863.

70. Board of Managers Minutes, April 4, 1864, Folder 13, Box 17, Part II: Women's Pennsylvania Branch, Pennsylvania Archives, MssCol 18781, New York Public Library Manuscripts and Archives Division, USSC Records.

71. Robert F. Ulle, "A History of St. Thomas' African Episcopal Church, 1794–1865" (PhD diss., University of Pennsylvania, 1986), 283. In 1855, the Pennsylvania Branch employed 830 wives and widows to sew garments at twice the rate offered by government contractors and their middlemen. United States Sanitary Commission, Philadelphia Branch, *Report of the General Superintendent 1866*, 34.

72. A list of the (white) visitors can be found in United States Sanitary Commission, Women's Pennsylvania Branch, *Report of the Proceedings of a Meeting of the Ladies and Ward Visitors of the Special Relief Committee, Held at the Rooms of the Committee on Monday, January 18th, 1864* (1864).

73. United States Sanitary Commission, Philadelphia Branch, *Report of the General Superintendent 1866*, 14.

74. "Western Sanitary Commission, St. Louis, Missouri," *North American Review*, April 1864, in William Greenleaf Eliot Papers, Missouri Historical Society, St. Louis.

75. *Daily Missouri Democrat*, January 23, 1863, January 24, 1863, and March 3, 1863.

76. Parsons, *Memoir of Emily Elizabeth Parsons*, 138–139.

77. "Freedmen and Refugees' Department of the Mississippi Valley Sanitary Fair," *U.S. Sanitary Commission Pamphlets*, a bound collection of various pamphlets and broadsides printed and circulated by the USSC, Missouri Historical Society, St. Louis.

78. Gerteis, *Civil War St. Louis*, chapter 7, offers a useful overview of the history and work of the WSC.

79. See Mary Ryan's *Cradle of the Middle Class: The Family in Oneida County, New York, 1790–1865* (Cambridge: Cambridge University Press, 1981), 210–218. While scholarship on women and the welfare state, and on maternalism, is considerable, most of it begins with the Gilded Age; commission women offer an important opportunity to understand the historical roots of activist women, the relationships they crafted with state functions, and their relationships with client populations.

80. United States Sanitary Commission, Philadelphia Branch, *Report of the General Superintendent of the Philadelphia Branch of the U.S. Sanitary Commission to the Executive Committee, January 1st, 1865* (Philadelphia: King & Baird, Printers, 1865), 13–14, for example.

81. *Sanitary Reporter*, December 1, 1863.

82. See Schultz, *Women at the Front*, 35–37; Samuel F. Jayne to Charlie, July 12, 1864, Samuel F. Jayne to Charlie, August 4, 1864, Jayne Papers, 1864, in James S. Schoff Civil War Collection, William L. Clements Library, University of Michigan, Ann Arbor; *Sanitary Commission Bulletin*, December 15, 1863; Hospital transport records, Item 930, p. 81, Folder 13, Box 4, Frederick Newman Knapp Papers, Massachusetts Historical Society, Boston; "New Orleans Soldiers Home and Brashear City Soldiers Rest," pp. 63–68, anonymous, n.d., Folder 1, Box 107, Section D: Special Relief Archives, Part IV: Historical Bureau Records, New York, NY, Archives, MssCol 22263, New York Public Library Manuscripts and Archives Division, USSC Records; A. M. Sperry to [illegible], Folder 15, Box 2, Part I: Letters and Reports, Army of the Potomac Archives, MssCol 18782, New York Public Library Manuscripts and Archives Division, USSC Records.

83. A. M. Sperry to [illegible], Folder 15, Box 2, Part I: Letters and Reports, Army of the Potomac Archives, MssCol 18782, New York Public Library Manuscripts and Archives Division, USSC Records. Sperry notes that the commission's employment of laundresses "has paid us well for the money invested."

84. Censer, *Papers of Frederick Law Olmsted*, 4:117–120, 4:271–313. For a critical assessment of his writings on the South, see Charles E. Beveridge and Charles Capen McLaughlin, eds., *The Papers of Frederick Law Olmsted* (Baltimore: Johns Hopkins University Press, 1981), 2:13–15.

85. The best overview of these events is offered in Censer, *Papers of Frederick Law Olmsted*, 4:3–25 and 4:271–313. Ware's report was printed by the commission and can be seen in Folder 6, Box 3 of the Frederick Newman Knapp Papers, Massachusetts Historical Society, Boston.

86. Laura Wood Roper, "Frederick Law Olmsted and the Port Royal Experiment," *Journal of Southern History* 31 (1965), 279.

87. Roper, "Frederick Law Olmsted," 280, 292–293.

88. Wormeley, *United States Sanitary Commission*.

89. The *Sanitary Commission Bulletin*, by the spring of 1864, reached about 14,000 readers; the *Sanitary Reporter*, as of the summer of 1863, printed 6,000 copies of each issue. Examples of reports of the conditions of former slaves are noted in the *Sanitary Reporter*, August 15, 1863, December 1, 1863, and November 14, 1864.

90. Tabular Statement of Disbursements, February 18–July 10, 1862, Folder 3, Box 1, Correspondence, Letters Received, 1862–1865, Part I: Letters and Reports, Department of North Carolina Archives, MssCol 18581, New York Public Library Manuscripts and Archives Division, USSC Records.

91. J. J. Delameter, Asst. Surg. Vols. & Chairman of the Board of Health at New Bern, to Henry Bellows, May 23, 1863, Vol. 1, pp. 105–106, Box 5, Part I: Standing Committee Records, New York, NY, Archives, MssCol 22263, New York Public Library Manuscripts and Archives Division, USSC Records.

92. Bellows to Dr. J. J. Delameter, Asst. Surg. Vols. & Chairman of the Board of Health of New Bern, May 23, 1863, enclosed in J. H. Douglas to Dr. Page, May 25, 1863, Letters and Reports, Folder 15, Box 2, Part I: Letters and Reports, Department of North Carolina, MssCol 18581, New York Public Library Manuscripts and Archives Division, USSC Records.

93. *Sanitary Commission Bulletin*, November 1, 1863.

94. Dr. J. Foster Jenkins & Miss Abby W. May to Henry W. Bellows, February 28 and 29, 1864, Folder 9.13, Box 9, Part II: Henry W. Bellows Papers, New York, NY, Archives, MssCol 22263, New York Public Library Manuscripts and Archives Division, USSC Records.

95. One of his many public lectures on behalf of freedmen's aid was noted in the *Christian Recorder*, October 14, 1865.

96. *Daily Missouri Democrat*, January 23, 1863.

97. See Attie, *Patriotic Toil*, chapter 4.

98. See, for example, the June and July 1865 correspondence between Louisa Schuyler and [illegible] Parrish, Folder 7, Letters Received, Washington and New York, Box 13, Part III: Committee Records, Women's Central Association of Relief Records, MssCol 22266, New York Public Library Manuscripts and Archives Division, USSC Records. Giesberg discusses the end of relief work in *Civil War Sisterhood*, chapter 6.

99. Building appraisal, October 7, 1865; Items Received by Jacob Shiperd, American Freedmen's Aid Commission, December 1, 1865, Closing accounts, 1865 August–1866 March, Folder 7, Box 122, Part I: Central Office, Washington, DC, Archives, MssCol 22261, New York Public Library Manuscripts and Archives Division, USSC Records; Minutes, Folder 4, Box 4, Part I: Standing Committee Records, New York, NY, Archives, MssCol 22263, New York Public Library Manuscripts and Archives Division, USSC Records; Col. Whittlesy to Agents of the Sanitary Commission, June 26, 1865, Col. E. Whittlesy to Doctor, November 22, 1865 and M. K. Hogan to Dr. J. Page, December 19, 1865, all in Folder 15, Box 2, Part I: Letters and Reports, Department of North Carolina Archives, MssCol 18581, New York Public Library Manuscripts and Archives Division, USSC Records. The Pennsylvania Branch donated

$1,616.20 worth of clothing, furnishings, and bedding; see United States Sanitary Commission, Philadelphia Branch, *Report of the General Superintendent 1866*, 71.

Chapter Three

1. James Hunt, *Anniversary Address Delivered before the Anthropological Society of London, January 5, 1864* (London: Trübner & Co., 1864). On the saturation of medical science with racial thought, see Christopher D. Willoughby, "Running Away from Praenomina: Samuel A. Cartwright, Medicine, and Race in the Antebellum South," *Journal of Southern History* 84 (2018): 579–614.

2. J. Marion Sims conducted experimental surgery without anesthesia on enslaved women in pursuit of a remedy for vesicovaginal fistula; Samuel Cartwright invented medical diagnoses to explain slave resistance and flight; Josiah Nott and Samuel George Morton, in addition to their work as physicians, were advocates of polygenesis and craniometry as empirical proof of Black inferiority; and biologist Louis Agassiz also advocated polygenesis. For an excellent overview of race and medicine in the antebellum South, see Marli Weiner and Mazie Hough, *Sex, Sickness, and Slavery: Defining Illness in the Antebellum South* (Urbana-Champaign: University of Illinois Press, 2012). On spirometry, anthropometry, phrenology, and other aspects of nineteenth-century scientific racism as well as their lasting impact on ideas about race, see Lundy Braun, *Breathing Race into Science: The Surprising Career of the Spirometer from Plantation to Genetics* (Minneapolis: University of Minnesota Press, 2014); John S. Haller Jr., *Outcasts from Evolution: Scientific Attitudes of Racial Inferiority, 1859-1900* (Urbana-Champaign: University of Illinois Press, 1971); and Paul H. D. Lawrie, "'Mortality as the Life Story of a People': Frederick L. Hoffman and Actuarial Narratives of African American Extinction, 1896–1915," *Canadian Review of American Studies* 43 (Winter 2013): 352–387.

3. See Bruce Dain, *A Hideous Monster of the Mind: American Race Theory in the Early Republic* (Cambridge, MA: Harvard University Press, 2002); Todd Savitt, *Medicine and Slavery: The Diseases and Health Care of Blacks in Antebellum Virginia* (Urbana-Champaign: University of Illinois Press, 1978), especially chapter 9; Harriet A. Washington, *Medical Apartheid: The Dark History of Medical Experimentation on Black Americans from Colonial Times to the Present* (New York: Harlem Moon Broadway Books, 2006), especially chapters 4 and 5; Gretchen Long, *Doctoring Freedom: The Politics of African American Medical Care in Slavery and Emancipation* (Chapel Hill: University of North Carolina Press, 2012), chapter 1; and Melissa N. Stein, *Measuring Manhood: Race the Science of Masculinity, 1830-1934* (Minneapolis: University of Minnesota Press, 2015), chapter 1.

4. Anthropological Society of America, *Uncivilized Races, Proving That Many Races of Men Are Incapable of Civilization. By an Appeal to the Most Eminent Scientific Naturalists, Explorers and Historians of All Ages. Being the Substance of a Paper Read before the Anthropological Society of America* (New York: Anthropological Society, 1868), 25. Stein, in *Measuring Manhood*, notes that many of the nineteenth-century "experts" on race lived in the North and also notes the importance of Philadelphia as a center for the production of ethnological work before the war (31). See also Long, *Doctoring Freedom*, chapter 1.

5. For example, in its review of the initial volumes of the surgeon general's multi-volume work, *The Medical and Surgical History of the War of the Rebellion 1861–1865*, the *Buffalo Medical and Surgical Journal* (16, no. 1 [1876–7]: 34–36) acclaimed "it has no rival in the world, in surgical literature; its compilation marks an era in scientific progress, in the medical record of our nation, in the professional advancement of the world. . . . To American surgery it is a monument more enduring than granite" (35). The *Northwestern Medical and Surgical Journal* (3, no. 12 [1873]: 484–485) proclaimed the work as "volumes through which the dead are made to relate their agonies . . . so complete and masterly a history has never before been published by any nation ot the medical aspect of its wars" (484) and "one of the grandest works of the age" (485). United States Surgeon General's Office, *The Medical and Surgical History of the War of the Rebellion (1861–1865)*, vol. 1: *Medical History, Part 1* [1870] and vol. 2, *Surgical History, Part 1* [1870] (Washington, DC: Government Printing Office, 1870–1883). During and after the war, authors, readers, publishers, and reviewers created a greatly expanded and newly popular literary marketplace. The Union Army's Medical Department and the U.S. Sanitary Commission alone published fifty war-related titles in the quarter-century following the war; prominent medical bibliographer John Shaw Billings noted that between 1860 and 1875, at least 436 medical books were published in the United States and seventy new medical journals began publishing ("Literature and Institutions," in *A Century of American Medicine, 1776–1876*, ed. Edward Clarke et al., 289–366 [Philadelphia: Henry C. Lea, 1876], 294). The Army Medical Museum became a popular spot for tourists visiting the nation's capital, including for veterans who wished to see the specimens they had "donated" during wartime surgeries; Robert S. Henry, *The Armed Forces Institute of Pathology: Its First Century, 1862–1962* (Washington, DC: Office of the Surgeon General, 1964), 57. Ann Fabian discusses the Amy Medical Museum and Smithsonian Civil War collections in *The Skull Collectors: Race, Science, and America's Unburied Dead* (Chicago: University of Chicago Press, 2010).

6. The receipt of over 1,000 submissions is noted in Elisha Harris to the Standing Committee, February 14, 1866, Folder 20.7, Box 127, General Correspondence, Section E: Medical Committee Archives, Part IV: Historical Bureau Records, New York, NY, Archives, MssCol 22263, New York Public Library Manuscripts and Archives Division, United States Sanitary Commission (USSC) Records. Powerful and newly intersecting social and cultural forces — brought together by the war — created and shaped this new medical publishing marketplace, one that gained substantial international cultural authority as well as popularity with medical institutions and lay readers. For one contemporary assessment of the impact of this literature, see *Johnson's New Universal Cyclopaedia: Scientific and Popular Treasury of Useful Knowledge* (New York: A.J. Johnson, 1877), vol. 4: "But a vast amount of facts not of immediate practical use, but of great scientific value, were collected by the bureau in matters of profound interest to students of anthropology, to life insurance, and to the whole science of vital statistics. . . . Its reports have made it known to the whole scientific world, and probably it has added more new and valuable facts to the science of vital statistics than any one contribution at any time" (79). The Sanitary Commission kept careful records of the universities, museums, government officials, learned societies, libraries, foreign governments, and individuals nationally and internationally to whom it

sent copies of its work; see, for example, B. A. Gould to Blatchford, May 4, 1866, Folder 13, Box 69, Part IV: Historical Bureau, New York, NY, Archives, MssCol 22263, New York Public Library Manuscripts and Archives Division, USSC Records. Reviews of commission and military medical and medical science publications were printed in such newspapers and periodicals as the *New York Times, Spectator, Chicago Tribune, Western and Southern Medical Recorder, Buffalo Medical and Surgical Journal, Independent Medical Investigator, American Journal of the Medical Sciences, American Literary Gazette and Publishers' Circular, Chicago Medical Examiner, Boston Medical and Surgical Journal, Medical and Surgical Reporter, Northwestern Medical and Surgical Journal, Round Table, Medical Examiner, Medical News, British Medical Journal, Journal of Social Science,* and *Philadelphia Medical Times.*

7. Henry Bellows, 1864 Address, Folder 1, Box 15, Part II: Henry W. Bellows Papers, New York, NY, Archives, MssCol 22263, New York Public Library Manuscripts and Archives Division, USSC Records.

8. The Sanitary Commission, for example, circulated, free of cost, thousands of pamphlets and booklets among army physicians during the war, creating an eager audience for their ongoing publication concern (as Benjamin Gould noted, those circulated works directed "public attention in some degree to the fact that the Comm. Is doing scientific work as well as charitable" (Benjamin Gould to Blatchford, November 25, 1865, Folder 2, Box 67, Part IV: Historical Bureau, New York, NY, Archives, MssCol 22263, New York Public Library Manuscripts and Archives Division, USSC Records.

9. See Maria Farland, "W.E.B. DuBois, Anthropometric Science, and the Limits of Racial Uplift," *American Quarterly* 4 (December 2006): 1017–1044, especially 1021–1023.

10. Here I draw on sociologist Owen Whooley's history of nineteenth-century American medicine, *Knowledge in the Time of Cholera: The Struggle over American Medicine in the Nineteenth Century* (Chicago: University of Chicago Press, 2012), in which he reminds us that "epistemological commitments precede facts, not the other way around" (11). See also Stephanie P. Browner, *Profound Science and Elegant Literature: Imagining Doctors in Nineteenth-Century America* (Philadelphia: University of Pennsylvania Press, 2005), chapter 6. The extensive scholarship on the history of racial ideologies and racial constructions in the United States provides an important starting point for the questions raised by this chapter. I have relied on Karen E. Fields and Barbara J. Fields, *Racecraft: The Soul of Inequality in American Life* (London: Verso Books, 2012); Nancy Stepan, *The Idea of Race in Science: Great Britain, 1800–1960* (London: Macmillan Press, 1982); and Jennifer L. Morgan, *Laboring Women: Reproduction and Gender in New World Slavery* (Philadelphia: University of Pennsylvania Press, 2004).

11. H. Glenn Penny aptly describes ethnology in late nineteenth-century Germany as a "public science" appealing to the "cosmopolitan interests of many autodidacts and educated elites" (228), in "The Civic Uses of Science: Ethnology and Civil Society in Imperial Germany," *Osiris* 17 (2002): 228–252.

12. See Oz Frankel, *States of Inquiry: Social Investigations and Print Culture in Nineteenth-Century Britain and the United States* (Baltimore: Johns Hopkins University Press, 2006), which very usefully overviews the history of nineteenth-century state

investigations in the United States and Great Britain; see also James H. Cassedy, "Numbering the North's Medical Events: Humanitarianism and Science in Civil War Statistics," *Bulletin of the History of Medicine* 66 (1992): 210–233.

13. L. P. Brockett, *The Philanthropic Results of the War in America Collected from Official and Authentic Sources* (New York: Sheldon & Co., 1864), and United States Sanitary Commission, *Hints for the Control and Prevention of Infectious Diseases in Camps, Transports, and Hospitals* (New York: Wm. C. Bryant & Co., 1863). These would later be collected and published as United States Sanitary Commission, *Military Medical and Surgical Essays Prepared for the United States Sanitary Commission 1862–1864*, vol. 1, nos. 1–60, and vol. 2, nos. 61–95 (Washington, DC: 1865).

14. Frederick Law Olmsted, *[Confidential] Report of the Secretary with Regard to the Probable Origin of the Recent Demoralization of the Volunteer Army at Washington and the Duty of the Sanitary Commission with Regard to Certain Deficiencies in the Existing Army Arrangements as Suggested Thereby* (Washington, DC: McGill & Witherow, Printers, 1861), 4. Unlike later commission investigations, this one relied almost entirely on qualitative evidence in the form of anecdote.

15. Bonnie E. Blustein, "'To Increase the Efficiency of the Medical Department': A New Approach to U.S. Civil War Medicine," *Civil War History* 33 (1987): 22–41; Frank Freemon, "Lincoln Finds a Surgeon General: William A. Hammond and the Transformation of the Union Army Medical Bureau," *Civil War History* 33 (1987): 5–21; Jeanie Attie, *Patriotic Toil: Northern Women and the American Civil War* (Ithaca, NY: Cornell University Press, 1998), 116; and William Quentin Maxwell, *Lincoln's Fifth Wheel: The Political History of the United States Sanitary Commission* (New York: Longmans, Green & Co., 1956), 122–143.

16. E. B. Elliott, *Preliminary Report on the Mortality and Sickness of the Volunteer Forces of the United States Government, during the Present War. Sanitary Commission, no. 46* (New York: Wm. C. Bryant & Co., Printers, 1862). Elliott presented his report to the International Statistical Congress in Berlin in 1863, which he published as *On the Military Statistics of the United States of America* (Berlin: R.V. Decker, 1863). On the bureau, see Charles Stillé, *History of the U.S. Sanitary Commission, Being the General Report of Its Work during the War of the Rebellion* (Philadelphia: J.B. Lippincott & Co., 1866), chapter 17.

17. In addition to Margaret Humphreys, *Intensely Human: The Health of the Black Soldier in the American Civil War* (Baltimore: Johns Hopkins University Press, 2008), see Richard M. Reid, ed., *Practicing Medicine in a Black Regiment: The Civil War Diary of Burt G. Wilder, 55th Massachusetts* (Amherst: University of Massachusetts Press, 2010), 1–39; J. H. Baxter, *Statistics, Medical and Anthropological, of the Provost-Marshal-General's Bureau, Derived from Records of the Examination for Military Service in the Armies of the United States during the Late War of the Rebellion, of over a Million Recruits, Drafted Men, Substitutes, and Enrolled Men: Compiled under Direction of the Secretary of War* (Washington, DC: Government Printing Office, 1875), part 3, 171–502 (containing reports of Surgeons of State Boards of Enrollment, with extensive commentary on the perceived anatomy and physiology of Black recruits); and Sanford B. Hunt, "The Negro as a Soldier," *Quarterly Journal of Psychological Medicine and Medical Jurisprudence* 1 (October 1867): 161–186. The General Correspondence files of the USSC Statistical

Bureau Archives offer extensive correspondence documenting the people and projects relating to the collection of data about African American soldiers. Many of the correspondents contributed to the material reported by Benjamin A. Gould in *Investigations in the Military and Anthropological Statistics of American Soldiers* (Cambridge, MA: Riverside Press, 1869), published by the U.S. Sanitary Commission.

18. This is a reference to the "Unknown Contraband File," Box 1172, Entry 225: Consolidated Correspondence Files, Record Group 92: Records of the Quartermaster General, National Archives and Records Administration (NARA), Washington, DC, in which requests for removal and burial of the corpses of both unidentified and identified African Americans from the streets, alleys, camps, and hospitals of wartime Washington, DC, are collected. Thanks to Kate Masur for pointing me to this material.

19. Teresa A. Goddu, "The Antislavery Almanac and the Discourse of Numeracy," *Book History* 12 (2009): 129–131. An important precedent to this use of military medical statistics in the service of racial ideology can be found decades earlier in Alexander Tulloch's 1838 study of medical data for Black and white British troops stationed in the West Indies. Tulloch's study endorsed the then-prevalent view that Black troops enjoyed racial advantages but also suffered from some racial susceptibilities to disease. His study was used (and historian Tim Lockley argues, misused) to support the notion that Black troops were racially distinct and therefore advantageous to use in the climates of the West Indies. Tulloch's report was circulated widely in the United States (including a copy forwarded to the U.S. surgeon general), and American ethnologists used Tulloch's work to support their claims that race was immutably inscribed on the human body. See Lockley, *Military Medicine and the Making of Race: Life and Death in the West India Regiments, 1795–1874* (New York: Cambridge University Press, 2020).

20. See Heather Lee Cooper, "Upstaging *Uncle Tom's Cabin*: African American Representations of Slavery on the Public Stage before and after the Civil War" (PhD diss., University of Iowa, 2017).

21. See, for example, Frederick L. Hoffman, *Race Traits and Tendencies of the American Negro* (New York: Macmillan Co., 1896); Charles B. Davenport and Albert G. Love, *The Medical Department of the United States Army in the World War*, vol. 15 of *Statistics, Part One: Army Anthropology* (Washington, DC: United States Government Printing Office, 1921); and Aleš Hrdlička, "Anthropology of the American Negro: Historical Notes," *American Journal of Physical Anthropology* 5 (April–June 1927): 205–221. Lundy Braun traces the use of spirometry in race science after Gould's use of the technique in "Spirometry, Measurement, and Race in the Nineteenth Century," *Journal of the History of Medicine and Allied Sciences* 2 (April 2005): 135–169; Farland explores Du Bois's critique of those data in "W.E.B. DuBois," 1021–1023. See also Frank Spencer, "Anthropometry," in *History of Physical Anthropology: An Encyclopedia*, vol. 1, ed. Frank Spencer, 80–90 (New York: Garland, 1997), which firmly places Gould's work in a long-lasting and significant history of racial classification and study.

22. Brooks's circular specifically asked for comments on Black soldiers' courage under fire, the quality and quantity of work they could perform, the kind of work Black men excelled at, and differences between Northern and Southern Blacks; United States War Department, *The War of the Rebellion: A Compilation of Official Records of the*

Union and Confederate Armies (Washington, DC: Government Printing Office, 1880–1901), series 1, vol. 28, part 1, 328–329. Brooks' reference to the "experiment" seems to ignore the fact that a regiment of Black South Carolinians had been serving for nearly a year already.

23. Whooley notes these as familiar modes of knowledge claims in *Knowledge in the Time of Cholera*, 45–47.

24. H. K. Neff to Surgeon G. H. Brinton, September 24, 1863, Folder N, 19th century Incoming Letters, OHA 25: Curatorial Records: Smithsonian Correspondence, Otis Historical Archives, National Museum of Health and Medicine (NMHM), Silver Spring, Maryland.

25. Woodward (1811–1887) enlisted as a surgeon in the 22nd Illinois, serving until July 1864, when he apparently gained appointment as a medical inspector in the Mississippi valley with the Sanitary Commission. See Finding Aid, Woodward Family papers, SC 2825, Abraham Lincoln Presidential Library, Springfield, IL.; and J. S. Newberry, *The U.S. Sanitary Commission in the Valley of the Mississippi, during the War of the Rebellion, 1861–1866* (Cleveland: Fairbanks, Benedict & Co., 1871), 160. Born in England, Woodward emigrated in 1823 and appears in the 1850 census as a physician, resident of Henry County, Illinois, and married with six children (Microfilm Roll 4, list number 341, *Registers of Vessels Arriving at the Port of New York from Foreign Ports, 1789–1919*, and Seventh Census of the United States, 1850, both accessed at Ancestry.com, May 19, 2015). The circular and the letter that Woodward used to instruct respondents can be found in Folder 1.2, Box 108, Section E: Medical Committee Archives, Part IV: Historical Bureau Records, New York, NY, Archives, MssCol 22263, New York Public Library Manuscripts and Archives Division, USSC Records.

26. B. Woodward to Dr. E. Harris, August 20, 1865, in Folder 1.2, Box 108, Section E: Medical Committee Archives, Part IV: Historical Bureau Records, New York, NY, Archives, MssCol. 22263, New York Public Library Manuscripts and Archives Division, USSC Records.

27. John Harley Warner, *The Therapeutic Perspective: Medical Practice, Knowledge, and Identity in America, 1820–1885* (Cambridge, MA: Harvard University Press, 1986), 11–82, and *Against the Spirit of System: The French Impulse in Nineteenth-Century American Medicine* (Princeton, NJ: Princeton University Press, 1998), chapter 7; Charles E. Rosenberg, "The Therapeutic Revolution: Medicine, Meaning, and Social Change in Nineteenth-Century America," *Perspectives in Biology and Medicine* 20 (1977): 485–506; and Whooley, *Knowledge in the Time of Cholera*, chapter 2.

28. See John Harley Warner, "The Fall and Rise of Professional Mystery: Epistemology, Authority, and the Emergence of Laboratory Medicine in Nineteenth-Century America," in *The Laboratory Revolution in Medicine*, ed. Andrew Cunningham and Perry Williams, 110–141 (Cambridge: Cambridge University Press, 1992); and Whooley, *Knowledge in the Time of Cholera*.

29. Browner, *Profound Science*, 182–186.

30. Dr. E. B. Wright to Dr. Woodward, n.d., Folder 9, Box 110, Section E: Medical Committee Archives, Part IV: Historical Bureau Records, New York, NY, Archives, MssCol 22263, New York Public Library Manuscripts and Archives Division, USSC Records.

31. The extant records include direct responses to the circular as well as Woodward's summaries of observations from several respondents. Woodward's "Observations on Injuries, and Repair" (on muscle development, feet, tread, legs, slouch, as well as rapid digestion, overwork, and vigor), Folder 4.4, and B. Woodward, "Reports on Diseases of Colored Troops" (on abdomen and size of colon, mental vigor, overwork, as well as susceptibility to disease), n.d., Folder 4.7, both in Box 111; Dr. O. M. Long, "Letter and Report from Dr. O. M. Long, New Orleans," n.d. (a great feeder; vigor), and "Dr. Pequette on Colored Soldiers" (endurance, overwork), November 13, 1865, both in Folder 10.11, Box 117; Dr. E. B. Wright to Dr. Woodward (a great feeder; physical and mental vigor), n.d., Folder 9, Box 110; Dr. Geo. L. Andrew, "Report to July 17 1865" (susceptibility to disease), and B. Woodward, "Regt. Surgeons' Notes on Colored Troops. B. W." (susceptibility to disease), n.d., both in Folder 1.6, Box 108; Dr. Russell, "The Negro in Hospital" (susceptibility to disease), Analytical index to surgical and medical reports and essays, Box 132; James Russell, "Report on Hospitals in Richmond, Norfolk, etc." (on vigor), n.d., item 338, and "Dr. Russell's Report [illegible] Hospital L'Overture" (endurance), both in Box 112, Section E: Medical Committee Archives, Part IV: Historical Bureau Records, New York, NY, Archives, MssCol 22263, New York Public Library Manuscripts and Archives Division, USSC Records.

32. Woodward's "Observations on Injuries, and Repair," Folder 4.4, Box 111, Section E: Medical Committee Archives, Part IV: Historical Bureau Records, New York, NY, Archives, MssCol 22263, New York Public Library Manuscripts and Archives Division, USSC Records.

33. Baxter, *Statistics, Medical and Anthropological*, 161–162. The examiners' responses are included on 171–502.

34. Baxter, *Statistics, Medical and Anthropological*, 270 ("facts"); 331 (historical or biblical fact); 359 ("universal opinion"); 173, 391 ("belief"); 237, 361 (familiarity with ethnology).

35. Baxter, *Statistics, Medical and Anthropological*, 390, 394, 449 (slavery as good training for soldiers); 285 (anatomical racism); 173 ("just enough animal"); 461 ("the usefulness of the horse"); 368–69 (specialized racial knowledge).

36. See Sharla M. Fett, *Working Cures: Healing, Health, and Power on Southern Slave Plantations* (Chapel Hill: University of North Carolina Press, 2002).

37. Deirdre Cooper Owens, *Medical Bondage: Race, Gender, and the Origins of American Gynecology* (Athens: University of Georgia Press, 2017), 77.

38. Baxter, *Statistics, Medical and Anthropological*. The few characterizations of Irish men are found on 192 (notes "abundant vitality" of Irish), 253–255 (impoverished and suffering from a poorer physique than Americans and other Europeans), 285 (like the English, inferior to the American), 314 ("intemperate, dirty, unhealthy"), 324–325 (lacking moral and intellectual qualifications for good soldiering), 369 (sometimes offering an excellent physique, like the Canadians), 448 ("brave and daring" but also "impulsive, impetuous, and rash").

39. "Address of H. W. Bellows, D. D. President to the Full Board of the United States Sanitary Commission at its session held in Washington D.C. Oct 25th 1864," Mss. Draft, Folder 1, Box 15, Part II: Henry W. Bellows Papers, New York, NY, Archives, MssCol 22263, New York Public Library Manuscripts and Archives Division, USSC Records.

40. The antebellum history of anthropometry is outlined in Haller, *Outcasts from Evolution*; Braun, "Spirometry, Measurement, and Race," 136–146; and Michael Tavel Clarke, "Andrometer," *Victorian Review* 34 (2008): 22–28. See also Michael Yudell, *Race Unmasked: Biology and Race in the Twentieth Century* (Ithaca, NY: Cornell University Press, 2014), 1–11; and Tracy Teslow, *Constructing Race: The Science of Bodies and Cultures in American Anthropology* (Cambridge: Cambridge University Press, 2014).

41. Ian Hacking, "Biopower and the Avalanche of Printed Numbers," *Humanities in Society* 5 (1992): 279–295.

42. James H. Cassedy, *American Medicine and Statistical Thinking, 1800–1860* (Cambridge, MA: Harvard University Press, 1984), 230, and "Numbering the North's Medical Events: Humanitarianism and Science in Civil War Statistics," *Bulletin of the History of Medicine* 66 (1992): 210–233.

43. Frankel, *States of Inquiry*, 144.

44. Frankel, *States of Inquiry*, 75. Among Frankel's many astute observations is his point that "nineteenth-century social inquiries were formalized in a culture that had already been conditioned to associate print with the rendering of facts, either in journalism, science, or, as importantly, the law" (11).

45. Gould, *Investigations*, 221, 218. On Gould's professional career, see George C. Comstock, "Biographical Memoir Benjamin Apthorp Gould, 1824–1896," in *National Academy of Sciences Biographical Memoir*, ed. National Academy of Sciences, 155–180 (Washington, DC: Government Printing Office, 1924).

46. Marc Rothenberg et al., eds., *The Papers of Joseph Henry* (Sagamore Beach, MA: Science History, 2004), 10:211–212. In 1858, the American Academy of Natural Sciences enthusiastically supported a similar proposal from physician and future USSC member S. Weir Mitchell to collect "physical statistics of our native born white race." Mitchell's project later gained the approval of the Smithsonian Institution. Perhaps this was the identical endeavor; see Academy of the Natural Sciences of Philadelphia, *Proceedings of the Academy of the Natural Sciences of Philadelphia, 1858* (Philadelphia: Printed for the Academy, 1859), 23, 26–27; S. Weir Mitchell to Oliver Wendell Holmes, [1859], cited in Cynthia J. Davis, *Bodily and Narrative Forms: The Influence of Medicine on Medical Literature, 1845–1915* (Stanford, CA: Stanford University Press, 2000), 199–200 (full date not provided); Nancy Cervetti, *S. Weir Mitchell, 1829–1914: Philadelphia's Literary Physician* (University Park, PA: Pennsylvania State University Press, 2012), 138; Oliver Wendell Holmes to Silas Weir Mitchell, March 8, 1860, S. Weir Mitchell Collection, Duke University Library, Durham, NC. On Olmsted's study, see Jane Turner Censer, ed., *The Papers of Frederick Law Olmsted* (Baltimore: Johns Hopkins University Press, 1986), 6:250n6, 681–683. On the Smithsonian study, see Censer, *Papers of Frederick Law Olmsted*, 4:51–52. Notably, on the eve of the war, Henry asserted that slavery was in accordance with both modern civilization and science and in 1862 refused to allow Frederick Douglass to lecture in a Smithsonian room; Robert V. Bruce, *The Launching of Modern American Science, 1846–1876* (New York: Alfred A. Knopf, 1987), 271, 275.

47. Rothenberg et al., *Papers of Joseph Henry*, 10:212.

48. Censer, *Papers of Frederick Law Olmsted*, 4:51–52, 6:250n6, and 6:681–683. In Form E, which was used only prior to Gould's move to measure Black soldiers, question 16 required inspectors to determine "from appearances and statements of the

subject" whether the soldier is "of American stock of three or more generations," followed up with questions about when he or his family had been born if outside the United States. Like Baxter, Gould understood nationality—which he understood that only whites held—as a subclass of race (*Investigations*, 226).

49. "Three or more distinct races of negroes are to be found in the Southern States" (Gould, *Investigations*, 297). On measurements of the Iroquois, see pages 308–311. The Statistical Bureau's efforts to obtained thousands of additional measurements among Dakota, Oneida, and Cherokee people are documented in the correspondence of examiners such as S. Buckley in Boxes 2 and 3, Letters Received, 1864 January–1869 October, and undated, Part I: Administrative Records, Statistical Bureau Archives, MssCol 18780, New York Public Library Manuscripts and Archives Division, USSC Records. By mid-July 1864, Gould was strenuously arguing in favor of appointing "a large force of inspectors" to investigate Black troops (B. A. Gould to Dr. J. Foster Jenkins, July 12, 1864, Folder 1, Box 10, Part I: Administrative Records, Statistical Bureau Archives, MssCol 18780, New York Public Library Manuscripts and Archives Division, USSC Records).

50. Gould, *Investigations*, 298, where we see this usage of "class" made explicit. See page 228 on his estimation of Quetelet.

51. Gould, *Investigations*, 246. Gould revered Quetelet as "the founder of statistical anthropology." However, not all of Gould's colleagues in the commission fully understood the statistical work Gould so valued. Writing to Gould after reading the completed volume, George Templeton Strong noted, "My favorite passage is that in which you allude to the fact that 'h = [triangle] × [over] nv [pie].' This is touching. I am sorry you are not a little more definite as to the '*Probable* Error of the Mean,' as I have always found the errors of mean people to vary with individual temperament so as to defy calculation. Seriously, though so much of the report is utterly beyond me, I can see that it embodies the results of numeric labor & analysis, & I fully believe what I hear from those more competent to judge than I am—that it is a most important contribution to science." G. T. Strong to B. A. Gould, April 15, 1869, Folder 22, Box 1, Part I: Administrative Records, Statistical Bureau Archives, MssCol 18780, New York Public Library Manuscripts and Archives Division, USSC Records.

52. Elisha Harris to Maj. Genl. Weitzel, May 28, 1865, Item 158, Box 109, Section E: Medical Committee Archives, Part IV: Historical Bureau Records, New York, NY, Archives, MssCol 22263, New York Public Library Manuscripts and Archives Division, USSC Records.

53. Elisha Harris to Maj. Genl. Weitzel, May 28, 1865, and Elisha Harris to B. A. Gould, October 26, 1865, Folder 8, Box 1, Part I: Administrative Records, Statistical Bureau Archives, MssCol 18780, New York Public Library Manuscripts and Archives Division, USSC Records. Gould held definitive ideas about the physiology of race— that the North American "race" was larger than the European, including and especially in brain size; that European immigrants gained a "lost manhood" on coming to the United States. See B. A. Gould to Dr. Elisha Harris, January 16, 1866, Box 119, Section E: Medical Committee Archives, Part IV: Historical Bureau Records, New York, NY, Archives, MssCol 22263, New York Public Library Manuscripts and Archives Division, USSC Records.

54. Elisha Harris to Dr. C. R. Agnew, July 22, 1865, Item 118, Box 109, Section E: Medical Committee Archives, Part IV: Historical Bureau Records, New York, NY, Archives, MssCol 22263, New York Public Library Manuscripts and Archives Division, USSC Records. The army and the commission became heated rivals for prominence, authority, and recognition in the realm of medical science; each claimed to offer the first, most complete, most accurate reports on and histories of wartime medicine.

55. S. B. Buckley to B. A. Gould, January 5, 1865, Box 2, Part I: Administrative Records, Statistical Bureau Archives, MssCol 18780, New York Public Library Manuscripts and Archives Division, USSC Records. Buckley was quoting a comment made to him by a military commander in the eastern theater.

56. The most useful sources for Gould's biography include Comstock, "Biographical Memoir Benjamin Apthorp Gould"; and Owen Gingerich, "Benjamin Apthorp Gould and the Founding of the Astronomical Journal," *Astronomy Journal* 117 (1999): 1–5.

57. Gould, *Investigations*, 221. Agassiz, a Swiss-born scientist, became intently involved in the American debates over race and was frank about his revulsion toward African Americans. In 1850 he commissioned a series of daguerreotypes of enslaved South Carolinian men and women, African-born, intent on producing evidence of racial types. See Brian Wallis, "Black Bodies, White Science: Louis Agassiz's Slave Daguerreotypes," *American Art* 9 (1995): 38–61.

58. The forms recording measurements of Black soldiers are in Boxes 109–120, Physical Examinations 1863 January–1866 May and undated, Part VII: Physical Examinations, Statistical Bureau Archives, MssCol 18780, New York Public Library Manuscripts and Archives Division, USSC Records. Michael Tavel Clarke explains of the apparatus: the andrometer "measured stature, neck width, shoulder width, waist size, leg length, and height to knee"; the "spirometer (a box with a gauge and breathing tube used to measure lung capacity), the goniometer (a sort of protractor with moveable arms that was eventually deemed unreliable), a dynamometer (a platform with a waist-high handlebar attached to a gauge for measuring strength in pulling upward), a platform-balance (a weight scale), calipers (used for measurements such as head width and distance between the nipples), and measuring tape (for measuring head and waist circumference, among other things)"; "Andrometer," 23, 24.

59. Gould, *Investigations*, 239.

60. Gould describes the history of the project in Gould, *Investigations*, 218–240. The forms recording measurements of Black soldiers are in Boxes 109–120, Part VII: Physical Examinations, Statistical Bureau Archives, MssCol 18780, New York Public Library Manuscripts and Archives Division, USSC Records. It should also be noted that Gould's *Investigations* offers several tables separating out for comparative purposes findings on Irish soldiers (age, stature, lifting strength, etc.). He offers no statement explaining why he offers the data and no conclusions about their significance.

61. Geo. A. Blake to Benj. Collins Esq., June 9, 1865, Box 1, Part I: Administrative Records, Statistical Bureau Archives, MssCol 18780, New York Public Library Manuscripts and Archives Division, USSC Records. Blake repeated this phrasing in other USSC correspondence, referring to "the length, breadth, thickness, capacity and comparative anatomy of several Ethiopians" in his letter to the office of the Statistical Department in Washington, DC, also on June 9, 1865 (Geo. A. Black to the Statistical

Department, June 9, 1865, Vol. 3, p. 42, Box 3, Part I: Main Office, Department of the Gulf, MssCol 18950, New York Public Library Manuscripts and Archives Division, USSC Records). The roster of examiners and clerks employed by the Statistical Bureau changed monthly; the largest number of examiners were employed in the spring of 1865 (Folder 17, Box 105, Part IV: USSC Staff Rosters, Accounts and Vouchers Archive, MssCol 18820, New York Public Library Manuscripts and Archives Division, USSC Records). Examiners were paid $100 per month (Samuel H. Stebbins to B. A. Gould, October 8, 1864, Folder 7, Box 1, Part I: Administrative Records, Statistical Bureau Archives, MssCol 18780, New York Public Library Manuscripts and Archives Division, USSC Records.

62. S. B. Buckley to B. A. Gould, December 1, 1864, December 6, 1864, and December 7, 1864, all in Folder 25; and S. B. Buckley to B. A. Gould, February 19, 1865, Folder 27, all in Box 2, Part I: Administrative Records, Statistical Bureau Archives, MssCol 18780, New York Public Library Manuscripts and Archives Division, USSC Records.

63. C. D. Lewis to B. A. Gould, February 20, 1865, Box 2, Part I: Administrative Records, Statistical Bureau Archives, MssCol 18780, New York Public Library Manuscripts and Archives Division, USSC Records.

64. James Russell to B. A. Gould, June 4, 1865, Box 3, Examiners, Letters Received, Statistical Bureau Archives, MssCol 18780, New York Public Library Manuscripts and Archives Division, USSC Records. Russell rated the pilosity of 2,129 Black soldiers on a scale he invented from 1 to 10; Gould, *Investigations*, 368–369. On race, pilosity, and manhood, see Stein, *Measuring Manhood*.

65. Thomas Furniss to B. A. Gould, March 17, 1866, Box 2, Part I: Administrative Records, Statistical Bureau Archives, MssCol 18780, New York Public Library Manuscripts and Archives Division, USSC Records.

66. B. A. Gould to Harris, December 25, 1865, Box 119, Section E: Medical Committee Archives, Part IV: Historical Bureau Records, New York, NY, Archives, MssCol 22263, New York Public Library Manuscripts and Archives Division, USSC Records.

67. William S. Baker to B. A. Gould, August 28, 1865, Folder 23, Box 2, Part I: Administrative Records, Statistical Bureau Archives, MssCol 18780, New York Public Library Manuscripts and Archives Division, USSC Records.

68. Thomas Furniss to B. A. Gould, February 19, 1866, April 10, 1866, and May 7, 1866, Box 2, and James Russell to B. A. Gould, April 14, 1865 (on records being stolen), Box 3, Part I: Administrative Records, Statistical Bureau Archives, New York Public Library Manuscripts and Archives Division, USSC Records.

69. H. T. Myers to B. A. Gould, May 10, 1866, and James Russell to B. A. Gould, October 9, 1865 (on refusing to disrobe), Box 3; Thomas Furniss to B. A. Gould, February 19, 1866 (on officers' orders), Box 2, Part I: Administrative Records, Statistical Bureau Archives, MssCol 18780, New York Public Library Manuscripts and Archives Division, USSC Records.

70. Thomas Furniss to B. A. Gould, March 17, 1866, Box 2, Part I: Administrative Records, Statistical Bureau Archives, MssCol 18780, New York Public Library Manuscripts and Archives Division, USSC Records.

71. James Russell to B. A. Gould, May 19, 1865, Box 3, Part I: Administrative Records, Statistical Bureau Archives, MssCol 18780, New York Public Library Manuscripts

and Archives Division, USSC Records. Russell's report of their average spirometer reading (131 inches) placed their lung capacity well below the averages for men of all races tested. Their lifting strength (248 pounds) approximated that of teenagers under the age of seventeen who were tested (Gould, *Investigations*, 471, 465). The eminent sports historian Professor Jan Todd (University of Texas at Austin) explained in a phone conversation with the author (October 10, 2020) that dynamometers were fairly popular devices; they were found in nineteenth-century gyms devoted to what was then called "health lifting," and they also were found at circus sideshows, fairs, and on city street corners where passersby could, for a penny, try their hand. See Jan Todd, *Physical Culture and the Body Beautiful: Purposive Exercise in the Lives of American Women, 1800–1870* (Macon, GA: Mercer University Press, 1998), especially chapter 7.

72. Elisha Harris to B. A. Gould, September 9, 1865, and October 26, 1865, Folder 8, Box 1, Part I: Administrative Records, Statistical Bureau Archives, MssCol 18780, New York Public Library Manuscripts and Archives Division, USSC Records.

73. The recruiting service in New York City, for example, came under attack by the *New York Times*, and surgeons feared the Sanitary Commission investigators would find further reason to criticize their work; see S. B. Buckley to B. A. Gould, January 6, 1865, Folder 26, Box 2, Part I: Administrative Records, Statistical Bureau, MssCol 18780, New York Public Library Manuscripts and Archives Division, USSC Records. Strategic secrecy about the location or transport of troops also contributed to the difficulties encountered by examiners.

74. William S. Baker to B. A. Gould, February 7, 1865, Folder 22, Box 2, Part I: Administrative Records, Statistical Bureau Archives, MssCol 18780, New York Public Library Manuscripts and Archives Division, USSC Records.

75. S. B. Buckley to B. A. Gould, February 26, 1865, Folder 28, Box 2, Part I: Administrative Records, Statistical Bureau Archives, MssCol 18780, New York Public Library Manuscripts and Archives Division, USSC Records.

76. H. T. Myers to B. A. Gould, May 10, 1865, Folder 33, Box 3, Part I: Administrative Records, Statistical Bureau Archives, MssCol 18780, New York Public Library Manuscripts and Archives Division, USSC Records.

77. James Russell to B. A. Gould, n.d., Folder 3.10, Box 3, General Corr., Part I, Statistical Bureau Archives, 1861–1869, MssCol 18780, New York Public Library Manuscripts and Archives Division, USSC Records.

78. George W. Avery to B. A. Gould, February 6, 1866, Folder 1, Box 2, Part I: Administrative Records, Statistical Bureau Archives, MssCol 18780, New York Public Library Manuscripts and Archives Division, USSC Records.

79. William S. Baker to B. A. Gould, March 26, 1865, Folder 22, Box 2, Part I: Administrative Records, Statistical Bureau Archives, MssCol 18780, New York Public Library Manuscripts and Archives Division, USSC Records.

80. S. B. Buckley to B. A. Gould, May 28, 1865, Folder 29, Box 2, Part I: Administrative Records, Statistical Bureau Archives, MssCol 18780, New York Public Library Manuscripts and Archives Division, USSC Records.

81. Gould notes these in *Investigations*, 228–229, 232–233, 270.

82. Gould, *Investigations*, 238.

83. Gould, *Investigations*, 320, 360.

84. Gould, *Investigations*, 297.

85. Gould, *Investigations*, 319.

86. Elisha Harris to B. A. Gould, n.d. [likely summer 1865], Folder 8, Box 1, Part I: Administrative Records, Statistical Bureau Archives, MssCol 18780, New York Public Library Manuscripts and Archives Division, USSC Records.

87. The authority that works like Gould's invested in racialized medicine could be seen in articles like "Hospital Observations upon Negro Soldiers," by Dr. A. W. Mc-Dowell, who had been stationed in Benton Barracks, St. Louis, during the war. Mc-Dowell reported, based on his observations of the living and autopsies performed on the deceased, that a substantial number of anatomical differences between African Americans and whites could be observed, from the size of the pectoral muscles to the size of the penis. Of those reported differences, he noted, "I present no opinions, but simply physical facts." *American Practitioner* (July 1874): 155–158.

88. United States Sanitary Commission Statistical Bureau, *Ages of U.S. Volunteer Soldiery* (Cambridge, MA: University Press, 1866).

89. Lucius Brown to Blatchford, May 7, 1866, Folder 13, Box 69, Section A: Office Correspondence, Part IV: Historical Bureau Correspondence, New York, NY, Archives, MssCol 22263, New York Public Library Manuscripts and Archives Division, USSC Records.

90. Henry W. Bellows to "My Dear Hale," November 7, 1866, pp. 62–63, Vol. 2 Box 4, Part I: Standing Committee Records, New York, New York Archives, MssCol 22263, New York Public Library Manuscripts and Archives Division, USSC Records.

91. Reviews were published in such newspapers and periodicals as the *New York Times, North American Review, Spectator, Chicago Tribune, Roundtable, American Literary Gazette and Publishers' Circular, Medical Examiner, Medical News, Chicago Medical Examiner, Boston Medical and Surgical Journal, Medical and Surgical Reporter, Northwestern Medical and Surgical Journal, Western and Southern Medical Reporter, Buffalo Medical and Surgical Journal, Independent Medical Investigator, American Journal of the Medical Sciences, British Medical Journal, Journal of Social Science*, and *Philadelphia Medical Times*.

92. Stillé, *History of the U.S. Sanitary Commission*, 465; Prospectuses, Folder 1, Box 79, Section A: Office Correspondence, Part IV: Historical Bureau Records, New York, NY, Archives; MssCol 22263, New York Public Library Manuscripts and Archives Division, USSC Records; Margaret Humphreys, *Marrow of Tragedy: The Health Crisis of the American Civil War* (Baltimore: Johns Hopkins University Press, 2013), 145–150.

93. The six-volume *Medical and Surgical History of the War of the Rebellion 1861–1865*, published by Surgeon General Joseph Barnes between 1870 and 1888, opens with an introduction that explains its approach to race, illness, and mortality: "The propriety of endeavoring to present separately such facts as it has been possible to collect, with regard to the sickness and mortality of Colored Soldiers, would appear too obvious to require extended remark in this place. Aside from all considerations of a scientific or historical nature, motives of humanity would seem to dictate that the statistics should be presented in the form most likely to render them serviceable as a contribution to our knowledge of the influence of race-peculiarities on disease. . . . The enlisted men of these regiments, however, included, besides persons of African descent, many of mixed African and European blood, and the returns afforded no available means for

discrimination" (part I, vol. 1, 13). The volumes resembled Gould's work in the assemblage of largely undigested tabulated numerical data (in part 1, vol. 1) and case reports grouped by categories of wounds and disease (in the remaining volumes). Although the numerical data are always separated by race, there are few inferences offered. The five later volumes, in which case reports of Black and white troops are intermingled, occasionally venture an explanation for information that seemed counterintuitive to contemporary racial thought. One example, in part 3, vol. 1, commented on the data about illness and mortality from malarial fevers and noted that the higher mortality rate among Black troops challenged the belief that people of African descent were not susceptible to malaria (6, 13). In part 3, vol. 2, there is also occasional reference to the stationing of Black troops in the least healthy regions as an explanation for the higher rates of disease (85). The higher mortality rate among Black troops from diarrheal disease and dysentery as well as consumption is speculated to be an artifact of Black men's homelessness: white soldiers were more often discharged due to serious illness, whereas men who enlisted out of slavery had no apparent home to return to—and were, it is speculated, kept in hospitals until their death, skewing the mortality rates among them (819). One of the most notable features of the volumes are the exhaustive footnotes, which trace reports on wounds and disease in the medical literature.

94. Hunt, "Negro as a Soldier," 40–54. The *Review* was published by the Anthropological Society of London, formed in 1863 specifically for the purposes of advancing racial science and to advance the role of racial scientists within the anthropological professions; see Afram Sera-Shriar, "Observing Human Difference: James Hunt, Thomas Huxley and Competing Disciplinary Strategies in the 1860s." *Annals of Science* 70 (2013): 461–491; and James Hunt, "Introductory Address on the Study of Anthropology," *Anthropological Review* 1 (May 1863): 1–20. Sandford Hunt's 1867 article received a positive notice in the widely circulated periodical, *The Nation* 5, no. 118 (October 3, 1867): 268–269.

95. United States Census Office, Department of the Interior, *Instructions to U.S. Marshals, Instructions to Assistants, Eighth Census, United States,—Act of Congress of Twenty-Third May, 1850* (Washington, DC: Geo. W. Bowman, Public Printer, 1860), 15; and Census Office, Department of the Interior, *Instructions to U.S. Marshals, Instructions to Assistants, Eighth Census, United States, —Act of Congress of Twenty-Third May, 1850* (Washington, DC: Geo. W. Bowman, Public Printer, 1860), 10.

Chapter Four

1. Historian Mark Harrison notes that one of the "most important advantages" enjoyed by British military surgeons in the century following 1750 was "the constant supply of fresh corpses for dissection, which enabled them to ground their clinical practice much more firmly upon post-mortem examinations." "Disease and Medicine in the Armies of British India, 1750–1830: The Treatment of Fevers and the Emergence of Tropical Therapeutics," in *British Military and Naval Medicine, 1600–1830*, ed. Geoffrey Hudson, 84–119 (Amsterdam: Rodopi, 2007), 89.

2. Michael Sappol finds that in the antebellum era "anatomy conferred epistemological credibility," in *A Traffic in Dead Bodies: Anatomy and Embodied Social Identity in Nineteenth-Century America* (Princeton, NJ: Princeton University Press, 2002), 55.

3. See Susan C. Lawrence, "Reading Civil War Medical Cases" and "Medical and Surgical Cases: Sources and Methods," both in *Civil War Washington*, ed. Susan C. Lawrence et al. (Lincoln: Center for Digital Research, University of Nebraska, 2006), at http://civilwardc.org/interpretations/narrative/rcwmc.php and http://civilwardc .org/texts/cases/about, respectively.

4. On dissection and autopsy, see Nystrom, ed., *The Bioarchaeology of Dissection and Autopsy in the United States* (New York: Springer, 2017); David C. Humphrey, "Dissection and Discrimination: The Social Origins of Cadavers in America, 1760–1915," *Bulletin of the New York Academy of Medicine* 49 (1973): 819–827; Sappol, *Traffic in Dead Bodies*; Edward C. Halperin, "The Poor, the Black, and the Marginalized as the Source of Cadavers in United States Anatomical Education," *Clinical Anatomy* 20, no. 5 (2007): 489–496; Daina Ramey Berry, *The Price for Their Pound of Flesh: The Value of the Enslaved, from Womb to Grave, in the Building of a Nation* (Boston: Beacon Press, 2017), 148–193; and Stephen C. Kenny, "The Development of Medical Museums in the Antebellum American South: Slave Bodies in Networks of Anatomical Exchange," *Bulletin of the History of Medicine* 87 (Spring 2013): 32–62. These and other scholars emphasize the relationships of power that dissection animated, particularly the dissector's transformation of human subjects into objects.

5. Berry introduces the concept of "ghost value" in *Price for Their Pound of Flesh*, 7.

6. Sappol, *Traffic in Dead Bodies*, 124.

7. Molly Rogers, *Delia's Tears: Race, Science, and Photography in Nineteenth-Century America* (New Haven, CT: Yale University Press, 2010), 221.

8. Sadiah Qureshi, in *Peoples on Display: Exhibitions, Empire, and Anthropology in Nineteenth-Century Britain* (Chicago: University of Chicago Press, 2011), argues persuasively that "human exhibitions" were not only popular spectacle but also engendered considerable scientific interest and investment.

9. Harriet A. Washington, *Medical Apartheid: The Dark History of Medical Experimentation on Black Americans from Colonial Times to the Present* (New York: Harlem Moon Broadway Books, 2006), 80–100; Jasmine Nichole Cobb, *Picture Freedom: Remaking Black Visuality in the Early Nineteenth Century* (New York: New York University Press, 2015); and Bernth Lindfors, ed., *Africans on Stage: Studies in Ethnological Show Business* (Bloomington: Indiana University Press, 1999).

10. Britt Rusert, *Fugitive Science: Empiricism and Freedom in Early African American Culture* (New York: New York University Press, 2017), 77.

11. Britt Rusert, "The Science of Freedom: Counterarchives of Racial Science on the Antebellum Stage," *African American Review* 45 (Fall 2012): 291–308; 292–293, quoting 293.

12. Benjamin Reiss, *The Showman and the Slave: Race, Death, and Memory in Barnum's America* (Cambridge, MA: Harvard University Press, 2010), 41–42.

13. The scholarship on Baartman is extensive; see Clifton Scully and Pamela Crais, *Sara Baartman and the Hottentot Venus: A Ghost Story and a Biography* (Princeton, NJ: Princeton University Press, 2010); and Natasha Gordon-Chipembere, ed., *Representation and Black Womanhood: The Legacy of Sara Baartman* (New York: Palgrave-McMillan, 2011).

14. Reiss, *Showman and the Slave*, 135.

15. Deirdre Cooper Owens, *Medical Bondage: Race, Gender, and the Origins of American Gynecology* (Athens: University of Georgia Press, 2017), 20.

16. This periodization is notably explored in Nicholas Bencel, Thomas David, and Dominic Thomas, eds., *The Invention of Race: Scientific and Popular Representations* (New York: Routledge, 2014), especially 6–8.

17. See Berry's *Price for their Pound of Flesh* for a compelling and exacting account of the commodification of Black bodies in life and in death.

18. This important distinction between objects and subjects comes from Shannon A. Novak, "Partible Persons or Persons Apart. Postmortem Interventions: Postmortem Interventions at the Spring Street Presbyterian Church, Manhattan," in *The Bioarcheology of Dissection and Autopsy in the United States*, ed. Kenneth C. Nystrom, 87–111 (New York: Springer, 2017).

19. Shauna Devine, *Learning from the Wounded: The Civil War and the Rise of American Medical Science* (Chapel Hill: University of North Carolina Press, 2014), 62–67.

20. Richard M. Reid, ed., *Recollections of a Medical Cadet: Burt Green Wilder* (Kent, OH: Kent State University Press, 2017), 15. Some military medical practitioners would publish pamphlets detailing their autopsy case records; see, for example, the pamphlet containing the case records of autopsies performed at the Baltimore's U.S. General Hospital, Surgeon in Charge: National U.S. Army General Hospital, *Observation Book Containing Certain Inductions and Classifications Ante Mortem and Post Mortems* (Baltimore: U.S. Army General Hospital Printing Office, [1865?].

21. Henrietta Stratton Jaquette, ed., *Letters of a Civil War Nurse: Cornelia Hancock, 1863–1865* (Lincoln: University of Nebraska Press, 1998), 63.

22. Reid, *Recollections of a Medical Cadet*, 70.

23. Acting assistant surgeon W. C. Minor, *Post Mortem Examinations Made at Knight U.S.A. General Hospital* (New Haven, CT: Knight Hospital Print, 1864).

24. Ira Spar, *New Haven's Civil War Hospital: A History of Knight U.S. General Hospital, 1862–1865* (Jefferson, NC: McFarland, 2013), 211; Ira Spar, *Civil War Hospital Newspapers* (Jefferson, NC: McFarland, 2017), 193.

25. Minor is the subject of Simon Winchester's nonfiction biography, *The Surgeon of Crowthorne: A Tale of Murder, Insanity, and the Making of the Love of Words* (New York: Harper Collins, 1998). See also "Local Legends: Broadmoor's Word-Finder," *BBC Legacies: Berkshire* (December 1, 2014, http://www.bbc.co.uk/legacies/myths_legends /england/berkshire/article_1.shtml), which suggests long-standing pyschosexual fixations. See also Jenny Blair, "A Tortured Soul Finds Redemption in Words," *Yale Medicine Magazine* (Winter 2009, https://medicine.yale.edu/news/yale-medicine-magazine /a-tortured-soul-finds-redemption-in-words/); and "William Chester Minor," Wikipedia, last modified May 2, 2022, https://en.wikipedia.org/wiki/William_Chester _Minor.

26. Edwin Bentley to Col. R. Abbott, Medical Director of Washington, August 19, 1865, and P. A. Jewett to Asst. Surgeon General E. H. Crane, February 28, 1872, in W. C. Minor, Per. Reports, Letters, Orders, Entry 561: Personal Papers of Medical Officers and Physicians, Record Group 94: Records of the Adjutant General's Office, 1780–1917, National Archives and Records Administration (NARA), Washington, DC. Professor James Dana declared him as having a thorough knowledge of anatomy

(Minor had worked as an anatomy demonstrator at Yale) and a thorough acquaintance with comparative anatomy; Professor James Dana (unaddressed reference letter), September 18, 1865, in same collection.

27. James D. Dana, letter of reference, September 18, 1865, Box 403, W. C. Minor Papers, Entry 561, Record Group 94: Records of the Adjutant General's Office, 1780–1917, NARA, Washington, DC.

28. Minor's case reports also were included in the U.S. Surgeon General's *Medical and Surgical History of the War of the Rebellion*, part III, vol. II, 784–785, for example.

29. Minor submitted those case reports to the Army Medical Museum; see Alfred A. Woodhull, *Catalogue of the Medical Section of the US Army Medical Museum* (Washington, DC: Government Printing Office, 1866), in the section "Medical and Microscopial," 63–67. See also Daniel S. Lamb, "A History of the United States Army Medical Museum, 1862–1917" (unpublished manuscript [1917], https://collections.nlm .nih.gov/catalog/nlm:nlmuid-12710920R-bk), 147.

30. Russell's full biography can be found in the finding aids for the Ira Russell Letters (MC 581), Special Collections Department, University of Arkansas Libraries, Fayetteville, and the Ira Russell Papers #4440, Southern Historical Collection, Wilson Library, University of North Carolina at Chapel Hill. On his military career, see "Ira Russell," Entry 561: Medical Officers Papers, Record Group 94: Records of the Adjutant General's Office, 1780–1917, NARA, Washington, DC. Margaret Humphreys, in *Intensely Human: The Health of the Black Soldier in the American Civil War* (Baltimore: Johns Hopkins University Press, 2008), comments on Russell's autopsies, that much of the data he collected seems pointless, apparently "directionless empiricism." I would disagree—he was looking for the biological definition of race and biological race difference.

31. William B. Atkinson, ed., *Physicians and Surgeons of the United States* (Philadelphia: Charles Robson, 1878), 310–311. See also Ira Russell, "The Sanitary Report of Benton Barracks Near St. Louis, Missouri; to the United States Sanitary Commission," Item 194, Folder 3.4, Box 110, Section E: Medical Committee Archives, Part IV: Historical Bureau Records, New York, NY, Archives, MssCol 22263, New York Public Library Manuscripts and Archives Division, United States Sanitary Commission (USSC) Records. Russell published "Cerebro-Spinal Meningitis as It Appeared among the Troops Stationed at Benton Barracks, Mo.," *Boston Medical and Surgical Journal*, 70, no. 16 (May 19, 1864), 309–313. He noted there that he had already published several articles in the *St. Louis Medical and Surgical Journal* on Black troops, although those articles are apparently not extant. See also Russell's "Vaccination in the Army," in *Sanitary Memoirs, Contributions to the Causation and Prevention of Disease, and to Camp Diseases*, ed. Austin Flint, 144–145 (New York: Hurd and Houghton, 1867). Russell also wrote on spurious vaccines, pneumonia, and measles.

32. By July 1865 he had conducted over 800 (Ira Russell to the Medical Committee, July 15, 1865, item 123, Folder 2.6, Box 109, and Ira Russell, "Autopsies of Colored Soldiers, 500 Cases, Classified and tabulated," Folder 10.4, Box 117, both in Part E: Medical Committee Archives, Part IV: Historical Bureau Records, New York, NY, Archives, MssCol 22263, New York Public Library Manuscripts and Archives Division, USSC Records. In his article "Hospital Reports: Benton Barracks," *St. Louis Medical and Surgical Journal* (March–April 1864): 121–128, Russell acknowledges fellow medical of-

ficers Drs. Martine, Shelly, and Dwelle for postmortem examinations (127). Furthermore, A. W. McDowell ("Hospital Observations upon Negro Soldiers," *American Practitioner* 9 [July 1874], 155–158) notes his service at Benton Barracks as well, and his "ample opportunities for observing United States colored soldiers in regard to their physical organization, their power of enduring disease or wounds, and for witnessing numerous autopsies" (155).

33. Margaret Humphreys offers additional information about Russell in *Intensely Human*.

34. Russell described the conditions provided for newly recruited Black troops at Benton Barracks a "disgrace to humanity." See Ira Russell to Col. H. Pile, Commanding Colored Recruits, January 6, 1864, Vol. 3, p. 35, Vol. 470/1219, 1220, Department of Missouri, entry 117, vol. 2 of 5, Record Group 393: Records of the U.S. Army Continental Commands, 1821–1920, part 4, NARA, Washington, DC. Nursing supervisor Emily Parsons, who worked under Russell, described him as a strong advocate for Black soldiers in *Memoir of Emily Elizabeth Parsons, Published for the Benefit of Cambridge Hospital* (Boston: Little, Brown & Co., 1880), 138–139.

35. Russell, "Sanitary Report of Benton Barracks Near St. Louis." A. M. McDowell, one of the hospital workers who performed autopsies for Russell's work, insisted that his work was not aimed at supporting the notion of polygenesis but asserted, "I present the truth as it was obvious to me, and I should be glad if others having like opportunities would do the same, and then possibly we might arrive nearer a solution of some of the difficult problems in reference to the negro" (155). At Benton Barracks, he reported, Black soldiers died easily and rapidly from pneumonia, and "autopsies explained the mystery" (156). Their chest muscles were large, but their lungs weighed far less than white men's. "Our autopsies too showed that his brain was smaller than the white man's" (156). "We weighed every brain in our post-mortem examinations, and just in exact proportion to the admixture of Caucasian blood did the weight increase. . . . I say nothing of relative intelligence. I present no opinions, but simply physical facts" (156). "The negro's liver was larger than the white man's." "The negro's lower bowel was smaller." The spleen was smaller. "The genital organs of the negro, especially true of the penis, were much larger than those of the white man" (157). "There is anatomically a marked difference between diseases in the black and white" (157), he reported.

36. Folder MM3067 (George Potts), Box 1297, Entry 15A: Court-Martial Case Files, 1809–1894, Record Group 153: Records of the Office of the Judge Advocate General (Army), NARA, Washington, DC.

37. Special Orders No. 178, April 21, 1865, Adjutant General's Office, Washington, DC.

38. Pension Certificate for Sarah Anderson, WC121303, Record Group 15: Records of the Veterans Administration, NARA, Washington, DC.

39. Folder MM3067 (George Potts), Box 1297, Entry 15A: Court-Martial Case Files, 1809–1894, Record Group 153: Records of the Office of the Judge Advocate General (Army), NARA, Washington, DC.

40. Folder MM3067 (George Potts), Box 1297, Entry 15A: Court-Martial Case Files, 1809–1894, Record Group 153: Records of the Office of the Judge Advocate General (Army), NARA, Washington, DC.

41. Folder MM3067 (George Potts), Box 1297, Entry 15A: Court-Martial Case Files, 1809–1894, Record Group 153: Records of the Office of the Judge Advocate General (Army), NARA, Washington, DC.

42. A cadaver can still "bleed" within six hours of death. Potts declared that it was untrue that there was any flow of blood.

43. Folder MM3067 (George Potts), Box 1297, Entry 15A: Court-Martial Case Files, 1809–1894, Record Group 153: Records of the Office of the Judge Advocate General (Army), NARA, Washington, DC.

44. Folder MM3067 (George Potts), Box 1297, Entry 15A: Court-Martial Case Files, 1809–1894, Record Group 153: Records of the Office of the Judge Advocate General (Army), NARA, Washington, DC.

45. Folder MM3067 (George Potts), Box 1297, Entry 15A: Court-Martial Case Files, 1809–1894, Record Group 153: Records of the Office of the Judge Advocate General (Army), NARA, Washington, DC. Potts's service record shows him to have been a some-what cranky fellow, and in a matter of months he attempted (unsuccessfully) to secure an honorable discharge for an exaggerated disability. George J. Potts, Service Record, Compiled Military Service Records of Volunteer Union Soldiers Who Served with the United States Colored Troops: Infantry Organizations, 20th through 25th (Folder 3, accessed June 19, 2020). Thomas P. Lowry and Jack D. Walsh concluded that Potts was improperly accused and court-martialed for performing a standard autopsy on Anderson's remains. They ventured that the charges had been brought against Potts because a squeamish assistant surgeon was appalled at the dissection and dismemberment that accompanied the autopsy and prompted the charges against a surgeon who was simply seeking to advance medical knowledge. See *Tarnished Scalpels: The Court-Martials of Fifty Union Surgeons* (Mechanicsburg, PA: Stackpole Books, 2000), 68–75.

46. *Harper's Weekly*, July 9, 1864. Two photographers recorded the hanging, which shows that the regiment and others witnessed the execution. See Franny Nuddle-man, *John Brown's Body: Slavery, Violence, and the Culture of War* (Chapel Hill: University of North Carolina Press, 2004), 144–149.

47. Jonathan Lande, "Trials of Freedom: African American Deserters during the U.S. Civil War." *Journal of Social History* 49 (2016): 693–709.

48. Affidavit by Henry Bush [aka Berry] and Franklin Weaver, August 22, 1867, in Sarah Anderson's pension file, WC121303, Record Group 15: Records of the Veterans Administration, NARA, Washington, DC.

49. Sappol, *Traffic in Dead Bodies*, 96–97.

50. Sally Brown to Mr. President, n.d. [1864], W-2 1865 (Record Group 94: Records of the Adjutant General's Office, 1780–1917, NARA, Washington, DC) accessed at the Freedmen and Southern Society Project, University of Maryland, as document B 132.

51. Julia Wilbur, Entry for April 13, 1864, Diary of Julia Wilbur, Quaker and Special Collections, Haverford College, transcriptions housed at "Alexandria During the Civil War: First Person Accounts," City of Alexandria, VA, https://www.alexandriava.gov/historic/civilwar/default.aspx?id=62774.

52. One undated logbook recording the reception of specimens classified by the AMM as "surgical specimens" included specimens from 379 African Americans, only 24 of them from soldiers; 153 were from women. MM8747, Index to Patients, Sur-

gical Section, Box 008, Series 001: Collection Logbooks, OHA 8: Museum Records: Curatorial Records, Otis Historical Archives, National Museum of Health and Medicine (NMHM), Silver Spring, MD.

53. Katherine Chilton, "'City of Refuge': Urban Labor, Gender, and Family Formation during Slavery and the Transition to Freedom in the District of Columbia, 1820–1875" (PhD diss., Carnegie Mellon University, 2009), 172, 195. See also the careful accounting offered in Robert Harrison, *Washington during the Civil War and Reconstruction: Race and Radicalism* (Cambridge: Cambridge University Press, 2011), 28–29, and more fully in Kenneth J. Winkle, *Lincoln's Citadel: The Civil War in Washington, D.C.* (New York: Norton, 2014).

54. Kristin Leigh Bouldin, "Is This Freedom?: Government Exploitation of Contraband Laborers in Virginia, South Carolina, and Washington, DC, during the American Civil War" (master's thesis, University of Mississippi, 2014), 67–78; and Zachary C. Lowe, "Meanings of Freedom: Virginia Contraband Settlements and Wartime Reconstruction" (master's thesis, College of William & Mary, 2003), 14–20. Chilton notes that, by summer of 1863, 4,700 African American men worked for the Washington and Alexandria quartermaster departments and another 11,000 labored in the field with the Army of the Potomac ("City of Refuge," 176).

55. Ashley Whitehead Luskey, "Inside the Civil War Defenses of Washington: An Interview with Steve T. Phan," *Gettysburg Compiler*, December 17, 2018, https://gettysburgcompiler.org/2017/12/18/inside-the-civil-war-defenses-of-washington-an-interview-with-steve-t-phan/.

56. Jill Newmark, "Contraband Hospital, 1862–1863: Health Care for the First Freedpeople," *Black Past*, March 28, 2012, https://www.blackpast.org/african-american-history/contraband-hospital-1862-1863-heath-care-first-freedpeople/; Chilton, "City of Refuge," 174–190; Capt. E. E. Camp to Brig. Genl. D. H. Rucker, July 31, 1863, enclosed in Act. Surgeon General W. K. Barnes to Brig. General M. C. Meigs, September 7, 1863, "Negroes Employed in Washington DC Hospitals," Consolidated Correspondence File, series 225, Central Records, Office of the Quartermaster General, Record Group 92: Records of the Office of the Quartermaster General, NARA, Washington, DC, published in Ira Berlin et al., eds., *The Wartime Genesis of Free Labor: The Upper South*, series 1, vol. 2 of *Freedom: A Documentary History of Emancipation, 1861–1867, Selected from the Holdings of the National Archives of the United States* (New York: Cambridge University Press, 1993), 303–305.

57. Surgeon R. O. Abbott to Brig. Genl. W. A. Hammond, September 4, 1863, enclosed in Act. Surgeon General W. K. Barnes to Brig. General M. C. Meigs, September 7, 1863, "Negroes Employed in Washington DC Hospitals," Consolidated Correspondence File, series 225, Central Records, Office of the Quartermaster General, Record Group 92: Records of the Office of the Quartermaster General, NARA, Washington, DC, published in Berlin et al., *Wartime Genesis of Free Labor: The Upper South*, 305–306.

58. Harrison, *Washington during the Civil War*, especially 34–39.

59. Bouldin, "Is This Freedom?" 67–78.

60. Tim Dennee, "A House Divided Still Stands: The Contraband Hospital and Alexandria's Freedmen's Aid Workers," Friends of Freedmen's Cemetery, 2011–2017,

www.freedmenscemetery.org/resources/documents/contrabandhospital.pdf, 7–8. See also Linda [Harriet Jacobs] to Mr. Garrison, "Life among the Contrabands," *Liberator*, September 5, 1862.

61. Camp Barker was described in New York Religious Society of Friends, "Report of a Committee of the Representatives of New York Yearly Meeting of Friends, upon the Condition and Wants of the Colored Refugees," *Friends' Review: A Religious, Literary and Miscellaneous Journal*, January 24, 1863, 325. Also see Lowe, "Meanings of Freedom," 14–20; and Chilton, "City of Refuge," 169. Some reports indicate that as many as 11,000 people passed through Camp Barker during the war (Harrison, *Washington during the Civil War*, 40).

62. Bouldin, "Is This Freedom?," 79.

63. Thomas Holt, Casandra Smith-Parker, and Rosalyn Terborg-Penn, *A Special Mission: The Story of Freedmen's Hospital, 1862–1962* (Washington, DC: Academic Affairs Division, Howard University, 1975), 3; and Ric Murphy and Timothy Stevens, *Section 27 and Freedman's Village in Arlington National Cemetery: The African American History of America's Most Hallowed Ground* (Jefferson, NC: McFarland, 2020), 74–75.

64. Chilton, "City of Refuge," 196; Holt et al., *Special Mission*, 5; Jean Fagan Yellin, ed., *The Harriet Jacobs Family Papers* (Chapel Hill: University of North Carolina, 2008), 2:535. Freedmen's Village, initially a simple encampment established on the former property of Robert E. Lee in the summer of 1863, was created as a rural village where, white military and civilian officials imagined, freed people would be safe, healthy, and labor successfully on government farms. Conditions deteriorated there, and the residents rejected the rigid rules and supervision with which the army and then the Freedmen's Bureau attempted to rule the residents. Also see U.S. National Park Service, "Freedman's Village," Arlington House, Robert E. Lee Memorial, November 3, 2019, https://www.nps.gov/arho/learn/historyculture/emancipation.htm.

65. For a thoughtful, digital history by Georgetown University historian Chandra Manning and her students, on the experience of slavery's refugees in wartime Washington, see Georgetown University History 396 Class, "Escaping Slavery, Building Diverse Communities: Stories of the Search for Freedom in the Capitol Region Since the Civil War," May 13, 2020, https://storymaps.arcgis.com/stories/98843655e3474b9 ab19a2afe25of0f22.

66. Murphy and Stevens, *Section 27 and Freedman's Village*, 75–91. Entry 577: Records Relating to Functions: Cemeteries; Burial Lists and Other Records Relating to Deceased Soldiers, Box 1, and Boxes 1–5 in Entry 581, Quartermaster Notifications, both in Record Group 92: Records of the Office of the Quartermaster General, NARA, Washington, DC, also contain numerous requests to the quartermaster office by bureau agents for the removal and burial of deceased freed people in 1867. Some of the requests were made to Lt. Col. Elias Greene, quartermaster of the Washington military district; others to his assistant quartermasters at offices across the city; some were requests to the U.S. undertaker from the quartermasters. I am indebted to Kate Masur for steering me toward these sources.

67. Samuel S. Bond, File N1294, Letters and their enclosures received by the Commission Branch of the Adjutant General's Office, 1863–70, Record Group 94: Records of the Adjutant General's Office, 1780–1917, NARA, Washington, DC.

68. Bond's former employers at the museum took issue with his effort to trade on his prior association with the museum, raising charges with the president of the Medical Association of the District of Columbia that Bond's advertisement was an attempt to gain "notoriety by misrepresentation." He suggested that the advertisement was a "grave offence against medical ethics requiring the discipline of the association." Letter from Woodward to Joshua Riley, October 5, 1867, OHA 28: Joseph Woodward Letterbooks, Otis Historical Archives, NMHM, Silver Spring, MD.

69. Daniel S. Lamb, "Some Reminiscences of Post Mortem Work," *Washington Medical Annals* 2, no. 6 (January 1904). 304.

70. Brian Spatola, "Daniel S. Lamb (1843–1929) of the Army Medical Museum," *Military Medicine* 181 (June 2016): 609–610; Rossiter Johnson, ed., s.v. "Lamb, Daniel Smith," in *Twentieth Century Biographical Dictionary* (Boston: Biographical Society, 1904), 6:307.

71. W. Montague Cobb described Lamb in this manner in 1958; "Daniel Smith Lamb. M.D., 1843–1929," *Journal of the National Medical Association* 50 (1958), 62. Augusta had been closely tied to the origins and development of Freedmen's Hospital as well as Howard University. Daniel S. Lamb, "Howard University Medical Department: A Historical, Biographical and Statistical Souvenir," College of Medicine Publications, Paper 1 (1900): 36–37, Digital Howard, https://dh.howard.edu/med_pub/1; and Heather M. Butts, "Alexander Thomas Augusta — Physician, Teacher, and Human Rights Activist," *Journal of the National Medical Association* 1 (January 2005): 106–109.

72. Amanda E. Bevers, "To Bind Up the Nation's Wounds: The Army Medical Museum and the Development of American Medical Science, 1862–1913" (PhD diss., University of California, San Diego, 2015), 97; "Adolph J. Schafhirt," *American Druggist and Pharmaceutical Record*, 43 (July–December 1903): 188.

73. Daniel S. Lamb, "The American Medical Museum, Washington, D.C." *Military Surgeon* 53 (1923), 110. In 1882, after the execution of President Garfield's assassin, Charles J. Guiteau, Ernst prepared the specimens from the body, including the head which he separated from the rest of the cadaver and embalmed (*New York Herald*, June 21, 1887).

74. Fred Schafhirt to Joseph Leidy, August 10, 1861, College of Physicians, Leidy Family Papers, Historical Medical Library at the College of Physicians of Philadelphia. I am obligated to Christopher Willoughby for sharing this letter and his work on Leidy with me.

75. Daniel S. Lamb, *The Army Medical Museum — A History* (Washington, DC: Beresford, 1916), 17. Frederick was reputed to engage in grave robbing to secure cadavers for the University of Pennsylvania; see Amy Liu, "Penn Used Bodies of Enslaved People for Teaching Purposes after Death, Student Research Reveals," *Daily Pennsylvanian*, December 10, 2018. https://www.thedp.com/article/2018/12/penn-slavery-project-ties-university-upenn-medicine. The Schafhirts emigrated from Germany to Philadelphia in 1847 and came to Washington in 1860. On Leidy's racist views, see Christopher D. Willoughby, "Race, Genitals, and Walt Whitman in Dr. Leidy's Lectures," *Fugitive Leaves*, April 13, 2017, https://histmed.collegeofphysicians.org/race-genitals-and-walt-whitman/.

76. Lamb, "History of the United States Army Medical Museum," 90–92; Lamb, *Army Medical Museum*, 17.

77. *The National Republican* (Washington, DC), June 5, 1861.

78. July 27, 1880, Frederic Schafhirt, Wills, Boxes 0067 Wagner, John J—0074 Buchly, Anthony, 1878-1881, Probate Records (District of Columbia), 1801-1920, accessed via Ancestry.com.

79. McBride, *Caring for Equality: A History of African American Health and Health Care* (Lanham, MD: Rowman and Littlefield, 2018). Lamb performed several hundred additional autopsies at the hospital between 1878 and 1909; his autopsies in 1865 and 1866 can be traced by examining the manuscript case record; Patricia S. Gindhart, "The Dead Shall Teach the Living," *Journal of the Washington Academy of Sciences* 79 (1989): 123-129.

80. Lamb, "History of the United States Army Medical Museum."

81. Lamb, "Some Reminiscences, 385; Lamb, "History of the United States Army Medical Museum," 149. After 1878, Lamb resumed making autopsies at the hospital, in all making more than 1,300.

82. Page 337, MM 8755 Medical Section II PS 1 Specimens 1-881, Renumbered as PS 7448-8330, Box 003, Series 001, OHA 8: Museum Records: Curatorial Records, Collection of Logbooks, Otis Historical Archives, NMHM, Silver Spring, MD.

83. Rogers, *Delia's Tears*, 220-221.

84. Pages 158, 259-261, 316, 330, Catalogue of the Surgical Section I, March 1864-November 1866; MM 8755 Medical Section II, OHA 8: Museum Records: Curatorial Records, Collection of Logbooks, Otis Historical Archives, NMHM, Silver Spring, MD. Fredric Schafhirt and William Chester Minor, as noted earlier, were among those whose dissections including making specimens from women's genitals and reproductive organs.

85. The Army Medical Museum kept manuscript logbooks for the receipt of each case and specimen; these logbooks were then transcribed into manuscript and then print catalogues. Many—but not all—then were noted in the U.S. Surgeon General's *Medical and Surgical History of the War of the Rebellion*. Dr. Mary Parsons, who attended Howard University's medical school and graduated in 1874 (and successfully protested to congress when she, another white female physician, and African American physician J. Ford Thompson were denied medical licenses by the District of Columbia), was among those who performed autopsies (38) on the deceased at Freedmen's Hospital and submitted specimens (44) and case reports to the Army Medical Museum. "Index of Names of the Person on Whom and the Physician for whom Autopsies were made," Autopsy Logbooks, Box 1, OHA 4: Curatorial Records: Autopsy Logbooks, 1866-1919, Otis Historical Archives, NMHM, Silver Spring, MD; Lamb, *Army Medical Museum*, 146, 150.

86. Butts, *African American Medicine*. For reasons unclear, the Army Medical Museum logbooks recording the receipt of medical, surgical, pathological, and comparative anatomical specimens note very few contributions by Black physicians during and immediately after the war.

87. Only one of the Black physicians appears at all in the Surgeon General's *Medical and Surgical History of the War of the Rebellion*. A. R. Abbott performed an amputation on a thirteen-year-old boy, John Thomas, who suffered frostbite up the knee of both legs; Thomas removed his left leg and the toes of his right foot, but the child died two

months after being admitted to Freedman's Hospital, in March 1866. The autopsy and preparation of several specimens was conducted by Bond (*Medical and Surgical History of the War of the Rebellion*, vol. 1, part 2, 259). Lamb's *Army Medical Museum*, which includes a list of all who contributed more than twenty-five specimens, does not include any of the Black physicians who served or were employed during the war (146–148).

88. Devine, *Learning from the Wounded*, 21. See also Erin Hunter McLeary, "Science in a Bottle: The Medical Museum in North America, 1860–1940" (PhD diss., University of Pennsylvania, 2001), 55

89. Michael Rhode, "An Army Museum or a National Collection? Shifting Interests and Fortunes at the National Museum of Health and Medicine," in *Medical Museums: Past, Present, Future*, ed. Samuel J.M.M. Alberti and Elizabeth Hallarn, 186–199 (London: Royal College of Surgeons of England, 2013), 188–199; McLeary, "Science in a Bottle," 33. Historian Amanda E. Bevers summarizes the implication of the museum's founding: the "Army Medical Museum, built to commemorate, celebrate and critique the battlefield medicine of the Civil War, laid the foundation for the development of medical science in the American context. The staff of the Army Medical Museum pioneered a uniquely American museological science practice during and after the war, by collecting, arranging, and analyzing specimens, case histories and statistics to produce cutting-edge medical knowledge" ("To Bind Up The Nation's Wounds," xi–xii). See also Devine, *Learning from the Wounded*, chapter 1; Lindsay Tuggle, *The Afterlives of Specimens: Science, Mourning, and Whitman's Civil War* (Iowa City, IA: University of Iowa Press, 2017).

90. See, for example, p. 32, Brinton to "My Dear Davis," December 26, 1862, Brinton, First Letter Book Series 1 #1, OHA 15: Curatorial Records: Letterbooks of the Curators, Otis Historical Archives, NMHM, Silver Spring, MD.

91. Typed transcript from *American Medical Times* 6 (May 23, 1863), 249; Folder: 1, 1863, Museum Records: Articles and Clippings, Box 1: 1863–1956, OHA 38, Otis Historical Archives, NMHM, Silver Spring, MD.

92. Brinton to Col. J. K. Barnes, August 24, 1863, Loose Outgoing Correspondence, 1862–1894, Records of the Curators, OHA 21: Outgoing Correspondence, Otis Historical Archives, NMHM, Silver Spring, MD. Despite Brinton's assertion, thousands of civilians visited the museum, and it was listed as a top sightseeing attraction by Mary Clemmer Ames in *Ten Years in Washington: Life and Scenes in the National Capital, as a Woman Sees Them* (Hartford, CT: A.D. Worthington & Co., 1873).

93. Otis to Professor Flowers, Curator of the Museum of the Royal College of Surgeons of London, November 4, 1864, Letterbooks of the Curators 1864–65, pp. 1–2, OHA 15: Curatorial Records: Letterbooks of the Curators, Otis Historical Archives, NMHM, Silver Spring, MD.

94. Otis to Dr. J. S. Martin, July 6, 1866, pp. 12–13, and Otis to William Wesley, May 24, 1867, p. 541, both in Letterbooks of the Curators 1866–67, Letters Sent, OHA 15: Curatorial Records: Letterbooks of the Curators, Otis Historical Archives, NMHM, Silver Spring, MD.

95. In his letter concerning the specimens to curator Brinton, Bontecou specifically refers to them as "heads (whole)." Robert B. Bontecou to Brinton, May 25, 1863

(South Carolina), OHA 13, Otis Historical Archives, NMHM, Silver Spring, MD; Brinton to Dr. Thomas M. Markoe, NY, March 4, 1863, First Letter Book Series 1 #1, Letters Sent, p. 59, OHA 15. Howard A. Kelly and Walter L. Burrage, s.v. "Bontecou, Reed Brockway (1824–1907)," in *American Medical Biographies* (Baltimore: Norman Remington, 1920), 123; Ron Coddington, "The Napoleon of Surgeons," *Faces of War*, May 4, 2013, http://facesofthecivilwar.blogspot.com/2013/05/the-napoleon -of-surgeons.html. See also Brinton to Surg. C. McDougall, Med. Dir., NY, February 23, 1863, and Brinton to Surgeon C. McDougall, Med. Dir., NY, March 4, 1863, First Letter Book Series 1 #1, Letters Sent, pp. 52, 60, OHA 15: Curatorial Records: Letterbooks of the Curators, Otis Historical Archives, NMHM, Silver Spring, MD. These letters document several efforts to reclaim specimens that remained in private hands or were illegally sold by enterprising hospital workers.

96. Kenny, "Development of Medical Museums," 32–62.

97. Samuel J. Redman, *Bone Rooms: From Scientific Racism to Human Prehistory in Museums* (Cambridge, MA: Harvard University Press, 2016), 7–9; Kenny, "Development of Medical Museums"; Sappol, *Traffic of Dead Bodies*; Ann Fabian, *The Skull Collectors: Race, Science, and America's Unburied Dead* (Chicago: University of Chicago Press, 2010).

98. I am grateful to my 2019 University of Iowa research assistant, Maya Buchanan (BA, University of Iowa, 2019) for her exacting research assistance investigating these sources.

99. Fabian, *Skull Collectors*, 183. See Otis to Lt. Col. Warren Webster, January 15, 1868, pp. 167–168, Letterbooks of the Curators July 1867–February 1869, Letters Sent, OHA 15: Curatorial Records: Letterbooks of the Curators, Otis Historical Archives, NMHM, Silver Spring, MD; and Lamb, "History of the United States Army Medical Museum," 43.

100. Otis to Brig. Gen. Eben Swift, January 16, 1869, pp. 558–559, Letterbooks of the Curators July 1867–February 1869, Letters Sent, OHA 15: Curatorial Records: Letterbooks of the Curators, Otis Historical Archives, NMHM, Silver Spring, MD.

101. "List of crania rec'd in exchange from the Smithsonian," January 25, 1869, US Army Medical Museum (AMM), Anatomical Section, Records Relating to Specimens Transferred to the Smithsonian Institution, #8-222 Box 1, National Anthropological Archives, Smithsonian Institution Suitland Annex, Suitland, MD. See also Redman, *Bone Rooms*, 26–36.

102. Lamb, "History of the United States Army Medical Museum," 50.

103. Tim Lockley, *Military Medicine and the Making of Race: Life and Death in the West India Regiments, 1795–1874* (New York: Cambridge University Press, 2020), 148–149; Fabian, *Skull Collectors*, 176–178.

104. Otis to [illegible], Letterbook # 3 of series 6, Outgoing Correspondence, July 1867–February 1869, OHA 15: Curatorial Records: Letterbooks of the Curators, Otis Historical Archives, NMHM, Silver Spring, MD; Ames, *Ten Years in Washington*, 185.

105. Otis to Doctor [illegible], January 20, 1871, Letters Sent, January 1871–October 1873, OHA 15: Curatorial Records: Letterbooks of the Curators, Otis Historical Archives, NMHM, Silver Spring, MD.

106. Of course, specimens also came in from across the nation: from military outposts, medical schools, and freedman's hospitals. The records of these acquisitions

are held at United States Army Medical Museum (AMM), Records Concerning Skeletal Material Transferred to the Smithsonian Institution, #8-222 Box 1, National Anthropological Archives, Smithsonian Institution Suitland Annex, Suitland, MD. Between 1808 and 1904, the Army Medical Museum would transfer its crania collection back to the Smithsonian ("United States Army Medical Museum, Anatomical Section, Records Relating to Specimens Transferred to the Smithsonian Institution," National Anthropological Archives, Smithsonian Institution, Suitland Annex. The National Museum of Health and Medicine also documented the crania transfer; see AMM Anatomical Section Logbooks (IV), MM8759-1 (1869-1875); MM8759-2 (1873-1879), MM8759-3 (1879-1888).

107. Folder SS 9249-9271, Box 021: Surgical Section, Series 001: Collection Logbooks, OHA 8: Museum Records: Curatorial Records, Collection of Logbooks, Otis Historical Archives, NMHM, Silver Spring, MD.

108. Lamb, "History of the United States Army Medical Museum," 150.

109. See, for example, Dr. O. H. Menees to John S. Billings, MD, October 25, 1888, Nashville, TN, and Dr. Rudolph Matas to Dr. J. L. Wortman [an anatomist at the Army Medical Museum] March 7, 1889, from NO, both in Folder M, as well as Dr. W. B. Towles to Dr. J. S. Billings, May 19, 1889, from Univ. of Va. At Charlottesville, Folder T, all in OHA 25: Curatorial Records: Smithsonian Correspondence, Otis Historical Archives, NMHM, Silver Spring, MD.

110. Surgeon General, *Medical and Surgical History of the War*, vol. 1, xiii.

111. Edwin Bentley, who supervised contraband hospitals in Alexandria, Virginia, for more than two years, similarly compiled a report of surgeries he had performed without any indication of interest in comparative anatomy; see Edwin Bentley, Surgical Reports, Alexandria, VA, 3rd Division, Folder A27-34, Box 2, Entry 621-B, File A, Records of the Record and Pension Office, Medical Records, Reports of Diseases and Individual Cases, 1841-1893 File A and Bound Manuscripts, 1861-1865, Record Group 94: Records of the Adjutant General's Office, 1780-1917, NARA, Washington, DC.

112. Otis to Asst. Surg. Edwin Bentley, July 11, 1866, p. 25, and Otis to Prof. Paul F. Eve, p. 26, Letterbooks of the Curators, 1866-67, OHA 8: Museum Records: Curatorial Records, Collection of Logbooks, Otis Historical Archives, NMHM, Silver Spring, MD.

113. McLeary, *Science in a Bottle*, 108; Londa Schiebinger, *Secret Cures of Slaves: People, Plants, and Medicines in the Eighteenth-Century Atlantic World* (Stanford, CA: Stanford University Press, 2017), 112-134.

114. Katherine Cober, "Dissecting Race: An Examination of Anatomical Illustration and the Absence of Non-white Bodies" (master's thesis, Dalhousie University, 2015), 1-2. Cober finds that even in late twentieth-century anatomical textbooks, non-whites are rarely portrayed in anatomical illustrations (in fact, only one of seven textbooks portrayed non-white women) (161). See also Kenny, "Development of Medical Museums," 61.

Chapter Five

1. See Carol Emberton, "'Cleaning Up the Mess': Some Thoughts on Freedom, Violence, and Grief," in *Beyond Freedom: Disrupting the History of Emancipation*, ed.

David W. Blight and Jim Downs, 136–144 (Athens: University of Georgia Press, 2017), for a thoughtful critique of the centering of white experiences in scholarly explorations of Civil War deaths.

2. Andrew K. Black, "In the Service of the United States: Comparative Mortality among African-American and White Troops in the Union Army," *Journal of Negro History* 79, no. 4 (1994): 317; Margaret Humphreys, *Intensely Human: The Health of the Black Soldier in the American Civil War* (Baltimore: Johns Hopkins University Press, 2008), 11.

3. Gaines M. Foster, "The Limitations of Federal Health Care for Freedmen, 1862–1868," *Journal of Southern History* 48 (August 1982): 351.

4. Herbert Aptheker, "Negro Casualties in the Civil War," *Journal of Negro History* 32 (1947): 10–80.

5. Drew Gilpin Faust, *This Republic of Suffering: Death and the American Civil War* (New York: Alfred A. Knopf, 2008), xi.

6. Figures adapted from "The Civil War by the Numbers," *American Experience: Death and the Civil War*, November 7, 2017, https://www.pbs.org/wgbh/american experience/features/death-numbers/.

7. Lt. Col. Theodore Barrett to the Officers and Men of the 62nd USCI, Ringgold Barracks, TX, January 4, 1866, pp. 124–127, Regimental Letter, Endorsement, and Order Book, 62nd USCI, Vol. 2, Book Records of Volunteer Union Organizations, E112–115, Record Group 94: Records of the Adjutant General's Office, 1780–1917, National Archives and Records Administration (NARA), Washington, DC.

8. Of course, Confederate soldiers were well-known for refusing to allow the retrieval or burial of Black soldiers and also for taking trophies from the bodies of Black soldiers, as noted in Simon Harrison, "Bones in the Rebel Lady's Boudoir: Ethnology, Race and Trophy-Hunting in the American Civil War," *Journal of Material Culture* 5 (2010): 397.

9. *Christian Recorder*, August 15, 1863.

10. On Black funerary and burial practices, see Periwinkle Initiative, *Memory and Landmarks: Report of the Burial Database Project of Enslaved Americans* (Ithaca, NY: Periwinkle Initiative, 2017), https://issuu.com/periwinkleinitiative/docs/flipbook; Karla F. C. Holloway, *Passed On: African American Mourning Stories* (Durham, NC: Duke University Press, 2003); and Ryan K. Smith, "Disappearing the Enslaved: The Destruction and Recovery of Richmond's Second African Burial Ground," *Buildings and Landscape: Journal of the Vernacular Architecture Forum* 27 (March 2020): 17–45.

11. *Christian Recorder*, May 10, 1862.

12. Elaine Nichols, ed., *The Last Miles of the Way: African-American Homegoing Traditions, 1890–Present* (Columbia: South Carolina State Museum, 1989); Lynn Rainville, *Hidden History: African American Cemeteries in Central Virginia* (Charlottesville: University of Virginia Press, 2014), chapter 5; Robert L. Blakely and Judith M. Harrington, "Grave Consequences: The Opportunistic Procurement of Cadavers at the Medical College of Georgia," in *Bones in the Basement: Postmortem Racism in Nineteenth-Century Medical Training*, ed. Robert L. Blakely and Judith M. Harrington, 162–183 (Washington, DC: Smithsonian Institution Press, 1997), 168–70; Holloway, *Passed On*.

13. *The North Star*, June 22, 1849. For an example of substantial investments in Black burial ground building among Charleston's free people of color, see Petition

11385602 [Charleston, SC, ca. 1856] in Race & Slavery Petitions Project, Digital Library on American Slavery, http://library.uncg.edu/slavery/petitions/details.aspx?pid=1627.

14. *The North Star*, June 8, 1849.

15. *Christian Recorder*, March 14, 1862, and October 8, 1864.

16. Rainville, *Hidden History*, 149–151.

17. Enslaved and free blacks in Richmond protested a law passed in the aftermath of the Nat Turned rebellion that prevented religious assemblies because it prevented them from conducting dignified burial services (see Petition 11683411, Race and Slavery Petitions Project, Digital Library on American Slavery, http://library.uncg.edu /slavery/petitions/details.aspx?pid=2683 [accessed December 6, 2019]. The petitioners protested that the consequence of the law was that "many coloured human beings are interred like brutes. . . ."). In1788, Black New Yorkers unsuccessfully petitioned the city's common council to protect the African Burial Ground; Benjamin Reiss, *The Showman and the Slave: Race, Death, and Memory in Barnum's America* (Cambridge, MA: Harvard University Press, 2010), 133.

18. Daina Ramey Berry, *The Price for Their Pound of Flesh: The Value of the Enslaved, from Womb to Grace, in the Building of a Nation* (Boston: Beacon Press), 148–193; Stephen C. Kenny, "The Development of Medical Museums in the Antebellum American South: Slave Bodies in Networks of Anatomical Exchange," *Bulletin of the History of Medicine* 87 (Spring 2013): 32–62; David C. Humphrey, "Dissection and Discrimination: The Social Origins of Cadavers in America, 1760–1915," *Bulletin of the New York Academy of Medicine* 49 (1973): 819–827; Ann Fabian, *The Skull Collectors: Race, Science, and America's Unburied Dead* (Chicago: University of Chicago Press, 2010); Robert L. Blakely and Judith M. Harrington, eds., *Bones in the Basement: Postmortem Racism in Nineteenth-Century Medical Training* (Washington, DC: Smithsonian Institution Press, 1997).

19. David R. Roediger, "And Die in Dixie: Funerals, Death, & Heaven in the Slave Community 1700–1865," *Massachusetts Review* 22 (Spring 1981): 164–165, and J. T. Roane, "Plotting the Black Commons," *Souls* 20 (2019): 245–246.

20. Petition 11683411 [Richmond, VA, December 17, 1834] in the Race & Slavery Petitions Project, Digital Library on American Slavery, http://library.uncg.edu/slavery /petitions/details.aspx?pid=2683. The petitioners protested that the consequence of the law was that "many coloured human beings are interred like brutes."

21. Douglas R. Egerton, "A Peculiar Mark of Infamy: Dismemberment, Burial, and Rebelliousness in Slave Societies," in *Mortal Remains: Death in Early America*, ed. Nancy Isenberg and Andrew Burstein, 149–160 (Philadelphia: University of Pennsylvania Press, 2003).

22. As late as 1807, municipal officials in Charleston worried about the number of dead bodies of the enslaved dumped in the harbor by owners trying to avoid burial fees. Mark S. Schantz, *Awaiting the Heavenly Country: The Civil War and America's Culture of Death* (Ithaca, NY: Cornell University Press, 2008), 131–132.

23. Federal Writers Project, *Slave Narratives: A Folk History of Slavery in the United States from Interviews with Former Slaves*, vol. 4: *Georgia*, part I, Willis Cofer, p. 207 (https://www.loc.gov/item/mesn041/), and part 3, Julia Larker, pp. 43–44 (https:// www.loc.gov/item/mesn043) Library of Congress, n.d.; Charles L. Perdue Jr.,

Thomas E. Barden, and Robert K. Phillips, eds., *Weevils in the Wheat: Interviews with Virginia Ex-Slaves* (Charlottesville: University of Virginia Press, 1976), 7, 289.

24. Federal Writers Project, *Slave Narratives*, vol. 7: *Kentucky*, Mary Wright, pp. 63, 65 quote (https://www.loc.gov/item/mesn070); Rainville, *Hidden History*, 51 53.

25. Stephanie M. H. Camp, *Closer to Freedom: Enslaved Women and Everyday Resistance in the Plantation South* (Chapel Hill: University of North Carolina Press, 2004).

26. Rainville, *Hidden History*, 2 9.

27. Petition 10682001 [Richmond, GA, ca. 1820], Race and Slavery Petitions Project, Digital Library on American Slavery, http://library.uncg.edu/slavery/petitions /details.aspx?pid=448.

28. Associated Press and NBC Washington Staff, "Evidence Shows U. Richmond Was Built over Slave Burial Site," 4 *NBC Washington*, January 22, 2020, https://www .nbcwashington.com/news/evidence-shows-u-richmond-was-built-over-slave -burial-site/2202692/. See also Smith, "Disappearing the Enslaved," 17–45.

29. Stephen J. Richardson, "The Burial Grounds of Black Washington: 1880–1919," *Records of the Columbia Historical Society* 52 (1989): 304–326.

30. It is important to note that extant archival and print sources offer limited documentation of Black ideas about wartime death and little documentation of the rituals and practices that accompanied the burial of Black soldiers and civilians.

31. Roane, "Plotting the Black Commons," 239–266.

32. Vincent Brown, *The Reaper's Garden: Death and Power in the World of Atlantic Slavery*. (Cambridge, MA: Harvard University Press, 2008). Kenneth C. Nystrom, in "The Bioarcheology of Structural Violence and Dissection in the 19th-century United States," *American Anthropologist* 116, no. 4 (2014): 765, refers to postmortem racism as "postmortem manifestations of social inequality." See also Kenny, "Development of Medical Museums," 49.

33. In an extract from the *Atlantic Monthly* republished in the *National Anti-Slavery Standard* of December 10, 1864.

34. Keith P. Wilson, *Campfires of Freedom: The Camp Life of Black Soldiers during the Civil War* (Kent, OH: Kent State University Press, 2002), 136–137. Armstrong commanded the 9th U.S.C.I.

35. *National Anti-Slavery Standard*, August 26, 1865.

36. Gooding's letters were printed in the New Bedford (MA) *Mercury*; this one was dated October 10, 1863. Virginia M. Adams, *On the Altar of Freedom: A Black Soldier's Civil War Letters from the Front, Corporal James Henry Gooding* (Amherst: University of Massachusetts Press, 1991), 69.

37. Bob Luke and John David Smith, *Soldiering for Freedom: How the Union Army Recruited, Trained, and Deployed the U.S. Colored Troops* (Baltimore: Johns Hopkins University Press, 2014), 75.

38. Ira Berlin, Joseph P. Reidy, and Leslie Rowland, eds., *The Black Military Experience*, series 2, book 1 of *Freedom: A Documentary History of Emancipation, 1861-1867, Selected from the Holdings of the National Archives of the United States* (New York: Cambridge University Press, 1982), 604–605.

39. Chaplain James B. Crane, Knight General Hospital, to Col. J. K. Barnes, January 31, 1864, Reports of Chaplains, Civil War E-F, Box 3 of 9, Entry 679, The Record &

Pension Office, Administrative Records, 1850–1912, Record Group 94: Records of the Adjutant General's Office, 1780–1917, NARA, Washington, DC.

40. Berlin et al., *Black Military Experience*, 652–653. Henry Clay Trumbull, in *War Memories of an Army Chaplain* (New York: Charles Scribner's Sons, 1898), offers detailed descriptions of soldier burials; see 203–232.

41. Jean Fagan Yellin, ed., *The Harriet Jacobs Family Papers* (Chapel Hill: University of North Carolina, 2008), 1:lxvii–lxviii.

42. Julia Wilbur, diary entry for May 15, 1863, February 5, 1864, May 5, 1864, and December 26, 1864; Diaries of Julia Wilbur, March 1860 to July 1866, Transcription, Quaker Collections, Haverford College, Haverford, PA.

43. Julia Wilbur, diary entry for May 15, 1863, February 5, 1864, May 5, 1864, and December 28, 1864; Diaries of Julia Wilbur, March 1860 to July 1866, Transcription, Quaker Collections, Haverford College, Haverford, PA.

44. Paula Tarnapol Whitacre, "'As American Citizens, We Have a Right. . . .': Death, Protest, and Respect in Alexandria, Virginia," *Journal of the Civil War Era: Muster*, November 16, 2021, https://www.journalofthecivilwarera.org/2021/11/as-american-citizens-we-have-a-right-death-protest-and-respect-in-alexandria-virginia/; Micki McElya, "The Politics of Mourning: Death and Honor in Arlington National Cemetery" (master's thesis, Harvard University, 2016), 103. Gladwin established Freedmen's Cemetery south of Alexandria for both Contraband and Black soldiers. Wilbur complained that at the first soldier's burial, May 5, 1864, for Private John Cooley, it was too brief and lacked proper ceremony. The cemetery was the burial ground used by L'Ouverture Hospital, opened in February 1864 with beds for 600. Dr. Edwin Bentley was head of all of Alexandria's hospitals, including this one, beginning in December 1864.

45. Julia Wilbur, diary entry for December 28, 1864; Diaries of Julia Wilbur, March 1860 to July 1866, Transcription, Quaker Collections, Haverford College, Haverford, PA.

46. Col. F. W. Geiger, March 3, 1864, General Order 6, HQ 3rd Ark. Vols. AD, Helena, Ark., Entry 112–115, Book Records of Volunteer Union Organizations, 56th USCT Infantry, Regimental Letter & Order Book 4, Record Group 94: Records of the Adjutant General's Office, 1780–1917, NARA, Washington, DC.

47. *National Anti-Slavery Standard*, July 22, 1865. Redpath's report elicited a response asserting that the Beaufort Soldier's Cemetery (later the Beaufort National Cemetery) included both Black and white dead; that respondent may not have realized that there were at least six cemeteries in the Charleston area (*National Anti-Slavery Standard*, August 26, 1865).

48. James Elton Johnson, "A History of Camp William Penn and Its Black Troops in the Civil War, 1863–1865" (PhD diss., University of Pennsylvania, 1999), 99.

49. *Christian Recorder*, August 20, 1864.

50. James G. Mendez, "A Great Sacrifice: Northern Black Families and Their Civil War Experience" (PhD diss., University of Illinois at Chicago, 2011), chapter 6, offers a valuable overview of these requests and asserts that Northern Black families made frequent inquiries as to the status of their kin (212). The holdings of the Freedmen and Southern Society Project at the University of Maryland (College Park, MD)

document such requests, including Eliza Blake to Stanton, March 7, 1865, RG 366, Box 348, B-112 (1865) [B 336]; Sarah Brown to Stanton, February 8, 1865, RG 366, Box 348, B-67 (1865) [B-338]; James Thomas Davis to Thomas, December 5, 1864 RG 366 Box 346 D-47 (1864) [B-341], and J. P. Creager to [Unknown], November 27, 1864 RG 366 Box 346 C-102 (1864) [B 340]. Extensive evidence of widows searching for information about their husbands' deaths while in the service can be found in Widow's Claims Register, Vol. 8, Army & Navy Agency Claim Agency, MssCol 18809, New York Public Library Manuscripts and Archives Division, United States Sanitary Commission (USSC) Records.

51. Vol. 1 of 7, Descriptive Book of 65th USCT, Book Records of Vol. Union Organizations, Record Group 94: Records of the Adjutant General's Office, 1780–1917, NARA, Washington, DC.

52. Vol. 8, Register 1(1864 May–1865 May), Box 157, Claim Registers, Army and Navy Agency Claims, MssCol 18809, New York Public Library Manuscripts and Archives Division, USSC Records.

53. The sample included pension records for the widows of fallen soldiers from the 24th, 25th, 29th, 61st, and 62nd U.S.C.I., recruited from the Mississippi valley, the border states of the Midwest, and the Middle Atlantic, who died during the war.

54. Apparently the surgeon general's office was overwhelmed by the requests for information they received from friends and families. A circular letter issued in June 1864 by the surgeon general's office sought to limit the provision of detailed information about a soldier's date and circumstances of death to legal claimants (in the case of pension applicants), ordering medical personnel to limit their responses to inquiries from anxious friends and family to confirming "the bare *fact* of death." William Grace, *The Army Surgeon's Manual for the Use of Medical Officers, Cadets, Chaplains, and Hospital Stewards Containing the Regulations of the Medical Department, All General Orders from the War Department and Circulars from the Surgeon-General's Office from January 1st, 1861, to April 1st, 1865* (New York: Baillière Brothers, 1865), 97, 198–199.

55. Bollet estimates that the costs for embalming ($30) and then shipping a body could easily exceed $75. *Civil War Medicine: Challenges and Triumphs* (Tucson, AZ: Galen Press, 2002), 465.

56. Berlin et al., *Black Military Experience*, 675–676. He remained buried at the Brownsville National Cemetery; John R. Neff, *Honoring the Civil War Dead: Commemoration and the Problem of Reconciliation* (Lawrence: University Press of Kansas, 2005), 45–46.

57. Noah Andre Trudeau, *Voices of the 55th: Letters from the 55th Massachusetts Volunteers, 1861–1865* (Dayton, OH: Morningside Press, 1996), 63.

58. *National Anti-Slavery Standard*, May 7, 1864.

59. Faust, *This Republic of Suffering*, 65.

60. Susan-Mary Grant, "Raising the Dead: War, Memory and American National Identity," *Nations and Nationalism* 11 (2005), 512.

61. Grant, "Raising the Dead," 482–483.

62. United States Sanitary Commission, *The Sanitary Commission of the U.S. Army, A Succinct History of its Works and Purposes* (New York: 1864), 105–107.

63. Rachel Williams, "The United States Christian Commission and the Civil War Dead," *U.S. Studies Online*, April 15, 2015, http://www.baas.ac.uk/usso/the-united -states-christian-commission-and-the-civil-war-dead/.

64. *The Sanitary Commission of the U.S. Army*, 105–106; Oliver Diefendorf, *General Orders of the War Department, Embracing the Years 1861, 1862 & 1863* (New York: Derby & Miller, 1864), 158; Erna Risch, *Quartermaster Support of the Army: A History of the Corps, 1775–1939* (Washington, DC: Quartermaster Historian's Office, 1962), 464.

65. *St. Louis Today*, May 27, 2015.

66. Vol. 115, Virginia: City Point National Cemetery, Entry 627: Records Re: Cemeterial Functions, Burial Registers of Military Post and national Cemeteries, ca. 1862–1960, Record Group 92: Records of the Quartermaster General, NARA, Washington, DC (accessed via Ancestry.com).

67. Risch, *Quartermaster Support*, 465, 248. In July, General Orders 212 instructed officers in the army's Invalid Corps to "see that the dead are properly buried" without further elaboration on what that entailed. Grace, *Army Surgeon's Manual*, 71.

68. Faust, *This Republic of Suffering*, 65.

69. Schantz, in *Awaiting the Heavenly Country*, notes that the massive battlefield mortality rates of the war—30 to 40 percent—had their parallels in the epidemics that struck the nation's cities. The yellow fever epidemics that struck New York City in 1849 and New Orleans in 1853 overwhelmed city officials with the need to improvise burial—the trenches they used to bury thousands of the dead would be deployed after major battles during the war (14–15).

70. Hospital Directory Archives, MssCol 19877, New York Public Library Manuscripts and Archives Division, USSC Records. The records are voluminous, and most pertain to white troops.

71. David Alan Rancy, "In the Lord's Army: The United States Christian Commission in the Civil War" (PhD diss., University of Illinois, 2001), 76.

72. Clipping, "The Sanitary Commission as Undertaker," Folder 23, January–April 1864, Box 1, Part One: Correspondence, etc., 1848–1889, Frederick Newman Knapp Papers, 1848–1904, Massachusetts Historical Society, Boston. Knapp's collection includes considerable materials related to documenting the burial and identification of the war dead for surviving families, without any mention of African American families. He served as head of the USSC's Special Relief department.

73. Relief Agent J. C. Hobbit to Dr. J. S. Newberry, November 22, 1862, Folder 5, 14–30 November 1864, Box 2, Part One: Correspondence, etc., 1848–1889, Frederick Newman Knapp Papers, 1848–1904, Massachusetts Historical Society, Boston.

74. Angela Y. Walston-Raji, "In Search of Quarantine Island," *The USCT Chronicle: Telling African American Civil War Stories, of Soldiers, Civilians, Contrabands, First Days of Freedom, and the Events That Led to Freedom*, December 14, 2013, http:// usctchronicle.blogspot.com/2013/12/in-search-of-quarantine-island.html.

75. August 20, 1864, from Morganzia, Henry Boltwood to Dr. Blake, Vol. 1, Box 2, Part 1: Main Office, Dept. of. the Gulf Archives, MssCol 18590, New York Public Library Manuscripts and Archives Division, USSC Records. The Classified Statement of Interments at Jefferson Barracks National Cemetery as of June 30, 1875, enumerated

1,071 Black soldiers buried there, 1,040 of them unknown. Classified Statement of Interments at Jefferson Barracks National Cemetery, June 30, 1875, Box 36, Jefferson Barracks, MO—Junction City, KY, Entry 576, General Correspondence and Reports Relating to National and Post Cemeteries ("Cemetery File"), Records Relating to Functions: Cemeterial, 1828–1829, 1865-ca. 1914, Record Group 92: Records of the Quartermaster General, NARA, Washington, DC.

76. U.S. Register of Colored Troops Deaths During the Civil War, 1861–1865, Records of the Adjutant General's Office, 1780s–1917, Record Group 94: Records of the Adjutant General's Office, 1780–1917, NARA, Washington, DC.

77. Lt. Col. David Branson to Lt. O. A. Rice, Morganzia, LA, August 31, 1864, pp. 39–40, Regimental Letter, Endorsement, and Order Book, 62nd USCI, Book Records of Volunteer Union Organizations, Vol. 2, E112–115, Record Group 94: Records of the Adjutant General's Office, 1780–1917, NARA, Washington, DC.

78. Russell, of course, was not the only white medical practitioner commodifying the bodies of Black soldiers after death—nor was he alone among those regarded at the time and now as sympathetic to Black soldiering. Burt Green Wilder, who would go on to become regimental surgeon for the 55th (Black) Massachusetts Regiment, was a medical cadet early in the war who dissected Black corpses at one of Washington's medical colleges and eagerly received the skeletal remains of another African American who had apparently been a patient at the military hospital at Judiciary Square; see Richard M. Reid, ed., *Recollections of a Medical Cadet: Burt Green Wilder* (Kent, OH: Kent State University Press, 2017), 75. Wilder, who would go on to become a recognized comparative anatomist at Cornell University, paid homage to racist ethnologist Louis Agassiz: Burt G. Wilder, "Louis Agassiz, Teacher," reprinted from *The Harvard Graduate's Magazine*, June 1907, [603–606], https://archive.org/details/louisagassizteacoowild/page/n3; and, in a festschrift celebrating his retirement from Cornell, Wilder's students published a collection of original research papers—including an essay epitomizing racist anthropology and comparative anatomy by Eugene Rollin Corson: "The Vital Equation of the Colored Race and Future in the United States," in *The Wilder Quarter-Century Book*, edited by Burt G. Wilder, 115–176 (Ithaca, NY: Comstock, 1893).

79. "U.S. Colored Soldiers interred in Jeff. Bks Mo Nat Cemetery," Jefferson Barracks, MO, 1834–1873, Consolidated Correspondence File, 1794–1890, Central Records, Record Group 92: Records of the Quartermaster General, NARA, Washington, DC.

80. Burial Registers can be found at *U.S., Burial Registers, Military Posts and National Cemeteries, 1862–1960*, accessible online via Ancestry.com.

81. Angela Locke Barton, "Shards of Medical History: Artifacts from the Point San Jose Hospital Medical Waste Pit" (paper presented at the 83rd Annual Meeting of the Society for American Archaeology, Washington, DC, 2018). Barton describes a waste pit studied by archaeologists at Fort Point, San Jose, California. See also Danika Fears, "Remains of Civil War Soldiers Found in 'Limb Burial Pit' Tell Tale of Bloody Battle," *Daily Beast*, June 20, 2018, https://www.thedailybeast.com/remains-of-civil-war-soldiers-found-in-limb-burial-pit-tell-tale-of-bloody-battle; and Becky Little, "Grisly Civil War Pit Reveals Bones of Severed Limbs," *History Channel*, June 22, 2018, https://web.archive.org/web/20180623011701/https://www.history.com/news/civil-war-burial-bones-severed-limbs.

82. There are additional reasons why Black soldiers were more likely than whites to be among the "unknown" dead. The 55th Massachusetts Volunteers, serving on the South Carolina barrier islands, performed extensive fatigue duty and in the first months lost twenty-three to disease; most were most laid to rest in a brigade cemetery that went undiscovered until 1987. Trudeau, *Voices of the 55th*, 16.

83. John R. Neff's otherwise valuable *Honoring the Civil War Dead* argues that the burial of African American soldiers in national cemeteries made these the first publicly funded integrated cemeteries (133), but he fails to note the disparity between marked and unmarked graves, and in making this assertion he fails to acknowledge the persistent segregation of Black from white graves. See Faust, "Battle over the Bodies: Burying and Reburying the Civil War Dead, 1865–1871," in *Wars within a War: Controversy and Conflict in the American Civil War*, ed. Joan Waugh and Gary Gallagher, 184–201 (Chapel Hill: University of North Carolina Press, 2009), 194.

84. Risch, *Quartermaster Support*, 465.

85. Grant, "Raising the Dead," 512–513.

86. McElya, "Politics of Mourning," 110.

87. McElya, "Politics of Mourning."

88. Classified Statements of Internment, June 1875, Pennsylvania, Box 55, General Correspondence and Reports Relating to National and Post Cemeteries ("Cemetery File"), 1865–c 1914, Entry 576, Record Group 92: Records of the Quartermaster General, NARA, Washington, DC.

89. Tennessee State Library and Archives Research and Collections, Federal Civil War Burial Sheets Project, https://www.tnsos.net/TSLA/BurialSheetsProject/index.php.

90. Medical History of Posts: Jefferson Barracks, vol. 143, pp. 77–78, Entry 547, Record Group 94: Records of the Adjutant General's Office, 1780–1917, NARA, Washington, DC.

91. Neff discusses Meigs's arguments in *Honoring the Civil War Dead*, 196–200.

92. McElya, "Politics of Mourning," 110–111.

93. Email correspondence, Dan Flees, Lead Cemetery Representative, Jefferson Barracks National Cemetery, September 21, 2017, to Leslie Schwalm (in author's possession).

94. Examples of the forms, "Classified Statement of Interments," can be seen in General Correspondence and Reports Relating to National and Post Cemeteries ("Cemetery File"), 1865–ca. 1914, Fredericksburg, VA—Gettysburg, PA, Box 30, Entry 576, Record Group 92: Records of the Quartermaster General, NARA, Washington, DC.

95. No Black soldier was buried at Gettysburg until 1884, and at that time, according to a local historian, the family of the white soldier adjacent removed his body in protest. Becca Stout, "African Americans Buried at Gettysburg," *Blog Divided*, June 11, 2018, http://housedivided.dickinson.edu/sites/blogdivided/2018/06/11/african-americans-in-gettysburg-national-cemetery/.

96. Capt. Horatio C. King, Acting Assistant Quartermaster of Contraband, Washington, DC, to Quartermaster James Moore, February 9, 1864, "Unknown Contraband negroes Also Known" file, Entry 225 Box 1172, Record Group 92: Records of the

Quartermaster General, NARA, Washington, DC. Temperatures were unusually cold that month, reaching below zero degrees Fahrenheit (Diary Entry February 18, 1864, Diary of Horatio Nelson Taft, 1861–1865, Library of Congress). The only requests for burial referring to whites pertained to the amputated limbs of white soldiers and officers, made by the medical officers at Judiciary Square Hospital.

97. *Daily National Republican* [Washington, DC], February 26, 1863; *Evening Star* [Washington, DC], December 4, 1863. These figures referred only to camps within the city, not those in Alexandria, Fairfax, on Mason's Island, or at Freedmen's Village in Arlington.

98. See the requests in folder "Freedmen's Hospital, 1865," Box 5, Entry 581: Records Relating to Functions: Cemeterial, 1828–1929, Quartermaster Notifications, 1863–1866, Record Group 92: Records of the Quartermaster General, NARA, Washington, DC. In reading hundreds of these requests for removal and interment, I have seen only a handful of requests where the family sought only a coffin, having located their own burial place. See also "Unknown Contraband negroes Also Known" file, E225, Box 1172, Record Group 92: Records of the Quartermaster General, NARA, Washington, DC. There is a smaller collection of similar requests preserved under "Camp Nelson" in Box 52, Entry 576, Records Relating to Functions: Cemeterial, 1828–1929, General Correspondence and Reports Relating to National and Post Cemeteries ("Cemetery File"), 1865–ca. 1914, Record Group 92: Records of the Quartermaster General, NARA, Washington, DC.

99. The quartermaster office printed forms that asked for name, age, and "length." See "Unknown Contraband negroes Also Known" file, E225, Box 1172, Record Group 92: Records of the Quartermaster General, NARA, Washington, DC. See also A. Q. Elias Greene to Major General M. C. Meigs, August 9, 1864, Folder "Contrabands (1864)," Box 399, Record Group 92: Records of the Quartermaster General, NARA, Washington, DC.

100. *Evening Star* [Washington, DC], January 16, 1864.

101. *Evening Star* [Washington, DC], January 15, 1866.

102. The requests are filed in 13 folders, Boxes 4 and 5, Entry 581: Records Relating to Functions: Cemeterial, 1828–1929, Quartermaster Notifications, 1863–1866, Record Group 92: Records of the Quartermaster General, NARA, Washington, DC.

103. Yellin, *Harriet Jacobs Family Papers*, 2:528–529.

104. Robert Harrison, *Washington during Civil War and Reconstruction: Race and Radicalism* (Cambridge: Cambridge University Press, 2011), 34–36; and Ira Berlin et al., eds., *The Wartime Genesis of Free Labor: The Upper South*, series 1, vol. 2 of *Freedom: A Documentary History of Emancipation, 1861–1867, Selected from the Holdings of the National Archives of the United States* (New York: Cambridge University Press, 1993), 243–244; *Evening Star* [Washington, DC], March 15, 1865; on white burials in 1864, *Evening Star*, November 14, 1864. Although I have been unable to track down the city common council minutes documenting this assignment of responsibility for the Black civilian war dead to the quartermaster office, that office did solicit proposals in June 1863 for the burial of soldiers but also those "under the protection of the United States" (*Evening Star*, June 10, 1863). The city provided both coffins and a burial site for white paupers

and smallpox victims without resources to cover the costs (*Evening Star*, January 20, 1864, and March 2, 1864. This distinction carried over to many arenas of life and death in the city. Deceased infants found in the city streets, if white, prompted investigation; Black infants were simply removed and buried (*Evening Star*, October 20, 1863).

105. *Evening Star*, April 27, 1863, and May 28, 1863.

106. Although those funds helped support the first year of the Freedman's Bureau's work in the city as well as the opening of Howard University, the majority of the reserved taxes were never distributed to the intended beneficiaries, a fact that plagued not only the tax system in Washington but throughout the South. Harrison, *Washington during Civil War and Reconstruction*, 37; Thavolia Glymph, "Black Women and Children in the Civil War: Archive Notes," in *Beyond Freedom: Disrupting the History of Emancipation*, ed. David W. Blight and Jim Downs, 121–135 (Athens: University of Georgia Press, 2017), 121–135; and Berlin et al., *Wartime Genesis of Free Labor: The Upper South*, 251–255.

107. *Daily National Republican* [Washington, DC], February 4, 1863.

108. Berlin et al., *Wartime Genesis of Free Labor: The Upper South*, 300, 363.

109. *The Liberator*, September 5, 1862.

110. Henrietta Stratton Jaquette, ed., *Letters of a Civil War Nurse: Cornelia Hancock, 1863–1865* (Lincoln: University of Nebraska Press, 1998), 46.

111. Arlington County (Va.) Book of Records Containing the Marriages and Deaths That Have Occurred within the Official Jurisdiction of Rev. A. Gladwin Together with Any Biographical or Other Reminiscences That May Be Collected, 1863–1869, p. 81, Arlington County (Va.) Reel 269, Local Government Records Collection, Arlington County Court Records, Library of Virginia, Richmond.

112. Steven J. Richardson, "The Burial Grounds of Black Washington, 1880–1919," *Records of the Columbia Historical Society, Washington, D.C.* 52 (1989): 304–326; Ric Murphy and Timothy Stephens, *Section 27 and Freedman's Village in Arlington National Cemetery: The African American History of America's Most Hallowed Ground* (Jefferson, NC: McFarland, 2020), chapter 11; Tim Dennee, "A District of Columbia Freedmen's Cemetery in Virginia? African-American Civilians Interred in Section 27 of Arlington National Cemetery, 1864–1867," Friends of Freedmen's Cemetery, April 11, 2018, http://www.freedmenscemetery.org/resources/resources.shtml; Tim Dennee, "A House Divided Still Stands: The Contraband Hospital and Alexandria Freedmen's Aid Workers," Friends of Freedmen's Cemetery, 2011–2017. www.freedmenscemetery.org/resources/documents/contrabandhospital.pdf; and Tim Dennee, "African-American Civilians and Soldiers Treated at Claremont Smallpox Hospital, Fairfax County, Virginia, 1862–1865," Friends of Freedmen's Cemetery, 2008–2015, http://www.freedmenscemetery.org/resources/documents/claremont.pdf, all available at the Friends of Freedmen's Cemetery website, https://www.freedmenscemetery.org /. According to Timothy Dennee, before 1864 more than 1,000 African Americans were buried at Union Cemetery in only four and a half months; and Harmony received 2,711 deceased refugees in a year and a half ("A District of Columbia Freedmen's Cemetery"). Dennee's exacting research has made an important contribution to the history of African Americans in the nation's capital.

113. Dennee, "A District of Columbia Freedmen's Cemetery in Virginia?" See also Sexton's Morning Reports, Arlington National Cemetery, 1865–1867, Box 1, Record Group 92: Records of the Quartermaster General, NARA, Washington, DC.

114. The history of Freedman's Village and Arlington Cemetery is carefully told by McElya in "Politics of Mourning."

115. Louis Gerteis, *From Contraband to Freedman: The Federal Policy Toward Southern Blacks* (Westport, CT: Greenwood Press, 1977), 121.

116. Berlin et al., *Wartime Genesis of Free Labor: The Upper South*, 182–183.

Conclusion

1. Harriet A. Washington, *Medical Apartheid: The Dark History of Medical Experimentation on Black Americans from Colonial Times to the Present* (New York: Harlem Moon Broadway Books, 2006); John S. Haller Jr., *Outcasts from Evolution: Scientific Attitudes of Racial Inferiority, 1859–1900* (Urbana-Champaign: University of Illinois Press, 1971), 62–63; Vanessa Northington Gamble, "Under the Shadow of Tuskegee: African Americans and Health Care," *American Journal of Public Health* 87 (November 1997): 1773–1778; Stephen Jay Gould, *The Mismeasure of Man* (New York: W.W. Norton, 1981).

2. Benjamin Gould to Blatchford, November 25, 1865, Folder 2, Box 67, Part IV: Historical Bureau Records, New York, NY, Archives, MssCol 22263, New York Public Library Manuscripts and Archives Division, United States Sanitary Commission (USSC) Records.

3. William D. McArdle, Frank L. Katch, and Victor L. Katch, "Introduction: A View from the Past," in *Exercise Physiology: Nutrition, Energy, and Human Performance*, ed. William D. McArdle, Frank I. Katch, and Victor L. Katch, xxxii–xliii (Baltimore: Walter Kluwer, 2015), xxxvii.

4. See, for example, W. J. Burt, "Anatomical and Physiological Differences between the White and Negro Races," *American Journal of Dental Science* 10, no. 7 (1876): 289–296; D. K Shute, "Racial Anatomical Peculiarities," *Medical Examiner and General Practitioner* 6 (August 1896), 154; and James Bardin, "The Psychological Factor in Southern Race Problems," *Popular Science Monthly* 83 (October 1913): 368–374.

5. Michael Omi and Howard Winant, *Racial Formation in the United States* (New York: Taylor and Francis, 2014), 3–4. The historian of medicine Lundy Braun describes the Civil War as a "turning point in the science of race differences" in *Breathing Race into Science: The Surprising Career of the Spirometer from Plantation to Genetics* (Minneapolis: University of Minnesota Press, 2014), 31.

6. Tim Lockley, *Military Medicine and the Making of Race: Life and Death in the West India Regiments, 1795–1874* (New York: Cambridge University Press, 2020); and Andrew D. Evans, *Anthropology at War: World War I and the Science of Race in Germany* (Chicago: University of Chicago Press, 2010). Thank you to my colleague H. Glenn Penny for steering me to the latter book.

7. Susan L. Smith, *Toxic Exposures: Mustard Gas and the Health Consequences of World War II in the United States* (New Brunswick, NJ: Rutgers University Press, 2017), 42–67.

8. Margaret Humphreys, *Intensely Human: The Health of the Black Soldier in the American Civil War* (Baltimore: Johns Hopkins University Press, 2008), xiii.

9. Chandra Manning, *Troubled Refuge: Struggling for Freedom in the Civil War* (New York: Knopf, 2016); Amy Murrell Taylor, *Embattled Freedom: Journeys through the Civil War's Refugee Camps* (Chapel Hill: University of North Carolina Press, 2018); and Jim Downs, *Sick from Freedom: African-American Illness and Suffering during the Civil War and Reconstruction* (New York: Oxford University Press, 2012).

10. Rana A. Hogarth, *Medicalizing Blackness: Making Racial Difference in the Atlantic World, 1780-1840* (Chapel Hill: University of North Carolina Press, 2017), xv.

11. Dierdre Cooper Owens and Sharla Fett, "Black Maternal and Infant Health: Historical Legacies of Slavery," *American Journal of Public Health* 109, no. 10 (2019): 1342-1345.

12. Owens and Fett, "Black Maternal and Infant Health," 1344. See also Jamila K. Taylor, "Structural Racism and Maternal Heath among Black Women," *Journal of Law, Medicine, and Ethics* 48 (2020): 506-517.

13. Lundy Braun, "Race Correction and Spirometry: Why History Matters," *Chest* 159, no. 4 (2021): 1670-1675; and Braun, *Breathing Race into Science.*

14. Dorothy E. Roberts, "The Arts of Medicine: Abolish Race Correction," *The Lancet* 397, no. 10268 (2021): 17-18, quote on 18. See her larger body of work, including *Fatal Invention: How Science, Politics, and Big Business Re-create Race in the Twenty-First Century* (New York: New Press, 2011), and *Killing the Black Body: Race, Reproduction, and the Meaning of Liberty* (New York: Vintage Books, 1999).

Bibliography

Primary Sources

Manuscript Collections

Arkansas
  Fayetteville
    University of Arkansas Libraries Special Collections Department
      Ira Russell Letters, MC 581
Maryland
  College Park
    University of Maryland
      Freedmen and Southern Society Project
  Silver Spring
    National Museum of Health and Medicine
      Otis Historical Archives
        OHA 4: Curatorial Records: Autopsy Logbooks, 1866–1919
        OHA 8: Museum Records: Curatorial Records, Collection of Logbooks
        OHA 13: Curatorial Records: Incoming Correspondence (Loose),
              1862–1894
        OHA 15: Curatorial Records: Letterbooks of the Curators
        OHA 21: Outgoing Correspondence
        OHA 25: Curatorial Records: Smithsonian Correspondence
        OHA 28: Joseph Woodward Letterbooks
        OHA 38: Museum Records: Articles and Clippings
  Suitland
    National Anthropological Archives
      United States Army Medical Museum (AMM), Records concerning skeletal
            material transferred to the Smithsonian Institution, National
            Anthropological Archives, Smithsonian Institution
Massachusetts
  Boston
    Massachusetts Historical Society
      Frederick Newman Knapp Papers
Michigan
  Ann Arbor
    University of Michigan William L. Clements Library
      James S. Schoff Civil War Collection
        Jayne Papers, 1864

Missouri
  St. Louis
    Missouri Historical Society
      William Greenleaf Eliot Papers
      U. S. Sanitary Commission Pamphlets
New York, New York
  New York Public Library Manuscripts and Archives Division
    United States Sanitary Commission (USSC) Records
      Accounts and Vouchers Archive, MssCol 18820
        Part IV: USSC Staff Rosters
      Army and Navy Claim Agency Records, MssCol 18809
        Part I: Army and Navy Claim Agency
          Section B: Claim Registers
            Widows' Pensions
      Army of the Potomac Archives, MssCol 18782
        Part I: Letters and Reports
      Department of the Gulf Archives, MssCol 18590
        Part I: Main Office
        Part II: Special Relief Department
      Department of North Carolina Archives, MssCol 18581
        Part I: Letters and Reports
      Hospital Directory Archives, MssCol 19877
      Maryland Archives, MssCol 18817
        Part I: Annapolis
      New England Women's Auxiliary Association Archives, MssCol 18579
        Part III: Supplies
      New York, NY, Archives, MssCol 22263
        Part I: Standing Committee Records
        Part II: Henry W. Bellows Papers
        Part IV: Historical Bureau Records
          Section A: Office Correspondence
          Section D: Special Relief Archives
          Section E: Medical Committee Archives
            General Correspondence
      Pennsylvania Archives, MssCol 18781
        Part II: Women's Pennsylvania Branch
      Statistical Bureau Archives, MssCol 18780
        Part I: Administrative Records
          Letters Received 1864 Jan.–1869 Oct., General Correspondence
        Part VII: Physical Examinations
      Washington, DC, Archives, MssCol 22261
        Part I: Central Office
        Part II: Special Relief Department
          Section C: Homes and Lodges

Women's Central Association for Relief Records, MssCol 22266
Part I: Numbered Documents
Part III: Committee Records
North Carolina
Chapel Hill
University of North Carolina Wilson Library
Southern Historical Collection
Ira Russell Papers #4440
Durham
Duke University Library
S. Weir Mitchell Collection
Pennsylvania
Philadelphia
The College of Physicians of Philadelphia Historical Medical Library
Leidy Family Papers
Haverford
Haverford College Quaker Collections
Diaries of Julia Wilbur, March 1860 to July 1866, Transcription
Washington, DC
Library of Congress, Manuscript Division
Diary of Horatio Nelson Taft, 1861–1865
National Archives
Record Group 15: Records of the Veterans Administration
Record Group 92: Records of the Office of the Quartermaster General
Record Group 94: Records of the Adjutant General's Office, 1780–1917
Record Group 153: Records of the Office of the Judge Advocate General (Army)
Record Group 393: Records of the U.S. Army Continental Commands, 1821–1920

Online Resources

Ancestry.com. Probate Records (District of Columbia), 1801–1920: July 27, 1880, Frederic Schafhirt, Wills, Boxes 0067; Wagner, John J—0074; Buchly, Anthony, 1878–1881, U.S., Burial Registers, Military Posts and National Cemeteries, 1862–1960.
City of Alexandria (Virginia). Alexandria during the Civil War: First Person Accounts. Including the diary of Julia Wilbur. https://www.alexandriava.gov/historic/civilwar/default.aspx?id=62774.
Civil War Washington. Center for Digital Research in the Humanities and University of Nebraska-Lincoln. http://civilwardc.org/interpretations/narrative/rcwmc.php and http://civilwardc.org/texts/cases/about.
Florida History Online, Wartime Letters from Seth Rogers, M.D., Surgeon of the First South Carolina . . . 1862–1863, transcribed by University of North Florida. https://www.unf.edu/floridahistoryonline/Projects/Rogers/index.html.
Friends of Freedmen's Cemetery. https://www.freedmenscemetery.org/.

Gilder Lehrman Institute of American History. History Resources: The Western Sanitary Commission Reports on Suffering in the Mississippi Valley, 1863. http://www.gilderlehrman.org/history-by-era/african-americans-and -emancipation/resources/western-sanitary-commission-reports-suff.

Howard University College of Medicine Publications. https://dh.howard.edu/med _pub/1.

The Race and Slavery Petitions Project. Part of Digital Library on Slavery. https:// library.uncg.edu/slavery/petitions/.

Published Primary Sources

Academy of the Natural Sciences of Philadelphia. *Proceedings of the Academy of the Natural Sciences of Philadelphia, 1858*. Philadelphia: Printed for the Academy, 1859.

Adams, Virginia M. *On the Altar of Freedom: A Black Soldier's Civil War Letters from the Front, Corporal James Henry Gooding*. Amherst: University of Massachusetts Press, 1991.

"Adolph J. Schafhirt." *American Druggist and Pharmaceutical Record* 43 (July–December 1903): 188.

American Social History Project/Center for Media and Learning. "The What Is It? Exhibit." *The Lost Museum Archive*, City University of New York, 2015. https:// lostmuseum.cuny.edu/archive/exhibit/what/.

Ames, Mary Clemmer. *Ten Years in Washington: Life and Scenes in the National Capital, as a Woman Sees Them*. Hartford, CT: A.D. Worthington & Co., 1873.

Anthropological Society of America. *Uncivilized Races, Proving That Many Races of Men Are Incapable of Civilization. By an Appeal to the Most Eminent Scientific Naturalists, Explorers and Historians of All Ages. Being the Substance of a Paper Read before the Anthropological Society of America*. New York: Anthropological Society, 1868.

Aptheker, Herbert. "Negro Casualties in the Civil War." *Journal of Negro History* 32 (1947): 10–80.

Atkinson, William B., ed. *Physicians and Surgeons of the United States*. Philadelphia: Charles Robson, 1878.

Bardin, James. "The Psychological Factor in Southern Race Problems." *Popular Science Monthly* 83 (October 1913): 368–374.

Baxter, J. H. *Statistics, Medical and Anthropological, of the Provost-Marshal-General's Bureau, Derived from Records of the Examination for Military Service in the Armies of the United States during the Late War of the Rebellion, of over a Million Recruits, Drafted Men, Substitutes, and Enrolled Men: Compiled under Direction of the Secretary of War*. Washington, DC: Government Printing Office, 1875.

Beveridge, Charles E., and Charles Capen McLaughlin, eds. *The Papers of Frederick Law Olmsted*. Baltimore: Johns Hopkins University Press, 1981.

Billings, John S. "Literature and Institutions." In *A Century of American Medicine, 1776-1876*, edited by Edward Clarke et al., 289–366. Philadelphia: Henry C. Lea, 1876.

Boynton, Charles Brandon. *History of the Great Western Sanitary Fair.* Cincinnati, OH: C.F. Vent & Co., 1864. Published anonymously.

Briggs, May S., ed. *The Ferguson-Jayne Papers, 1826-1938.* 2 vols. Davenport, NY: Davenport Historical Society, 1981.

Brockett, L. P. *Heroines of the Rebellion: Or, Woman's Work in the Civil War: A Record of Heroism, Patriotism, and Patience.* Philadelphia: Edgewood, 1867.

———. *The Philanthropic Results of the War in America Collected from Official and Authentic Sources.* New York: Sheldon & Co., 1864.

Bumstead, Freeman J., et al. *Report of a Committee of the Associate Medical Members of the United States Sanitary Commission, on the Subject of Venereal Diseases, with Special References to Practice in the Army and Navy.* Washington, DC: Printed for Circulation by the United States Sanitary Commission, 1863.

Burt, W. J. "Anatomical and Physiological Differences between the White and Negro Races." *American Journal of Dental Science* 10, no. 7 (1876): 289-296.

Censer, Jane Turner, ed. *The Papers of Frederick Law Olmsted.* Baltimore: Johns Hopkins University Press, 1986.

Cobb, W. Montague. "Daniel Smith Lamb. M.D., 1843-1929." *The Journal of the National Medical Association* 50 (January 1958): 62-65.

Colyer, Vincent. *Report of the Services Rendered by the Freed People to the United States Army, in North Carolina, in the Spring of 1862, after the Battle of Newbern.* New York: Vincent Colyer, 1864.

Comstock, George C. "Biographical Memoir Benjamin Apthorp Gould, 1824-1896." In *National Academy of Sciences Biographical Memoir,* edited by the National Academy of Sciences, 155-180. Washington, DC: Government Printing Office, 1924.

Corson, Eugene Rollin. "The Vital Equation of the Colored Race and Future in the United States." In *The Wilder Quarter-Century Book,* edited by Burt G. Wilder, 115-176. Ithaca: Comstock Publishing Co., 1893.

Diefendorf, Oliver. *General Orders of the War Department, Embracing the Years 1861, 1862 & 1863.* New York: Derby & Miller, 1864.

"Editorial: The Medical and Surgical Results of the War." *Buffalo Medical and Surgical Journal* 16 (1876-7): 34-36.

Elliott, E. B. *Preliminary Report on the Mortality and Sickness of the Volunteer Forces of the United States Government, During the Present War.* Sanitary Commission, no. 46. New York: Wm. C. Bryant & Co., Printers, 1862.

———. *On the Military Statistics of the United States of America.* Berlin: R.V. Decker, 1863.

Davenport, Charles B., and Albert G. Love. *The Medical Department of the United States Army in the World War.* Vol. 15 of *Statistics, Part One: Army Anthropology.* Washington, DC: United States Government Printing Office, 1921.

Du Bois, W. E. B. "The Negro in Africa and America by Joseph Alexander Tillinghast." *Political Science Quarterly* 18 (December 1903): 695-697.

———, ed. *The Health and Physique of the Negro American. Report of a Social Study Made under the Direction of Atlanta University; Together with the Proceedings of the Eleventh Conference for the Study of the Negro Problems, Held at Atlanta University, on May the 29th, 1906* (Atlanta, GA: Atlanta University Press, 1906).

Federal Writers Project. *Slave Narratives: A Folk History of Slavery in the United States from Interviews with Former Slaves*. Vol. 4: *Georgia*, Part 1, Willis Cofer, https://www.loc.gov/item/mesn041/; Vol. 4, *Georgia*, Part 3, Julia Larker, https://www.loc.gov/item/mesn043; Vol. 7: *Kentucky*, Mary Wright, https://www.loc.gov/item/mesn070. Library of Congress, n.d.

Giesberg, Judith, ed. *Emilie Davis's Civil War: The Diaries of a Free Black Woman in Philadelphia, 1863-1865*. University Park: Pennsylvania State University Press, 2014.

Gladding, H. G., and Frederick A. Farely. *History of the Brooklyn and Long Island Fair, February 22, 1864*. Brooklyn: Union Steam Presses, 1864.

Gould, Benjamin A. *Investigations in the Military and Anthropological Statistics of American Soldiers*. Cambridge, MA: Riverside Press, 1869.

Grace, William. *The Army Surgeon's Manual for the Use of Medical Officers, Cadets, Chaplains, and Hospital Stewards Containing the Regulations of the Medical Department, All General Orders from the War Department and Circulars from the Surgeon-General's Office from January 1st, 1861, to April 1st, 1865*. New York: Baillière Brothers, 1865.

Henry, Robert S. *The Armed Forces Institute of Pathology: Its First Century, 1862-1962*. Washington, DC: Office of the Surgeon General, 1964.

Hoffman, Frederick L. *Race Traits and Tendencies of the American Negro*. New York: Macmillan Co., 1896.

Hrdlička, Aleš. "Anthropology of the American Negro: Historical Notes." *American Journal of Physical Anthropology* 5 (April–June 1927): 205–221.

Hunt, James. *Anniversary Address Delivered before the Anthropological Society of London, January 5, 1864*. London: Trübner & Co., 1864.

——. "Introductory Address on the Study of Anthropology." *Anthropological Review* 1 (May 1863): 1–20.

Hunt, Sanford B. "The Negro as a Soldier." *Quarterly Journal of Psychological Medicine and Medical Jurisprudence* 1 (October 1867): 161–186.

Jacobs, Harriet [Linda Brent]. "Life among the Contrabands." *Liberator*, 5 September 1862, 3.

Jaquette, Henrietta Stratton, ed. *Letters of a Civil War Nurse: Cornelia Hancock, 1863-1865*. Lincoln: University of Nebraska Press, 1998.

Johnson, Rossiter, ed. *Twentieth Century Biographical Dictionary of Notable Americans*. Vols. 1–10. Boston: Biographical Society, 1904.

Jones, Rufus S. "Letter from Sergeant-Major Rufus S. Jones, 8th U.S. Colored Troops," *Christian Recorder*, May 7, 1864.

Kelly, Howard A., and Walter L. Burrage. *American Medical Biographies*. Baltimore: The Norman Remington Co., 1920.

Ladies' Union Association of Philadelphia. *Report of the Ladies' Union Association of Philadelphia, Formed July 20th, 1863, for the Purpose of Administering Exclusively to the Wants of the Sick and Wounded Colored Soldiers*. Philadelphia: G.T. Stockdale, 1867.

Lamb, Daniel S. "The American Medical Museum, Washington, D.C." *Military Surgeon* 53 (1923): 89–140.

————. *The Army Medical Museum—A History*. Washington, DC: Beresford, 1916.

————. "A History of the United States Army Medical Museum, 1862–1917." Unpublished manuscript [1917]. https://collections.nlm.nih.gov/catalog /nlm:nlmuid-12710920R-bk.

————. "Howard University Medical Department: A Historical, Biographical and Statistical Souvenir." College of Medicine Publications, 1 (1900). Digital Howard, https://dh.howard.edu/med_pub/1.

————. "Some Reminiscences of Post Mortem Work." *Washington Medical Annals* 2, no. 6 (January 1904): 383–390.

Livermore, Mary A. *My Story of the War: A Woman's Narrative of Four Years Personal Experience as Nurse in the Union Army, and in Relief Work at Home, in Hospitals, Camps, and at the Front, during the War of the Rebellion. With Anecdotes, Pathetic Incidents, and Thrilling Reminiscences Portraying the Lights and Shadows of Hospital Life and the Sanitary Service of the War.* Hartford, CT: A.D. Worthington & Co., 1889.

Matas, Rudolph. *The Surgical Peculiarities of the American Negro: A Statistical Inquiry Based upon the Records of the Charity Hospital of New Orleans, La., Decennium 1884-'94.* Philadelphia: [no identified publisher], 1896.

McDowell, A. W. "Hospital Observations upon Negro Soldiers." *American Practitioner* (July 1874): 155–158.

Miller, Kelly. "A Review of Hoffman's Race Traits and Tendencies of the American Negro." *American Negro Academy, Occasional Papers.* Washington, DC: The Academy, 1897.

Minor, W. C. *Post Mortem Examinations Made at Knight U.S.A. General Hospital.* New Haven, CT: Knight Hospital Print, 1864.

N. "Honor to Whom Honor Is Due." *Liberator*, December 16, 1864.

National U.S. Army General Hospital. *Observation Book Containing Certain Inductions and Classifications Ante Mortem and Post Mortems.* Baltimore: U.S. Army General Hospital Printing Office, [1865?].

Newberry, J. S. *The U.S. Sanitary Commission in the Valley of the Mississippi, during the War of the Rebellion, 1861-1866.* Cleveland: Fairbanks, Benedict & Co., 1871.

New York Religious Society of Friends. "Report of a Committee of the Representatives of New York Yearly Meeting of Friends, upon the Condition and Wants of the Colored Refugees." *Friends' Review: A Religious, Literary and Miscellaneous Journal,* January 24, 1863.

Olmsted, Frederick Law. *[Confidential] Report of the Secretary with Regard to the Probable Origin of the Recent Demoralization of the Volunteer Army at Washington and the Duty of the Sanitary Commission with Regard to Certain Deficiencies in the Existing Army Arrangements as Suggested Thereby.* Washington, DC: McGill & Witherow, Printers, 1861.

Parsons, Emily. *Memoir of Emily Elizabeth Parsons, Published for the Benefit of Cambridge Hospital.* Boston: Little, Brown & Co., 1880.

Race & Slavery Petitions Project, Digital Library on American Slavery, University of North Carolina at Greensboro. https://library.uncg.edu/slavery/petitions/. Petition 10682001 [Richmond, GA, ca. 1820], http://library.uncg.edu/slavery

/petitions/details.aspx?pid=448; Petition 11385602 [Charleston, SC, ca 1856], http://library.uncg.edu/slavery/petitions/details.aspx?pid=1627; Petition 11683411 [Richmond, VA, December 17, 1834], http://library.uncg.edu/slavery/petitions/details.aspx?pid=2683.

Reid, Richard M., ed. *Practicing Medicine in a Black Regiment: The Civil War Diary of Burt G. Wilder, 55th Massachusetts*. Amherst: University of Massachusetts Press, 2010.

———, ed. *Recollections of a Civil War Medical Cadet: Burt Green Wilder*. Kent, OH: Kent State University Press, 2017.

"Reviews and Book Notices: *The Medical and Surgical Results of the War of the Rebellion*." *Northwestern Medical and Surgical Journal* 3, no. 12 (1873): 484–485.

Richardson, Stephen J. "The Burial Grounds of Black Washington: 1880–1919." *Records of the Columbia Historical Society* 52 (1989): 304–326.

Ripley, C. Peter, ed. *The Black Abolitionist Papers*. Chapel Hill: University of North Carolina Press, 1992.

Ripley, William Z. *The Races of Europe: A Sociological Study*. New York: D. Appleton, 1899.

Rosecrans, W. S. "Art. VIII: Annual Report of the Western Sanitary Commission for the Years Ending July 1862, and July 1863; Circular of Mississippi Valley Sanitary Fair, to Be Held in St. Louis, May 17th, 1864." *North American Review* 98 (April 1864): 519–530.

Rothenberg, Marc, et al., eds. *The Papers of Joseph Henry*. Vol. 10: *The Smithsonian Years: January 1858–December 1865*. Sagamore Beach, MA: Science History, 2004.

Russell, Ira. "Cerebro-Spinal Meningitis as It Appeared among the Troops Stationed at Benton Barracks, Mo." *Boston Medical and Surgical Journal* 70 (May 19, 1964): 309–313.

———. "Hospital Reports: Benton Barracks." *St. Louis Medical and Surgical Journal* (March–April 1864): 121–128.

———. "Vaccination in the Army." In *Sanitary Memoirs, Contributions to the Causation and Prevention of Disease, and to Camp Diseases*, edited by Austin Flint, 144–145. New York: Hurd and Houghton, 1867.

Schultz, Adolphe H. "Biographical Memoir of Aleš Hrdlička." *National Academy of Sciences of the United States of America Biographical Memoirs* 23 (1944): 305–338.

Seaver, Jay W. *Anthropometry and Physical Examination: A Book for Practical Use in Connection with Gymnastic Work and Physical Education*. New Haven, CT: Press of the O. A. Gorman Co., 1896.

Shute, D. K. "Racial Anatomical Peculiarities." *Medical Examiner and General Practitioner* 6 (August 1896): 123–132.

Steiner, Lewis. "Report on the Operations of the Eastern Department." *Sanitary Commission Bulletin* (November 1, 1863): 4–10.

Stillé, Charles. *History of the United States Sanitary Commission, Being the General Report of Its Work during the War of the Rebellion*. Philadelphia: J.B. Lippincott & Co., 1866.

———. *The Sanitary Commission of the United States Army: A Succinct Narrative of Its Works and Purposes*. New York: Published for the Benefit of the United States Sanitary Commission, 1864.

Surgeon General's Office. "Circular No. 2, May 21, 1862." National Library of Medicine Digital Collections. http://resource.nlm.nih.gov/101534229.

Tillinghast, Joseph Alexander. "The Negro in Africa and America." *Publications of the American Economic Association* 3 (May 1902): 403–637.

Trumbull, Henry Clay. *War Memories of an Army Chaplain*. New York: Charles Scribner's Sons, 1898.

Union League Club. *Report of the Committee on Volunteering, Presented October 18th, 1864*. New York: Union League Club, 1864.

United States Census Office, Department of the Interior. *Instructions to Assistant Marshals, Act of May 23, 1850*. Washington, DC: Government Printing Office, 1870

———. *Instructions to U.S. Marshals, Instructions to Assistants, Eighth Census, United States, —Act of Congress of Twenty-Third May, 1850*. Washington, DC: Geo. W. Bowman, Public Printer, 1860.

United States Sanitary Commission. *The Book of Bubbles, A Contribution to the New York Fair, in Aid of the Sanitary Commission*. New York: Endicott & Co, 1864.

———. *Documents of the U.S. Sanitary Commission*. 2 vols. New York: 1866.

———. *Hints for the Control and Prevention of Infectious Diseases in Camps, Transports, and Hospital*. New York: Wm. C. Bryant & Co., 1863.

———. *Military Medical and Surgical Essays Prepared for the United States Sanitary Commission 1862–1864*. Washington, DC: 1865.

———. *The Sanitary Commission of the U.S. Army, A Succinct History of its Works and Purposes*. New York: 1864.

United States Sanitary Commission, Boston Branch. *Report Concerning the Special Relief Service of the U.S. Sanitary Commission in Boston, Mass. for the Year Ending March 31, 1864*. Boston: Prentiss & Deland, 1864.

United States Sanitary Commission, Philadelphia Branch. *Report of the General Superintendent of the Philadelphia Branch of the U.S. Sanitary Commission to the Executive Committee, January 1st, 1865*. Philadelphia: King & Baird, Printers, 1865.

———. *Report of the General Superintendent of the Philadelphia Branch of the U.S. Sanitary Commission to the Executive Committee, January 1st, 1866*. Philadelphia: King & Baird, Printers, 1866.

United States Sanitary Commission Statistical Bureau. *Ages of U. S. Volunteer Soldiery*. New York: 1866.

United States Sanitary Commission, Women's Pennsylvania Branch. *Report of the Proceedings of a Meeting of the Ladies and Ward Visitors of the Special Relief Committee, Held at the Rooms of the Committee on Monday, January 18th, 1864*. [1864].

United States Surgeon General's Office. *The Medical and Surgical History of the War of the Rebellion 1861–1865*. 6 Vols. Washington, DC: Government Printing Office, 1870–1883.

United States War Department. *The War of the Rebellion: A Compilation of Official Records of the Union and Confederate Armies*. Washington, DC: Government Printing Office, 1880–1901.

Weld, Charles Richard. "History of the Royal Society; with the Memoirs of the Presidents." *British Quarterly Review* 39 (January–April 1864): 105–110.

Western Sanitary Commission. *Final Report of the Western Sanitary Commission, from May 9th, 1864, to December 31st, 1865*. St. Louis: R.F. Studley & Co., 1866.

Wilder, Burt Green, "Louis Agassiz, Teacher." *Harvard Graduate's Magazine,* June 1907, [603–606]. https://archive.org/details/louisagassizteacoowild/page/n3.

White, Andrew Dickson. *The Annual Report of the Women's Pennsylvania Branch, U.S. Sanitary Commission, Present April 1, 1864.* Philadelphia: Henry B. Ashmead, Book and Job Printer, 1864.

Women's Central Association of Relief. *Second Annual Report of the Women's Central Association of Relief, No. 10, Cooper Union, New York.* New York: William S. Dorr, Book & Job Printer, 1863.

Woodhull, Alfred A. *Catalogue of the Medical Section of the US Army Medical Museum.* Washington, DC: Government Printing Office, 1866.

Wormeley, Katharine Prescott. *The United States Sanitary Commission, A Sketch of Its Purposes and Its Work.* Boston: Little, Brown & Co., 1863.

Yellin, Jean Fagan, ed. *The Harriet Jacobs Family Papers,* 2 vols. Chapel Hill: University of North Carolina, 2008.

Newspapers and Journals

The American Journal of the Medical Sciences
The American Literary Gazette and Publishers' Circular
Anti-Slavery Standard
Atlantic Monthly
The Boston Medical and Surgical Journal
The British Medical Journal
The British Quarterly Review
The Buffalo Medical and Surgical Journal
The Chicago Tribune
The Chicago Medical Examiner
Christian Recorder
Daily National Republican (Washington, DC)
Daily Missouri Democrat
Evening Star
Harper's Weekly

The Independent Medical Investigator
The Journal of Social Science
The Liberator
The Medical Examiner
Medical News
The Medical and Surgical Reporter
National Anti-Slavery Standard
The New York Times
The North Star
The Northwestern Medical and Surgical Journal
The Philadelphia Medical Times
The Round Table
Sanitary Commission Bulletin
The Spectator
Weekly Anglo African
The Western and Southern Medical Recorder

Secondary Sources

Adams, Virginia M. *On the Altar of Freedom: A Black Soldier's Civil War Letters from the Front, Corporal James Henry Gooding.* Amherst: University of Massachusetts Press, 1991.

Associated Press and NBC Washington Staff. "Evidence Shows U. Richmond Was Built Over Slave Burial Site." 4 *NBC Washington,* January 22, 2020. https://www .nbcwashington.com/news/evidence-shows-u-richmond-was-built-over-slave -burial-site/2202692/.

Attie, Jeanie. *Patriotic Toil: Northern Women and the American Civil War*. Ithaca, NY: Cornell University Press, 1998.

Barrett, James R., and David Roediger. "Inbetween Peoples: Race, Nationality and the 'New Immigrant' Working Class." *Journal of American Ethnic History* 16, no. 3 (1997): 3–44.

Barton, Angela Locke. "Shards of Medical History: Artifacts from the Point San Jose Hospital Medical Waste Pit." Paper presented at the 83rd Annual Meeting of the Society for American Archaeology, Washington, DC, 2018.

Bay, Mia. *The White Image in the Black Mind: African-American Ideas about White People, 1830–1925*. Oxford: Oxford University Press, 2000.

Bencel, Nicholas, Thomas David, and Dominic Thomas, eds. *The Invention of Race: Scientific and Popular Representations*. New York: Routledge, 2014.

Berlin, Ira, Steven F. Miller, Joseph P. Reidy, and Leslie S. Rowland, eds. *The Wartime Genesis of Free Labor: The Upper South*. Series 1, Vol. 2 of *Freedom: A Documentary History of Emancipation, 1861–1867, Selected from the Holdings of the National Archives of the United States*. New York: Cambridge University Press, 1993.

Berlin, Ira, Joseph P. Reidy, and Leslie Rowland, eds. *The Black Military Experience*. Series 2, Book 1, of *Freedom: A Documentary History of Emancipation, 1861–1867, Selected from the Holdings of the National Archives of the United States*. New York: Cambridge University Press, 1982.

Berry, Daina Ramey. *The Price for Their Pound of Flesh: The Value of the Enslaved, from Womb to Grave, in the Building of a Nation*. Boston: Beacon Press, 2017.

Beveridge, Charles E., and Charles Capen McLaughlin, eds. *The Papers of Frederick Law Olmsted*. Baltimore: Johns Hopkins University Press, 1981.

Bevers, Amanda E. "To Bind Up the Nation's Wounds: The Army Medical Museum and the Development of American Medical Science, 1862–1913." PhD diss., University of California, San Diego, 2015.

Black, Andrew K. "In the Service of the United States: Comparative Mortality among African-American and White Troops in the Union Army." *Journal of Negro History* 79, no. 4 (1994): 317–333.

Blair, Jenny. "A Tortured Soul Finds Redemption in Words." *Yale Medicine Magazine*, Winter 2009, https://medicine.yale.edu/news/yale-medicine-magazine/a-tortured-soul-finds-redemption-in-words/.

Blakely, Robert L., and Judith M. Harrington, eds. *Bones in the Basement: Postmortem Racism in Nineteenth-Century Medical Training*. Washington, DC: Smithsonian Institution Press, 1997.

———. "Grave Consequences: The Opportunistic Procurement of Cadavers at the Medical College of Georgia." In *Bones in the Basement: Postmortem Racism in Nineteenth-Century Medical Training*, edited by Robert L. Blakely and Judith M. Harrington, 162–183. Washington, DC: Smithsonian Institution Press, 1997.

Blight, David W., and Jim Downs, eds. *Beyond Freedom: Disrupting the History of Emancipation*. Athens: University of Georgia Press, 2017.

Blustein, Bonnie E. "'To Increase the Efficiency of the Medical Department': A New Approach to U.S. Civil War Medicine." *Civil War History* 33 (1987): 22–41.

Bollet, Alfred Jay. *Civil War Medicine: Challenges and Triumphs*. Tucson, AZ: Galen Press, 2002.

Bouldin, Kristin Leigh. "Is This Freedom?: Government Exploitation of Contraband Laborers in Virginia, South Carolina, and Washington, D.C. during the American Civil War." Master's thesis, University of Mississippi, 2014.

Braun, Lundy. *Breathing Race into Science: The Surprising Career of the Spirometer from Plantation to Genetics*. Minneapolis: University of Minnesota Press, 2014.

———. "Race Correction and Spirometry: Why History Matters." *Chest* 159, no. 4 (2021): 1670–1675.

———. "Spirometry, Measurement, and Race in the Nineteenth Century." *Journal of the History of Medicine and Allied Sciences* 2 (April 2005): 135–169.

Bremner, Robert H. *The Public Good: Philanthropy and Welfare in the Civil War Era*. New York: Knopf, 1980.

Brookes, Daphne A. *Bodies in Dissent: Spectacular Performances of Race and Freedom, 1850–1910*. Durham, NC: Duke University Press, 2006.

Brown, Vincent. *The Reaper's Garden: Death and Power in the World of Atlantic Slavery*. Cambridge, MA: Harvard University Press, 2008.

Browner, Stephanie P. *Profound Science and Elegant Literature: Imagining Doctors in Nineteenth-Century America*. Philadelphia: University of Pennsylvania Press, 2005.

Bruce, Robert V. *The Launching of Modern American Science, 1846–1876*. New York: Alfred A. Knopf, 1987.

Butts, Heather M. "Alexander Thomas Augusta—Physician, Teacher, and Human Rights Activist." *Journal of the National Medical Association* 1 (January 2005): 106–109.

Camp, Stephanie M. H. *Closer to Freedom: Enslaved Women and Everyday Resistance in the Plantation South*. Chapel Hill: University of North Carolina Press, 2004.

Cassedy, James H. *American Medicine and Statistical Thinking, 1800–1860*. Cambridge, MA: Harvard University Press, 1984.

———. "Numbering the North's Medical Events: Humanitarianism and Science in Civil War Statistics." *Bulletin of the History of Medicine* 66 (1992): 210–233.

Cervetti, Nancy. *S. Weir Mitchell, 1829–1914: Philadelphia's Literary Physician*. University Park, PA: Pennsylvania State University Press, 2012.

Chilton, Katherine. "'City of Refuge': Urban Labor, Gender, and Family Formation during Slavery and the Transition to Freedom in the District of Columbia, 1820–1875." PhD diss., Carnegie Mellon University, 2009.

Clarke, Michael Tavel. "Andrometer." *Victorian Review* 34 (2008): 22–28.

Cobb, Jasmine Nichole. *Picture Freedom: Remaking Black Visuality in the Early Nineteenth Century*. New York: New York University Press, 2015.

Cobb, W. Montague. "Daniel Smith Lamb. M.D., 1843–1929." *Journal of the National Medical Association* 50 (1958): 62–65.

Cober, Katherine. "Dissecting Race: An Examination of Anatomical Illustration and the Absence of Non-white Bodies." Master's thesis, Dalhousie University, 2015.

Coddington, Ron. "The Napoleon of Surgeons." *Faces of War*, May 4, 2013, http://facesofthecivilwar.blogspot.com/2013/05the-napoleon-of-surgeons.html.

Connolly, Brian, and Marisa J. Fuentes. "Introduction: From Archives of Slavery to Liberated Futures." *History of the Present* 6 no. 2 (2016), 105–116.

Cooper, Heather Lee. "Upstaging *Uncle Tom's Cabin*: African American Representations of Slavery on the Public Stage before and after the Civil War." PhD diss., University of Iowa, 2017.

Crais, Clifton, and Pamela Scully. *Sara Baartman and the Hottentot Venus: A Ghost Story and a Biography*. Princeton, NJ: Princeton University Press, 2010.

Dain, Bruce. *A Hideous Monster of the Mind: American Race Theory in the Early Republic.* Cambridge, MA: Harvard University Press, 2002.

Daniels, Daryl Keith. "African Americans at the Yale University School of Medicine, 1810–1960." MD diss., Yale University School of Medicine, 1991.

Davidson, Jane P. *The Bone Sharp: The Life of Edward Drinker Cope*. Philadelphia: Academy of Natural Sciences of Philadelphia, 1997.

Davis, Cynthia J. *Bodily and Narrative Forms: The Influence of Medicine on Medical Literature, 1845–1915*. Stanford, CA: Stanford University Press, 2000.

De la Cova, Carlina. "Army Health Care for Sable Soldiers during the American Civil War." In *Bioarcheology of Women and Children in Times of War*, edited by Debra L. Martin and Caryn Tegmeyer, 129–148. Basel, Switzerland: Springer International, 2017.

Dennee, Tim. "African-American Civilians and Soldiers Treated at Claremont Smallpox Hospital, Fairfax County, Virginia, 1862–1865." Friends of Freedmen's Cemetery, 2008–2015. http://www.freedmenscemetery.org/resources/documents/claremont.pdf.

———. "A District of Columbia Freedmen's Cemetery in Virginia? African Americans Interred in Section 27 of Arlington National Cemetery, 1864–1867." Friends of Freedmen's Cemetery, 2011–2016. http://www.freedmenscemetery.org/resources/documents/arlington-section27.pdf.

———. "A House Divided Still Stands: The Contraband Hospital and Alexandria's Freedmen's Aid Workers." Friends of Freedmen's Cemetery, 2011–2017. www.freedmenscemetery.org/resources/documents/contrabandhospital.pdf.

DeRoche, Andrew J. "Freedom without Equality: Maine Civil War Soldiers' Attitudes about Slavery and African Americans." *UCLA Historical Journal* 16 (1996): 24–38.

Desmond, Jane. *Staging Tourism: Bodies on Display from Waikiki to Sea World*. Chicago: University of Chicago Press, 1999.

Devine, Shauna. *Learning from the Wounded: The Civil War and the Rise of American Medical Science*. Chapel Hill: University of North Carolina Press, 2014.

Downs, Jim. *Sick from Freedom: African-American Illness and Suffering during the Civil War and Reconstruction*. New York: Oxford University Press, 2012.

Egerton, Douglas R. "A Peculiar Mark of Infamy: Dismemberment, Burial, and Rebelliousness in Slave Societies." In *Mortal Remains: Death in Early America*, edited by Nancy Isenberg and Andrew Burstein, 149–160. Philadelphia: University of Pennsylvania Press, 2003.

Emberton, Carol. "'Cleaning up the Mess': Some Thoughts on Freedom, Violence, and Grief." In *Beyond Freedom: Disrupting the History of Emancipation*, edited by

David W. Blight and Jim Downs, 136–144. Athens: University of Georgia Press, 2017.

Evans, Andrew D. *Anthropology at War: World War I and the Science of Race in Germany*. Chicago: University of Chicago Press, 2010.

Fabian, Ann. *The Skull Collectors. Race, Science, and America's Unburied Dead*. Chicago: University of Chicago Press, 2010.

Farland, Maria. "W.E.B. DuBois, Anthropometric Science, and the Limits of Racial Uplift." *American Quarterly* 4 (December 2006): 1017–1044.

Faulkner, Carol. *Women's Radical Reconstruction: The Freedmen's Aid Movement*. Philadelphia: University of Pennsylvania Press, 2006.

Faust, Drew Gilpin. "Battle over the Bodies: Burying and Reburying the Civil War Dead, 1865–1871." In *Wars within a War: Controversy and Conflict in the American Civil War*, edited by Joan Waugh and Gary Gallagher, 184–201. Chapel Hill: University of North Carolina Press, 2009.

———. *This Republic of Suffering: Death and the American Civil War*. New York: Alfred A. Knopf, 2008.

Fears, Danika. "Remains of Civil War Soldiers Found in 'Limb Burial Pit' Tell Tale of Bloody Battle." *Daily Beast*, June 20, 2018. https://www.thedailybeast.com/remains -of-civil-war-soldiers-found-in-limb-burial-pit-tell-tale-of-bloody-battle.

Fett, Sharla M. *Working Cures: Healing, Health, and Power on Southern Slave Plantations*. Chapel Hill: University of North Carolina Press, 2002.

Fields, Barbara. "Whiteness, Racism, and Identity." *International Labor and Working-Class History* 60 (Fall 2001): 48–56.

Fields, Karen E., and Barbara J. Fields. *Racecraft: The Soul of Inequality in American Life*. London: Verso Books, 2012.

Finley, Randy. "In War's Wake: Health Care and Arkansas Freedmen, 1863–1868." *Arkansas Historical Quarterly* 51 (Summer 1992): 135–163.

Forbes, Ella. *African American Women during the Civil War*. New York: Garland, 1998.

Foster, Gaines M. "The Limitations of Federal Health Care for Freedmen, 1862–1868." *Journal of Southern History* 48 (August 1982): 349–372.

Frankel, Oz. *States of Inquiry: Social Investigations and Print Culture in Nineteenth-Century Britain and the United States*. Baltimore: Johns Hopkins University Press, 2006.

Freemon, Frank. "Lincoln Finds a Surgeon General: William A. Hammond and the Transformation of the Union Army Medical Bureau." *Civil War History* 33 (1987): 5–21.

Fuentes, Marisa J. "A Violent and Violating Archive: Black Life and the Slave Trade." *Black Perspectives*, March 7, 2017. https://www.aaihs.org/a-violent-and-violating -archive-black-life-and-the-slave-trade/.

———. *Dispossessed Lives: Enslaved Women, Violence, and the Archive*. Philadelphia: University of Pennsylvania Press, 2016.

Gamble, Vanessa Northington. *Making a Place for Ourselves: The Black Hospital Movement, 1920–1945*. New York: Oxford University Press, 1995.

———. "Under the Shadow of Tuskegee: African Americans and Health Care." *American Journal of Public Health* 87 (November 1997): 1773–1778.

Georgetown University History 396 Class. "Escaping Slavery, Building Diverse Communities: Stories of the Search for Freedom in the Capitol Region Since the Civil War." May 13, 2020. https://storymaps.arcgis.com/stories/98843655e3474b9 ab19a2afe250f0f22.

Gerteis, Louis. *Civil War St. Louis*. Lawrence: University Press of Kansas, 2001.

———. *From Contraband to Freedman: The Federal Policy Toward Southern Blacks*. Westport, CT: Greenwood Press, 1977.

Giesberg, Judith. *Civil War Sisterhood: The U.S. Sanitary Commission and Women's Politics in Transition*. Boston: Northeastern University Press, 2000.

Gilmore, Ruth Wilson. "Fatal Couplings of Power and Difference: Notes on Racism and Geography." *Professional Geographer* 54, no. 1 (2002): 15–24.

Gindhart, Patricia S. "The Dead Shall Teach the Living." *Journal of the Washington Academy of Sciences* 79 (1989): 123–129.

Gingerich, Owen. "Benjamin Apthorp Gould and the Founding of the Astronomical Journal." *Astronomy Journal* 117 (1999): 1–5.

Glatthaar, Joseph T. "The Costliness of Discrimination: Medical Care for Black Troops in the Civil War." In *Inside the Confederate Nation: Essays in Honor of Emory M. Thomas*, edited by Leslie J. Gordon and John C. Inscoe, 251–271, Baton Rouge: Louisiana State University Press, 2005.

———. *Forged in Battle: The Civil War Alliance of Black Soldiers and White Officers*. New York: Free Press, 1990.

Glymph, Thavolia. "Black Women and Children in the Civil War: Archive Notes." In *Beyond Freedom: Disrupting the History of Emancipation*, edited by David W. Blight and Jim Downs, 121–135. Athens: University of Georgia Press, 2017.

Goddu, Teresa A. "The Antislavery Almanac and the Discourse of Numeracy." *Book History* 12 (2009): 129–131.

Gordon-Chipembere, Natasha, ed. *Representation and Black Womanhood: The Legacy of Sara Baartman*. New York: Palgrave-McMillan, 2011.

Gould, Stephen Jay. *The Mismeasure of Man*. New York: W.W. Norton, 1981.

Grant, Susan-Mary. "Raising the Dead: War, Memory and American National Identity." *Nations and Nationalism* 11 (2005): 509–529.

Greenwood, Janette Thomas. *First Fruits of Freedom: The Migration of Former Slaves and Their Search for Equality in Worcester, Massachusetts, 1862–1900*. Chapel Hill: University of North Carolina Press, 2009.

Hacking, Ian. "Biopower and the Avalanche of Printed Numbers." *Humanities in Society* 5 (1992): 279–295.

Haller, John S., Jr. *Outcasts from Evolution: Scientific Attitudes of Racial Inferiority, 1859–1900*. Urbana-Champaign: University of Illinois Press, 1971.

Halperin, Edward C. "The Poor, the Black, and the Marginalized as the Source of Cadavers in United States Anatomical Education." *Clinical Anatomy* 20, no. 5 (2007): 489–495.

Harrison, Mark. "Disease and Medicine in the Armies of British India, 1750–1830: The Treatment of Fevers and the Emergence of Tropical Therapeutics." In *British Military and Naval Medicine, 1600–1830*, edited by Geoffrey Hudson, 84–119. Amsterdam: Rodopi, 2007.

Harrison, Robert. *Washington during Civil War and Reconstruction: Race and Radicalism*. Cambridge: Cambridge University Press, 2011.

Harrison, Simon. "Bones in the Rebel Lady's Boudoir: Ethnology, Race and Trophy-Hunting in the American Civil War." *Journal of Material Culture* 5 (2010): 385–401.

Hartman, Saidiya. "Venus in Two Acts." *Small Axe* 26, no. 2 (June 2008): 1–14.

Helton, Laura, Justin Leroy, Max Mishler, Samantha Seeley, and Shauna Sweeney. "The Question of Recovery: Slavery, Freedom, and the Archive." *Social Text* 33, no. 4 (2015): 1–18.

Heng, Geraldine. *The Invention of Race in the European Middle Ages*. New York: Cambridge University Press, 2018.

Henry, Robert. *The Armed Forces Institute of Pathology: Its First Century, 1862–1962*. Washington, DC: Office of the Surgeon General, 1964.

Hogarth, Rana A. "A Case Study in Charleston: Impressions of the Early National Slave Hospital." In *Medicine and Healing in the Age of Slavery*, edited by Sean Morey Smith and Christopher D. E. Willoughby, 143–164. Baton Rouge: Louisiana State University Press, 2021.

———. *Medicalizing Blackness: Making Racial Difference in the Atlantic World, 1780–1840*. Chapel Hill: University of North Carolina Press, 2017.

Holloway, Karla F. C. *Passed On: African American Mourning Stories*. Durham, NC: Duke University Press, 2003.

Holt, Thomas, Casandra Smith-Parker, and Rosalyn Terborg-Penn. *A Special Mission: The Story of Freedmen's Hospital, 1862–1962*. Washington, DC: Academic Affairs Division, Howard University, 1975.

Hovenkamp, Herbert. "Social Science and Segregation before Brown." In *Critical White Studies: Looking behind the Mirror*, edited by Richard Delgado and Jean Stefanic, 199–209. Philadelphia: Temple University Press, 1997.

Hoy, Suellen. *Chasing Dirt: The American Pursuit of Cleanliness*. New York: Oxford University Press, 1996.

Humphrey, David C. "Dissection and Discrimination: The Social Origins of Cadavers in America, 1760–1915." *Bulletin of the New York Academy of Medicine* 49 (1973): 819–827.

Humphreys, Margaret. *Intensely Human: The Health of the Black Soldier in the American Civil War*. Baltimore: Johns Hopkins University Press, 2008.

———. *Marrow of Tragedy: The Health Crisis of the American Civil War*. Baltimore: Johns Hopkins University Press, 2013.

Isenberg, Nancy, and Andrew Burstein, eds. *Mortal Remains: Death in Early America*. Philadelphia: University of Pennsylvania Press, 2003.

Johnson, James Elton. "A History of Camp William Penn and Its Black Troops in the Civil War, 1863–1865." PhD diss., University of Pennsylvania, 1999.

Kantrowitz, Stephen. *More Than Freedom: Fighting for Black Citizenship in a White Republic, 1829–1889*. New York: Penguin, 2012.

Keane, Jennifer. "A Comparative Study of White and Black American Soldiers during the First World War." *Annales de démographie historique* 103 (2002): 71–90.

Kenny, Stephen C. "The Development of Medical Museums in the Antebellum American South: Slave Bodies in Networks of Anatomical Exchange." *Bulletin of the History of Medicine* 87 (Spring 2013): 32–62.

———. "'A Dictate of Both Interest and Mercy': Slave Hospitals in the Antebellum South." *Journal of the History of Medicine and Allied Sciences* 65 (2009): 1–47.

Kuritz, Hyman. "The Popularization of Science in Nineteenth-Century America." *History of Education Quarterly* 21, no. 3 (1981): 259–274.

Lande, Jonathan. "Trials of Freedom: African American Deserters during the U.S. Civil War." *Journal of Social History* 49 (2016): 693–709.

Lass, Virginia Jeans, ed. *Wartime Washington: The Civil War Letters of Elizabeth Blair Lee*. Urbana: University of Illinois Press, 1999.

Lawrence, Susan C. "Medical and Surgical Cases: Sources and Methods." In *Civil War Washington*, ed. Susan C. Lawrence, Elizabeth Lorang, Kenneth M. Price, and Kenneth J. Winkle, Lincoln: Center for Digital Research, University of Nebraska, 2006. http://civilwardc.org/texts/cases/about.

———. "Reading Civil War Medical Cases." In *Civil War Washington*, ed. Susan C. Lawrence, Elizabeth Lorang, Kenneth M. Price, and Kenneth J. Winkle, Lincoln: Center for Digital Research, University of Nebraska, 2006. http://civilwardc.org/interpretations/narrative/rcwmc.php.

Lawrie, Paul H. D. "'Mortality as the Life Story of a People': Frederick L. Hoffman and Actuarial Narratives of African American Extinction, 1896–1915." *Canadian Review of American Studies* 43 (Winter 2013): 352–387.

Lawson, Melinda. *Patriotic Fires: Forging a New American Nationalism in the Civil War North*. Lawrence: University of Kansas Press, 2002.

Lindfors, Bernth, ed. *Africans on Stage: Studies in Ethnological Show Business*. Bloomington: Indiana University Press, 1999.

Little, Becky. "Grisly Civil War Pit Reveals Bones of Severed Limbs." *History Channel*, June 22, 2018. https://web.archive.org/web/20180623011701/https://www.history.com/news/civil-war-burial-bones-severed-limbs.

Liu, Amy. "Penn Used Bodies of Enslaved People for Teaching Purposes after Death, Student Research Reveals." *Daily Pennsylvanian*, December 10, 2018. https://www.thedp.com/article/2018/12/penn-slavery-project-ties-university-upenn-medicine.

"Local Legends: Broadmoor's Word-Finder," *BBC Legacies: Berkshire*, December 1, 2014, https://www.bbc.co.uk/legacies/myths_legends/england/berkshire/article_1.shtml.

Lockley, Tim. *Military Medicine and the Making of Race: Life and Death in the West India Regiments, 1795–1874*. New York: Cambridge University Press, 2020.

Lombardo, Paul A. "Anthropometry, Race, and Eugenic Research: 'Measurements of Growing Negro Children' at the Tuskegee Institute, 1932–1944." In *The Uses of Humans in Experiment*, edited by Erika Dyck and Larry Stewart, 215–239. Boston: Brill Rodopi, 2016.

Long, Gretchen. *Doctoring Freedom: The Politics of African American Medical Care in Slavery and Emancipation*. Chapel Hill: University of North Carolina Press, 2012.

Lowe, Zachary C. "Meanings of Freedom: Virginia Contraband Settlements and Wartime Reconstruction." Master's thesis, College of William & Mary, 2003.

Lowry, Tom, and Jack D. Welsh. *Tarnished Scalpels: The Court-Martials of Fifty Union Surgeons*. Mechanicsburg, PA: Stackpole Books, 2000.

Luke, Bob, and John David Smith. *Soldiering for Freedom: How the Union Army Recruited, Trained, and Deployed the U.S. Colored Troops*. Baltimore: Johns Hopkins University Press, 2014.

Luskey, Ashley Whitehead. "Inside the Civil War Defenses of Washington: An Interview with Steve T. Phan," *Gettysburg Compiler*, December 18, 2017. https://gettysburgcompiler.org/2017/12/18/inside-the-civil-war-defenses-of-washington-an-interview-with-steve-t-phan/.

Macdonald, Sharon, ed. *The Politics of Display: Museums, Science, Culture*. New York: Routledge, 2010.

Manning, Chandra. *Troubled Refuge: Struggling for Freedom in the Civil War*. New York: Knopf, 2016.

———. *What This Cruel War Was Over: Soldiers, Slavery, and the Civil War*. New York: Vintage Civil War Library, 2008.

Manning, Chandra, and Georgetown University History 396 Students. "Escaping Slavery, and Building Diverse Communities: Stories of the Search for Freedom in the Capital Region since the Civil War." May 13, 2020. https://storymaps.arcgis.com/stories/98843655e3474b9ab19a2afe250f0f22.

Maxwell, William Quentin. *Lincoln's Fifth Wheel: The Political History of the United States Sanitary Commission*. New York: Longmans, Green & Co., 1956.

McArdle, William D., Frank L. Katch, and Victor L. Katch. "Introduction: A View from the Past," in *Exercise Physiology: Nutrition, Energy, and Human Performance*, edited by William D. McArdle, Frank I. Katch, and Victor L. Katch, xxxii–xliii. Baltimore: Walter Kluwer, 2015.

McBride, David. *Caring for Equality: A History of African American Health and Health Care*. Lanham, MD: Rowman and Littlefield, 2018.

McElya, Micki. "The Politics of Mourning: Death and Honor in Arlington National Cemetery.", Master's thesis, Harvard University, 2016.

McLeary, Erin Hunter. "Science in a Bottle: The Medical Museum in North America, 1860–1940." PhD diss., University of Pennsylvania, 2001.

Meier, Kathryn Shively. "U.S. Sanitary Commission Physicians and the Transformation of American Health Care." In *So Conceived and So Dedicated: Intellectual Life in the Civil War-Era North*, edited by Lorien Foote and Kanisorn Wongsrichanalai, 19–40. New York: Fordham University Press, 2015.

Mendez, James G. "A Great Sacrifice: Northern Black Families and Their Civil War Experience." PhD diss., University of Illinois at Chicago, 2011.

Miller, Edward A., Jr. "Angel of Light: Helen L. Gilson, Army Nurse," *Civil War History* 43 (March 1997): 17–37.

Milroy, Elizabeth. "Avenue of Dreams: Patriotism and the Spectator at Philadelphia's Great Central Sanitary Fair." In *Making and Remaking Pennsylvania's Civil War*, edited by William Blair and William Pencak, 23–57. University Park: Pennsylvania State University Press, 2001.

Morgan, Jennifer L. *Laboring Women: Reproduction and Gender in New World Slavery*. Philadelphia: University of Pennsylvania Press, 2004.

Murphy, Ric, and Timothy Stephens. *Section 27 and Freedman's Village in Arlington National Cemetery: The African American History of America's Most Hallowed Ground*. Jefferson, NC: McFarland, 2020.

Neff, John R. *Honoring the Civil War Dead: Commemoration and the Problem of Reconciliation*. Lawrence: University Press of Kansas, 2005.

Newby, I. A. *Jim Crow's Defense: Anti-Negro Thought in America, 1900–1930*. Baton Rouge: Louisiana State University Press, 1965.

Newman, Louise Michele. *White Women's Rights: The Racial Origins of Feminism in the United States*. New York: Oxford University Press, 1999.

Newman, Richard S. "All's Fair: Philadelphia and the Sanitary Fair Movement during the Civil War." *Pennsylvania Heritage* (Summer 2013): 56–65.

Newmark, Jill. "Contraband Hospital, 1862–1863: Health Care for the First Freedpeople." *Black Past*, March 28, 2012. https://www.blackpast.org/african -american-history/contraband-hospital-1862-1863-heath-care-first-freedpeople/.
———. "Face to Face with History." *Prologue* 41 (Fall 2009): 22–25.

Nichols, Elaine, ed. *The Last Miles of the Way: African-American Homegoing Traditions, 1890–Present*. Columbia: South Carolina State Museum, 1989.

Novak, Shannon A. "Partible Persons or Persons Apart: Postmortem Interventions at the Spring Street Presbyterian Church, Manhattan." In *The Bioarcheology of Dissection and Autopsy in the United States*, edited by Kenneth C. Nystrom, 87–111. New York: Springer, 2017.

Nuddleman, Franny. *John Brown's Body: Slavery, Violence, and the Culture of War*. Chapel Hill: University of North Carolina Press, 2004.

Nystrom, Kenneth C., ed. *The Bioarcheology of Dissection and Autopsy in the United States*. New York: Springer, 2017.
———. "The Bioarcheology of Structural Violence and Dissection in the 19th-century United States," *American Anthropologist* 116, no. 4 (2014): 765–779.

Omi, Michael, and Howard Winant. *Racial Formation in the United States*. New York: Taylor and Francis, 2014.

Owens, Deirdre Cooper. *Medical Bondage: Race, Gender, and the Origins of American Gynecology*. Athens: University of Georgia Press, 2017.

Owens, Deirdre Cooper, and Sharla Fett. "Black Maternal and Infant Health: Historical Legacies of Slavery." *American Journal of Public Health* 109, no. 10 (2019): 1342–1345.

Pandora, Katherine. "Popular Science in National and Transnational Perspective: Suggestions from the American Context." *Isis* 100, no. 2 (2009): 346–358.

Park, Roberta J. "'Taking Their Measure in Play, Games, and Physical Training': The American Scene, 1870s to World War I." *Journal of Sports History* 33 (2006): 193–217.

Parrish, William E. "The Western Sanitary Commission." *Civil War History* 36 (March 1990): 17–35.

Pearl, Sharrona. "White, with a Class-Based Blight: Drawing Irish Americans." *Eire-Ireland* 44, nos. 3 and 4 (2009): 171–199.

Penny, H. Glenn. "The Civic Uses of Science: Ethnology and Civil Society in Imperial Germany." *Osiris* 17 (2002): 228–252.

Perdue, Charles L., Jr., Thomas E. Barden, and Robert K. Phillips, eds. *Weevils in the Wheat: Interviews with Virginia Ex-Slaves.* Charlottesville: University of Virginia Press, 1976.

Periwinkle Initiative. *Memory and Landmarks: Report of the Burial Database Project of Enslaved Americans.* Ithaca, NY: Periwinkle Initiative, 2017. https://issuu.com /periwinkleinitiative/docs/flipbook.

Peterson, Carla L. *Black Gotham: A Family History of African Americans in Nineteenth-Century New York City.* New Haven, CT: Yale University Press, 2011.

Pfatteicher, Sarah K. A. "Rebecca Lee Crumpler." In *African American Lives,* edited by Henry Louis Gates Jr. and Evelyn Brooks Higginbotham, 199–200. New York: Oxford University Press, 2004.

Public Broadcasting Service. "The Civil War by the Numbers." *American Experience: Death and the Civil War,* November 7, 2017, https://www.pbs.org/wgbh /americanexperience/features/death-numbers/.

Qureshi, Sadiah. *Peoples on Display: Exhibitions, Empire, and Anthropology in Nineteenth-Century Britain.* Chicago: University of Chicago Press, 2011.

Rainville, Lynn. *Hidden History: African American Cemeteries in Central Virginia.* Charlottesville: University of Virginia Press, 2014.

Rancy, David Alan. "In The Lord's Army: The United States Christian Commission in the Civil War." PhD diss., University of Illinois, 2001.

Redkey, Edwin S., ed. *A Grand Army of Black Men: Letters from African-American Soldiers in the Union Army, 1861–1865.* Cambridge: Cambridge University Press, 1992.

Redman, Samuel J. *Bone Rooms: From Scientific Racism to Human Prehistory in Museums.* Cambridge, MA: Harvard University Press, 2016.

Reiss, Benjamin. *The Showman and the Slave: Race, Death, and Memory in Barnum's America.* Cambridge, MA: Harvard University Press, 2010.

Rhode, Michael. "An Army Museum or a National Collection? Shifting Interests and Fortunes at the National Museum of Health and Medicine." In *Medical Museums: Past, Present, Future,* edited by Samuel J.M.M. Alberti and Elizabeth Hallarn, 186–199. London: Royal College of Surgeons of England, 2013.

Richardson, Steven J. "The Burial Grounds of Black Washington, 1880–1919." *Records of the Columbia Historical Society, Washington, D.C.* 52 (1989): 304–326.

Ripley, C. Peter, ed. *The Black Abolitionist Papers.* Chapel Hill: University of North Carolina Press, 1992.

Risch, Erna. *Quartermaster Support of the Army: A History of the Corps, 1775–1939.* Washington, DC: Quartermaster Historian's Office, 1962.

Roane, J. T. "Plotting the Black Commons," *Souls* 20 (2019): 239–266.

Roberts, Dorothy E. "The Arts of Medicine: Abolish Race Correction." *The Lancet* 397, no. 10268 (2021): 17–18.

———. *Fatal Invention: How Science, Politics, and Big Business Re-create Race in the Twenty-First Century.* New York: New Press, 2011.

———. *Killing the Black Body: Race, Reproduction, and the Meaning of Liberty.* New York: Vintage Books, 1999.

Roediger, David R. "And Die in Dixie: Funerals, Death, & Heaven in the Slave Community 1700–1865." *Massachusetts Review* 22 (Spring 1981): 163–183.

Rogers, Molly. *Delia's Tears: Race, Science, and Photography in Nineteenth-Century America*. New Haven, CT: Yale University Press, 2010.

Roper, Laura Wood. "Frederick Law Olmsted and the Port Royal Experiment." *Journal of Southern History* 31 (1965): 272–284.

Rosenberg, Charles E. "The Therapeutic Revolution: Medicine, Meaning, and Social Change in Nineteenth-Century America." *Perspectives in Biology and Medicine* 20 (1977): 485–506.

Rothenberg, Marc, et al., eds. *The Papers of Joseph Henry*. Sagamore Beach, MA: Science History Publications, 2004.

Rusert, Britt. *Fugitive Science: Empiricism and Freedom in Early African American Culture*. New York: New York University Press, 2017.

_____. "New World: The Impact of Digitization on the Study of Slavery." *American Literary History* 29, no. 2 (2017): 267–286.

———. "The Science of Freedom: Counterarchives of Racial Science on the Antebellum Stage." *African American Review* 45 (Fall 2012): 291–308.

Ryan, Mary. *Cradle of the Middle Class: The Family in Oneida County, New York, 1790–1865*. Cambridge: Cambridge University Press, 1981.

Salmon, Emily Jones. "J.D. Harris (ca. 1833–1884)." *Encyclopedia Virginia*, December 22, 2021, https://www.encyclopediavirginia.org/Harris_Joseph_D_c_1833-1884.

Sappol, Michael. *A Traffic in Dead Bodies: Anatomy and Embodied Social Identity in Nineteenth-Century America*. Princeton, NJ: Princeton University Press, 2002.

Savitt, Todd. *Medicine and Slavery: The Diseases and Health Care of Blacks in Antebellum Virginia*. Urbana-Champaign: University of Illinois Press, 1978.

Schantz, Mark S. *Awaiting the Heavenly Country: The Civil War and America's Culture of Death*. Ithaca, NY: Cornell University Press, 2008.

Schiebinger, Londa. *Secret Cures of Slaves: People, Plants, and Medicines in the Eighteenth-Century Atlantic World*. Stanford: Stanford University Press, 2017.

Schoeberlein, Robert W. "A Fair to Remember: Maryland Women in Aid of the Union." *Maryland Historical Society* 90 (1995): 467–488.

Schultz, Jane E. "African American Men in the Union Medical Service." *Mercy Street Revealed* Blog, February 21, 2017, http://www.pbs.org/mercy-street/blogs/mercy-street-revealed/african-american-men-in-the-union-medical-service/.

———. "Seldom Thanked, Never Praised, and Scarcely Recognized: Gender and Racism in Civil War Hospitals." *Civil War History* 48 (2002): 220–236.

———. *Women at the Front: Hospital Workers in Civil War America*. Chapel Hill: University of North Carolina Press, 2004.

Schwalm, Leslie A. "A Body of 'Truly Scientific Work': The U.S. Sanitary Commission and the Elaboration of Race in the Civil War Era." *Journal of the Civil War Era* 8 (2018): 647–676.

———. "Surviving Wartime Emancipation: African Americans and the Cost of Civil War." *Journal of Law, Medicine and Ethics* 39 (Spring 2011): 21–27.

Scully, Pamela, and Clifton Crais. "Race and Erasure: Sara Baartman and Hendrik Cesars in Cape Town and London." *Journal of British Studies* 47 (2008): 301–323.

Sears, Richard. *Camp Nelson, Kentucky: A Civil War History*. Lexington: University Press of Kentucky, 2002.

Selby, Kelly D. "The 27th United States Colored Troops: Ohio Soldiers and Veterans." PhD diss., Kent State University, 2008.

SenGutpa, Gunja. *From Slavery to Poverty: Racial Origins of Welfare in New York, 1840-1918*. New York: New York University Press, 2009.

Sera-Shriar, Afram. "Observing Human Difference: James Hunt, Thomas Huxley and Competing Disciplinary Strategies in the 1860s." *Annals of Science* 70 (2013): 461-491.

Sharpe, Christina. *In the Wake: On Blackness and Being*. Durham, NC: Duke University Press, 2016.

Smith, John David. "Let Us All Be Grateful That We Have Colored Troops That Will Fight." In *Black Soldiers in Blue: African American Troops in the Civil War Era*, edited by John David Smith, 1-77. Chapel Hill: University of North Carolina Press, 2002.

Smith, Ryan K. "Disappearing the Enslaved: The Destruction and Recovery of Richmond's Second African Burial Ground." *Buildings and Landscape: Journal of the Vernacular Architecture Forum* 27 (March 2020): 17-45.

Smith, Sean Morey, and Christopher D. E. Willoughby, eds. *Medicine and Healing in the Age of Slavery*. Baton Rouge: Louisiana State University Press, 2021.

Smith, Susan L. *Toxic Exposures: Mustard Gas and the Health Consequences of World War II in the United States*. New Brunswick, NJ: Rutgers University Press, 2017.

Sorisio, Carolyn. *Fleshing Out America: Race, Gender, and the Politics of the Body in American Literature, 1833-1879*. Athens: University of Georgia Press, 2002.

Spar, Ira. *Civil War Hospital Newspapers*. Jefferson, NC: McFarland, 2017.

———. *New Haven's Civil War Hospital: A History of Knight U.S. General Hospital, 1862-1865*. Jefferson, NC: McFarland, 2013.

Spatola, Brian. "Daniel S. Lamb (1843-1929) of the Army Medical Museum." *Military Medicine*, 181 (June 2016): 609-610.

Spencer, Frank. "Anthropometry." In *History of Physical Anthropology: An Encyclopedia*, vol. 1, edited by Frank Spencer, 80-90. New York: Garland, 1997.

———, ed. *History of Physical Anthropology: An Encyclopedia*. New York: Garland, 1997.

Stein, Melissa N. *Measuring Manhood: Race the Science of Masculinity, 1830-1934*. Minneapolis: University of Minnesota Press, 2015.

Stepan, Nancy. *The Idea of Race in Science: Great Britain, 1800-1960*. London: Macmillan Press, 1982.

Stout, Becca. "African Americans Buried at Gettysburg." *Blog Divided*, June 11, 2018, http://housedivided.dickinson.edu/sites/blogdivided/2018/06/11/african -americans-in-gettysburg-national-cemetery.

Taylor, Amy Murrell. *Embattled Freedom: Journeys through the Civil War's Refugee Camps*. Chapel Hill: University of North Carolina Press, 2018.

Taylor, Brian M. "'To Make the Union What It Ought to Be': African Americans, Civil War Military Service, and Citizenship." PhD diss., Georgetown University, 2015.

Taylor, Jamila K. "Structural Racism and Maternal Health among Black Women." *Journal of Law, Medicine, and Ethics* 48 (2020): 506-517.

Tennessee State Library and Archives Research and Collections. Federal Civil War Burial Sheets Project. https://www.tnsos.net/TSLA/BurialSheetsProject/index.php.

Teslow, Tracy. *Constructing Race: The Science of Bodies and Cultures in American Anthropology*. Cambridge: Cambridge University Press, 2014.

Tetrault, Lisa. *The Myth of Seneca Falls: Memory and the Women's Suffrage Movement, 1848-1898*. Chapel Hill: University of North Carolina Press, 2014.

Todd, Jan. *Physical Culture and the Body Beautiful: Purposive Exercise in the Lives of American Women, 1800-1870*. Macon, GA: Mercer University Press, 1998.

Trudeau, Noah Andre, ed. *Voices of the 55th: Letters from the 55th Massachusetts Volunteers, 1861-1865*. Dayton, OH: Morningside Press, 1996.

Tuggle, Lindsay. *The Afterlives of Specimens: Science, Mourning, and Whitman's Civil War*. Iowa City, IA: University of Iowa Press, 2017.

Turner, Sasha. "The Nameless and the Forgotten: Maternal Grief, Sacred Protection, and the Archive of Slavery." *Slavery and Abolition* 38, no. 2 (2017), 232-250.

Ulle, Robert F. "A History of St. Thomas' African Episcopal Church, 1794-1865." PhD diss., University of Pennsylvania, 1986.

U.S. National Park Service. "Freedman's Village." Arlington House, Robert E. Lee Memorial (November 3, 2019), https://www.nps.gov/arho/learn/historyculture/emancipation.htm.

Valencius, Conevery Bolton, David I. Spanagel, Emily Pawley, Sara Stidstone Gronim, and Paul Lucier. "Science in Early America: Print Culture and the Sciences of Territoriality." *Journal of the Early Republic* 36 (2016): 73-123.

Wallis, Brian. "Black Bodies, White Science: Louis Agassiz's Slave Daguerreotypes." *American Art* 9 (1995): 38-61.

Walton-Raji, Angela Y. "In Search of Quarantine Island." *USCT Chronicle*, December 14, 2013, http://usctchronicle.blogspot.com/2013/12/in-search-of-quarantine-island.html.

Warner, John Harley. *Against the Spirit of System: The French Impulse in Nineteenth-Century American Medicine*. Princeton, NJ: Princeton University Press, 1998.

———. "The Fall and Rise of Professional Mystery: Epistemology, Authority, and the Emergence of Laboratory Medicine in Nineteenth-Century America." In *The Laboratory Revolution in Medicine*, edited by Andrew Cunningham and Perry Williams, 110-141. Cambridge: Cambridge University Press, 1992.

———. *The Therapeutic Perspective: Medical Practice, Knowledge, and Identity in America, 1820-1885*. Cambridge, MA: Harvard University Press, 1986.

Warren, Robert Penn. *The Legacy of the Civil War*. Lincoln, NE: Bison Books, 1998. Reprinted with an introduction by Howard Jones. First published in 1961 by Random House (New York).

Washington, Harriet A. *Medical Apartheid: The Dark History of Medical Experimentation on Black Americans from Colonial Times to the Present*. New York: Harlem Moon Broadway Books, 2006.

Waugh, Joan, and Gary Gallagher, eds. *Wars within a War: Controversy and Conflict in the American Civil War*. Chapel Hill: University of North Carolina Press, 2009.

Weiner, Marli, and Mazie Hough. *Sex, Sickness, and Slavery: Defining Illness in the Antebellum South*. Urbana-Champaign: University of Illinois Press, 2012.

Whitacre, Paula Tarnapol. "'As American Citizens, We Have a Right. . . .'; Death, Protest, and Respect in Alexandria, Virginia." *Journal of the Civil War Era: Muster*, November 16, 2021. https://www.journalofthecivilwarera.org/2021/11/as -american-citizens-we-have-a-right-death-protest-and-respect-in-alexandria -virginia/.

White, Kellee. "The Sustaining Relevance of W. E. B. Du Bois to Health Disparities Research." *DuBois Review* 8 (2011): 285–293.

Whooley, Owen. *Knowledge in the Time of Cholera: The Struggle over American Medicine in the Nineteenth Century*. Chicago: University of Chicago Press, 2012.

"William Chester Minor." Wikipedia. Last modified May 2, 2022. https://en .wikipedia.org/wiki/William_Chester_Minor.

Williams, David. *A People's History of the Civil War*. New York: Free Press, 2005.

Williams, Rachel. "The United States Christian Commission and the Civil War Dead." *U.S. Studies Online*, April 15, 2015, http://www.baas.ac.uk/usso/the -united-states-christian-commission-and-the-civil-war-dead/.

Willoughby, Christopher D. "'His Native, Hot Country:' Racial Science and Environment in Antebellum American Medical Thought." *Journal of the History of Medicine and Allied Sciences* 3 (2017): 328–351.

———. "Race, Genitals, and Walt Whitman in Dr. Leidy's Lectures." *Fugitive Leaves*, April 13, 2017, https://histmed.collegeofphysicians.org/race-genitals-and -walt-whitman/.

———. "Running Away from Praenomina: Samuel A. Cartwright, Medicine, and Race in the Antebellum South." *Journal of Southern History* 84 (2018): 579–614.

Wilson, Keith P. *Campfires of Freedom: The Camp Life of Black Soldiers during the Civil War*. Kent, OH: Kent State University Press, 2002.

Winchester, Simon. *The Surgeon of Crowthorne: A Tale of Murder, Insanity, and the Making of the Love of Words*. New York: Harper Collins, 1998.

Winkle, Kenneth J. *Lincoln's Citadel: The Civil War in Washington, D.C.* New York: Norton, 2014.

Young, Robert J. C. *Colonial Desire: Hybridity in Theory, Culture, and Race*. London: Routledge, 1995.

Yudell, Michael. *Race Unmasked: Biology and Race in the Twentieth Century*. Ithaca, NY: Cornell University Press, 2014.

Index

Abbott, Anderson R., 17, 87, 111, 168n87

abolitionists, xii, 5, 9, 12–17 passim, 29, 31, 67, 74, 101, 109, 119

African American/s:

—civilian burial customs, 69, 95–99, 103–4, 172n10, 172n13

—deceased: treatment of (civilians, free and enslaved), 4, 11, 51, 69, 80–102 passim, 109–14, 173n17

—educators, 4–5

—enslaved, xi, xii, 19, 55, 63, 70, 71, 96–99, 119

—free northern (antebellum), 4–5, 31

—refugees from slavery ("contraband"), 31–47 passim, 51, 63, 69–70, 80–83, 100–102, 109–18 passim, 133n33, 142n61

—soldiers and regiments, 3, 14–20, 29–41 passim, 46, 51–69 passim, 72–79, 94, 99–109 passim, 113–17, 158n93

—specific regiments: First Louisiana Native Guard, 94; 20th U.S. Colored Infantry, 63; 23rd U.S. Colored Infantry, 76–79; 24th U.S. Colored Infantry, 176n53; 25th U.S. Colored Infantry, 176n53; 28th U.S. Colored Infantry, 102, 103; 29th U.S. Colored Infantry, 176n53; 32nd U.S. Colored Infantry, 101; 33rd U.S. Colored Infantry, 16; 43rd U.S. Colored Infantry, 104; 50th U.S. Colored Infantry, 100; 56th U.S. Colored Infantry, 101; 54th Massachusetts, 16; 55th Massachusetts Infantry, 105; 56th U.S. Colored Infantry, 101, 105; 60th U.S. Colored Infantry, 16, 18;

61st U.S. Colored Infantry, 176n53; 62nd U.S. Colored Infantry, 94, 176n53; 65th U.S. Colored Infantry, 131n5; 67th, U.S. Colored Infantry, 107; 81st U.S. Colored Infantry, 63

—streetcar protests, 17, 34–35,41

—mortality, 8, 18, 44, 65, 75, 82, 93–94, 107–8, 118, 119. *See also* Black physicians; burial: military interment; cemeteries; Civil War pensions; crania; crania collections; nurses; U.S. Sanitary Commission; "Unknown Contraband Negroes Also Known"; women: refugees from slavery; women's war work

Agassiz, Louis, 10, 48, 60, 70, 85, 146n2, 155n57, 178n78

Allen, John, 16

amalgamationists, 31, 139n30

Anderson, Private Benjamin; family; comrades, 76, 79, 164n45

The Anglo-African, 35, 140n37

anthropology, 5–9 passim, 54, 60, 65–67, 115, 129n27, 159n94, 178n78

anthropometry, 4, 7–9, 55–58 passim, 64–65, 116

archives, xi–xii, 49, 70, 109

Armstrong, Col. Samuel, 99, 174n34

Army Medical Museum, 4, 48, 71, 75, 77, 78, 81–92 passim, 168nn85–86

Augusta, Alexander, 17, 84, 87, 111, 133n33, 167n71

authorship, 49, 73

autopsies, 72, 74, 83, 85–86, 91, 107

autopsy reports: published, 71, 73, 83, 91, 161n20, 161n25, 168n84

Avery, George W., 63

Baartman, Saartjie, 71
Baker, Theodore J., 17
Baltimore, Maryland, 17, 28, 34, 80,
    108, 138n25, 161n20
Banneker, Institute, 5
Barnum, 11, 62, 71, 130n37
Bassett, Ebenezer, 138n25
Baxter, J. H., 8, 54, 56, 92
Bay, Mia, 5
Bellows, Henry Whitney, 23, 44, 46, 49,
    57, 66, 136n5
benevolence, 22, 23, 25, 27, 36, 39, 41,
    44, 135n4
Bethel, Bennet, 76–78
biomedical racism, xi, 1–6 passim,
    11–19 passim, 44–55 passim, 67,
    71–80 passim, 85–93 passim, 115–120,
    146n2, 150n19, 152n31, 158n93;
    practice: resistance to, 16, 19, 36–37,
    67, 75. See also autopsies; dissection
Bird, Sergeant John, 104
Black Americans. See African Americans
Black extinction, 4
Black physicians (and Army surgeons).
    See Augusta, Alexander; Creed,
    Cortland V. R.; Baker, Theodore J.;
    Abbott, Anderson R.; Boseman,
    Benjamin A.; DeGrasse, John Van
    Surly; Ellis, William Baldwin; Harris,
    J. D.; Powell, William P.; Purvis,
    Charles Burleigh; Rapier, John H.;
    Revels, Willis R.; Taylor, Charles H.;
    Tucker, Alpheus W.
Black "superbodies," 56
Blackwell, Elizabeth, 22–23, 25
Blumenbach, Johann, 84
Boaz, Franz, 8
Bond, Samuel S., 82–86, 91, 167n68,
    168–169n87
Bontecou, Reed B., 88, 169–170n95
Book of Bubbles, The, 29–30
Boseman, Benjamin A., 17, 133n27
Boston, 5, 26, 34, 36, 39, 140n44,
    141nn55–56
Bowditch, Henry Pickering, 8

Bowers, Mrs. Thomas J., 33
brain, 51, 62, 67, 74, 77, 154n53, 163n35
Bremner, Robert H., 26
Briggs, Charles E., 16, 132n16
Broca, Paul, 8
Brockett, L. P., 27
Brooklyn (NY), 35, 138n26, 141n54,
    142n65
Brooks, Major T. B., 52–53, 56,
    150–51n22
Brown, Vincent, 99, 174n32
Buddy, E., 33
burial: military interment, 69–70
    passim, 86, 93–95, 99–109
Burnett, Dr. S. M., 91

Cailloux, Andre, 94
Camp Nelson (KY), 62, 108
Camp William Penn (PA), 101
Cassedy, James, 57
cemeteries: Arlington National (D.C),
    100, 108, 113, 175n44; City Point
    National (VA), 37–38, 42, 63, 105, 108;
    Contraband, 113; Friends of Freed-
    man's, 165n60, 175n44; Gettysburg
    National, 179n95; Harmony Cem-
    etery, 111; Jefferson Barracks
    National Cemetery, 177–78n75;
    Jefferson National Cemetery, 105,
    107, 108; Lebanon Cemetery (PA),
    108; Mount Olivet, 113; Mount
    Pleasant, (D.C.), 113; Mount Zion,
    (D.C.), 113; Nashville (TN), 108; Olive
    (PA), 96; Quarantine Island (MO),
    106; Soldiers Cemetery, (SC), 99,
    175n47; Union, 181n112
Cherokee, 154. See also indigenous
    people
Chew, Mrs. John, 33
Chilton, Katherine, 81, 165n54
Christian Commission, 103, 105
Christian Recorder, The, 96–97, 102,
    140n37
Christianson, C., 33
circus, 11, 70, 156–57n71

citizenship, xi, 3, 13, 21–22, 27, 28, 36, 48, 99, 118, 131n4
City Point (VA), 37–38, 42, 63, 105, 108, 140n44
Civilians: Black, 36, 40–42, 44–45, 93, 95, 101, 113, 118
Civil War memory, 36, 95, 103, 140n34, 174n40
Civil War pensions: nurses' applications, 133n33; widows' applications, 79, 101–3; U.S. Sanitary Commission Army and Navy Claims Agency, 25, 37, 47
Cleveland (OH), 26, 28, 33, 140n40, 141n51
Cober, Katherine, 92, 171n114
Collins, Ellen, 31–32, 46, 138–139n30
Colored Women's Loyal League (Philadelphia), 32–33, 35–36
Congress, 13, 50, 58, 81, 168n85
Contraband Relief Association (Wash., D.C.), 28
Contraband Relief Society (St. Louis, MO), 40
Cooley, Private John, 100, 175n44
Cope, Edward Drinker, 8, 128–29n22
Craft, William, 5
crania, 11, 84, 88, 90
crania collections, 11, 90–91, 101, 115, 170n101, 170–71n106
craniology, 48, 70
craniometry, 4, 57, 64, 84, 146n2
Creed, Cortland V. R., 17
Curtis, Edward, 89

Daina Ramey Berry, 4, 11, 69, 97, 125n4, 160n4
Dakota, 154n49. See also indigenous people
Darwin, Charles, 8
Davenport, Charles, 8
DeGrasse, John Van Surly, 17
Detroit, 26, 30, 138n29, 138–39n30
Devine, Shauna, 72, 126–127n7
discrimination: racial, 3, 9, 13–15, 17, 65, 74, 93, 158–59n93

dissection, 11, 69–74 passim, 77–80, 83, 86–91 passim, 95, 107, 112, 159n1, 164n4, 168n84
Dorsey, Mrs. Thomas, 33
Douglass, Frederick, 5, 96, 153n46
Douglass, Sarah Mapps, 5, 142n62
Downs, Jim, 118, 172n1
Drummond, E., 33
DuBois, W. E. B., 129–30n31, 150n21

Ellis, William Baldwin, 17
emancipation, 1–3 passim, 7, 9, 35, 36, 46–50 passim, 56, 110, 116–19 passim
engineers: U.S. Army, 51, 66
enlistment examinations, 3, 13–15, 18–19, 35–38, 48–51 passim, 54, 56–66, 100, 104
ethnology, 2, 5, 48, 55, 60, 65, 84, 90, 128n22, 148n11
eyewitness accounts and observations, 14, 48, 51–53, 55, 74, 86, 113, 152n31, 158n87, 162–63n32

Fabian, Ann, 89–90, 147n5
Farland, Maria, 9, 150n21
fatigue labor, 3, 14–15, 52, 55, 117, 179n82
Faulkner, Carol, 31–32, 139n33
federal census and race, 67, 139n33
Forten, Sergeant Major Robert Bridges, 104
Forten, William, 138n25
Fortress Monroe (VA), 43, 81
Freedmen's Aid, 29, 30–32, 37, 41, 43, 45–46, 140n44
Freedmen's Bureau (Bureau of Refugees, Freedmen and Abandoned Lands), 4–5, 46–47, 90, 110, 118, 139n33, 166n64
Freedmen's Hospital (Wash., D.C.), 84–85, 87, 91, 112, 168n85

Gage, Francis, 29
Galloway, L., 33
Galton, Frances, 8

General Orders No. 75 (Sept. 11, 1861), 105

Gibbons, Mrs., 33

Giesberg, Judith, 27, 122, 136n7, 139n34

Gilson, Helen, 37, 142n61

Gladwin, Reverend Albert, 100

Glidden, George, 90

Goines, L., 33

Gooding, Sergeant James Henry, 99–100

Gould, Benjamin Apthorp (president, U.S. Sanitary Commission Statistical Bureau), 58–66 passim, 115, 128n17, 148n8, 150n21, 153n48, 154n53, 155n60, 158n87

grave-robbers ("resurrectionists"), 97, 166n66, 167n75

Greene, Elias (Wash., D.C.), 112, 166n66, 180n99

Greenwood, Janette, 34

gynecology, 2, 56

Hammond, Surgeon General William, 71, 78, 87, 89

Hancock, Cornelia, 72, 113

Harris, Elisha, 59, 63, 65, 147n6, 155n54

Harris, J. D., 17

Henry, Joseph (Smithsonian president), 58–60, 153n46

Heth, Joyce, 71

Higginson, Thomas W., 16, 99

Hinton, Miss Ada, 33

Hoffman, Frederick, 4, 8–9

hospitals, 17–18, 25, 26, 34–45 passim, 69, 72–75, 80, 85–91 passim, 100, 106–13 passim; segregation, 18, 36–37, 45, 87, 93–95, 141n51, 171n111; slave hospitals, 134n42

hospital stewards, 7, 18, 80, 84, 86–87

hospital workers, 17–18, 42, 69, 81–82, 85, 95, 117, 133n33, 163n35, 170n95

Howard, Cinta, 85

Howard University, 84, 91, 181n106

Hrdlicka, Ales, 8, 129n27

human remains: value of, 1, 4, 11, 68–72 passim, 79–80, 83, 86, 89 passim, 97–98, 107

Humphreys, Margaret, 15, 17, 117, 126–127n7, 132n22, 162n30, 163n33

Hunt, Sanford B., 9, 66

Hygeia Hospital (VA), 88

indigenous people: anthropometry, 6, 59, 63–64, 90–91, 154n49. See also Cherokee; Dakota; Iroquois; Oneida

Investigations in the Military and Anthropological Statistics of American Soldiers (1869), 65–66, 150n17

Irish Americans, 56

Iroquois, 59, 153n49; See also indigenous people

Jacobs, Harriet, 101, 112–13

Jayne, Samuel F., 37, 142n61

Johnson, Private William, 79

Johnston, Private Willis, 103

Keckley, Elizabeth, 28

Kenny, Stephen, 89

Ladies Aid Association (Norfolk, VA), 35

Ladies' Committee for the Relief of Sick Soldiers (New York City), 140n44

Ladies Union Aid Association (St. Louis, MO), 40

Lamb, Daniel S., 82

Leidy, Joseph, 84–85, 167n75

Liberator, The, 16, 112

life insurance companies, 25, 50, 66

Lincoln, 13, 44, 80, 137n31

Linnaean taxonomy, 48

Long, Gretchen, 5

Mann, Maria, 113

Manning, Chandra, 118, 166n65

masculinity, 26, 128n18; and authority, 7; idealized manhood, 27, 56, 146n4, 154n53

Matas, Rudolph, 8

Maxwell, William, 23
May, Abby, 46
McElya, Micki, 109, 182n114
measuring apparatus, 57–58, 60, 63, 64,
    119, 155n58, 157n71
*Medical and Surgical History of the War of
    the Rebellion*, 87, 91, 147n5, 158n93,
    168n85
medical authority, 49
medical practitioners, 2–7 passim, 10,
    14, 48–54 passim, 64, 69–72, 80,
    91–93, 112, 114; lay, 4–5
medical racism. *See* biomedical racism
Medical Society of the District of
    Columbia, 84
medical specimens, 11, 71, 83, 87–88, 95
medical theories, 10, 53–54, 64, 115, 118
Meigs, Montgomery, 108
military death regulations, 94, 101,
    104–5, 176n54
Miller, C., 33
Miller, Kelly, 8–9
Minor, William Chester, 73–74, 79–80,
    83, 161n25, 162n29
Minton, Mrs., 33
modernity, 2, 10, 20, 28, 36, 51, 94,
    101–5 passim, 116–17, 136n7
Morris Island (SC), 52
Morton, Samuel, 48, 67, 84, 90, 146n2
museums, 1, 11, 70–71, 88–90, 97, 169n89

Nashville (TN), 40, 41, 108, 133n33
New Bedford (MA), 36, 141n56, 174n36
New Berne (NC), 37, 44, 45, 111, 113
New England Women's Auxiliary
    Association (NEWAA). *See* U.S.
    Sanitary Commission
New Orleans (LA), 65, 94, 177n69
Nott, Josiah, 48, 84, 91, 146n2
nurses, 5, 17–18, 44–46, 72, 133n33

Olmsted, Frederick Law, 43–44, 58–59
Oneida, 154. *See also* indigenous people
Otis, George, 90, 92
Owens, Deirdre Cooper, 56, 119, 126n3

Page, J. W., 37
Parsons, Emily Elizabeth, 17, 163n34
Parsons, Mary, 168n85
Philadelphia, 80, 83–84, 95–96, 101, 104,
    108, 146n4
Potts, George J., 76–79
Powell, William P., 17, 87, 111
print culture, 4, 58, 70; medical, 10, 49
proslavery ideology, 7, 16, 48
Purnell, Jane Tobia, 103
Purvis, Charles Burliegh, 17, 87, 111

questionnaires, 9, 52–53, 58
Quetelet, Adolphe, 57, 154n51

race: and classifications schemes, 6, 10,
    22, 47–68 passim, 74–75, 89, 90–91,
    115–117; and citizenship, 7, 13, 21–22,
    27, 28, 36, 48; cultural history of, 1–3,
    29–30, 49, 64–66, 70–71; historiciza-
    tion of, 9–11, 54, 55, 57; and inter-
    changeability of bodies, 1, 85, 92; and
    spectacle, 11, 16, 62, 70–72, 89, 97;
    visual culture of, 28–29, 70, 92. *See also*
    biomedical racism; race formation;
    racial categories; racial knowledge;
    scientific racism; racism; Statistics
race formation/racemaking: and
    emancipation, 1–3, 7, 9, 13, 27, 43–44,
    48–49, 56, 67–68, 116; in historical
    context, xii, 1–11, 21–26 passim, 57,
    59, 69–71, 84, 90–91, 96–99, 115–20;
    northern white investments in, xi–xii,
    1–2, 5–13, 18–28 passim, 30–36
    passim, 41–43, 46, 56–59, 68–71, 95,
    108–18 passim; and slavery, xii, 2–3,
    7, 9–13 passim, 21–22, 48, 67–75
    passim, 98–99, 114, 119
racial categories: ascribed anatomical
    characteristics, 12, 14, 49–51, 55–57,
    60–62, 64, 74, 91, 112, 115–16;
    gendered, 6–7, 27, 56, 62; sexualized,
    73–74, 86; whiteness, 4–9 passim, 15,
    21–39 passim, 40–59 passim, 62, 68,
    74, 75, 92, 115–18

racial knowledge: as a professional commodity, xii–xiii, 1–4, 7–10, 16, 48–53 passim, 70–80 passim, 82–83, 85, 116–17

racial science/scientific racism, xi, 2–4, 5–12 passim, 48–49, 52, 60, 67–71 passim, 77, 84–86, 115–20 passim; and comparative anatomy, 1, 8, 11, 48, 57, 59, 69–74, 85–92 passim, 97, 178n78; critiques of, 5, 8–9, 28, 36–37, 49, 54, 62–63, 119–20; ties to empiricism, 1, 2, 10, 49–53, 57–59, 64–67, 75, 92, 115, 116. *See also* anthropometry; crania; crania collections; craniology; craniometry; ethnology

racism, and abolition, 2, 9, 16–17, 74–75; criticism of, 30, 32, 39, 74–75. *See also* biomedical racism; Black physicians; U.S. Army

Rapier, John H., Jr., 17, 87, 111

Reconstruction, 7, 31, 68

Redman, Samuel, 89

Redpath, James, 101

Revels, William, 39

Revels, Willis R., 17, 87

Ripley, William Zebina, 8

Roane, J. T., 99

Roediger, David, 98

Rogers, Molly, 70

Rogers, Seth, 16

Rusert, Britt, 5, 70

Russell, Ira, 74–76, 162n30; autopsies, dissections, and anatomization of Black soldiers, 80, 107; publications, 74

sanitary fairs. *See* U.S. Sanitary Commission

Sappol, Michael, 70, 79, 89

Schafhirt, Adolphe J., 82, 84–86, 91

Schafhirt, Ernst, 84

Schafhirt, Frederic, 84, 89, 168n84

Schultz, Jane, 18, 42

Schureman, Elizabeth A., 95–96

Schuyler, Louisa, 46

Sebastian, Mrs. F., 33

Sims, J. Marion, 48, 146n2

slave owners, 83, 97–98, 102

slavery, 2–3, 7–13 passim, 40–48 passim, 56, 75, 86, 94, 97–99, 109–10, 114–19 passim; archives and records, xi–xiii

slave trade, 11, 63, 69–70, 97, 130n37

Smith, Dr. James McCune, 5

Smith, John David, 13

Smithsonian Institution, 58–59, 65, 68, 85, 90, 128n97, 153n46

social surveys, 6, 8, 11, 14, 51–56, 58, 66–67, 88

South Carolina, 16, 30, 43–44, 52–53, 59, 99; Charleston, 101, 172n13, 173, 22, 175n47

statistical thinking ("numerical discourse"), 1, 6, 49–51 passim, 57, 59, 64–65, 147n6, 150n19, 154n51, 158n93

Statistics, Medical and Anthropological, of the Provost Marshal General's Bureau, 54–56. *See also* J. H. Baxter

Steggerda, Morris, 8

Stein, Melissa, 5, 128n18

St. Louis, MO, 18–19, 28–31 passim, 34–35, 40, 46, 105, 107, 138n25, 139n31, 163n35

suffrage: women's, 32

Taylor, Charles H., 17

Tillinghast, Joseph Alexander, 8

Tilmon, Mrs. Sarah, 31–32

Tucker, Alpheus W., 17, 87, 111

"Unknown Contraband Negroes Also Known," 51, 109–13, 150n18

U.S. Army, 8, 10, 12, 18, 30–31, 36–38, 52, 65. *See also* African Americans: soldiers and regiments; Army Medical Museum; U.S. Army Medical Department; U.S. Army Quartermaster Department

U.S. Army Medical Department, 1, 10, 21, 23–26, 48–51 passim, 53, 59, 66,

78, 147n5. *See also* Army Medical Museum; Black physicians

U.S. Army Provost Marshal's Bureau survey, 54–56. *See also* J. H. Baxter; *Statistics, Medical and Anthropological, of the Provost Marshal General's Bureau*

U.S. Army Quartermaster Department: employment of Black civilians and refugees from slavery, 46, 82, 111–12, 165n54; responsibility for civilian burials, 109–114, 166n66, 180n99, 180n104; responsibility for military burials, 101, 105, 108–9, 177n75

U.S. Sanitary Commission, 5–6, 12–13, 21–28. *See also* Henry Bellows; Dr. Elizabeth Blackwell; Ellen Collins; Benjamin Apthorp Gould; Frederick Law Olmstead; Benjamin Woodward

—and Army Medical Department, 10–13, 23, 25, 50, 66

—Black auxiliaries: Boston Colored Ladies' Sanitary Commission, 36, 141n55; Ladies' Sanitary Commission of the African Episcopal Church of St. Thomas, 28, 32–33, 35–36, 140n44, 141n55; Colored Women's Loyal League, 28, 32; Cleveland, 28

—and biomedical racism, 8, 21–22, 48–49, 53–54, 66–67, 72, 115–17

—and Black soldiers, 36–40, 46–51, 53–54, 56–68, 102–3, 106, 107, 132n20

—and freedmen's aid movement, 31–32, 34, 43–44

—gender conflict within, 22–25, 26–28

—*Investigations in the Military and Anthropological Statistics of American Soldiers*, 7–9, 58–66

—medical print culture, 50

—misogynoir, 26–36, 137n20, 138–139n30, 140n37

—racially exclusive, 25–32, 35–40

—and refugees from slavery, 41–46

—relief work and race, 25–27, 36–40, 41–47

—Sanitary Fairs, 26, 28–36, 137n21, 138nn25–26, 138n29, 141n51, 141nn55–56, 142n57

—scientific racism, 5–6, 57–67, 115–17

—unaffiliated Black Sanitary Organizations, 32–36

—white auxiliaries: New England Women's Auxiliary Association (NEWAA), 25; Women's Central Association for Relief (WCAR); 23–26, 32, 39, 136n7; Women's Pennsylvania Branch, 25, 28, 32, 34, 37, 39, 40, 47, 143n71, 145n91

—Women's Council, 28

Wells, Augustus, 103–4
Wells, Martha, 103–4
Western Sanitary Commission (St. Louis), 31, 40–41, 46, 139n31
White, Garland H., 102
Wilbur, Julia, 80, 101, 137n19
Wilder, Burt Green, 72, 132n20, 178n78
Williamsburg (NY), 35
women: refuges from slavery, 31–32, 41–42, 80–82, 86, 100–102, 107, 109–14, 118
Women: white, racial hegemony, 2, 7, 17–22 passim, 25–34, 36–43, 46–47 passim, 68, 117
Women's war work, 3, 7, 17–29 passim, 30–47, 63, 81, 111, 117–18; Black, 3, 17–18, 21, 27–36 passim, 39–40, 42, 63, 81, 140n37; white, 7, 17, 21–32 passim, 35–43 passim, 46–47, 117–18
Woodward, Benjamin, 14, 53–54, 56, 66–67, 151n25
Worcester (MA), 34

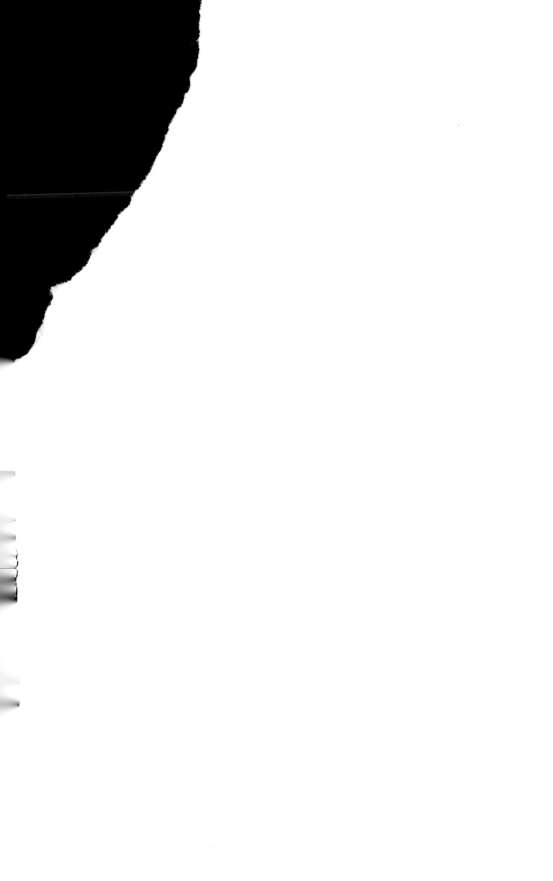

CPSIA information can be obtained
at www.ICGtesting.com
Printed in the USA
BVHW030709260223
659229BV00001B/21

9 781469 672687